610.73072   CRO

W £18.62

Research into Practice

Accession no.
010...

D0333905

ET LIBRARY

WITHDRAWN
FROM
STOCK

JET LIBRARY

Research into Practice

Essential skills for reading and applying research in nursing and health care

Edited by

Patrick Crookes
Senior Lecturer, Department of Nursing,
University of Wollongong, Australia

Sue Davies
Lecturer in Nursing,
Department of Gerontological and Continuing Care Nursing,
University of Sheffield, UK

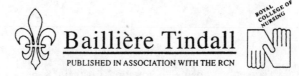

Baillière Tindall

PUBLISHED IN ASSOCIATION WITH THE RCN

Edinburgh London New York Philadelphia St Louis Sydney Toronto 1998

BAILLIERE TINDALL
An imprint of Harcourt Publishers Limited

 is a registered trademark of Harcourt Publishers Limited

© Harcourt Publishers Limited 1998

All rights reserved. No part of this publication may be reproduced, stored in a retrieval system or transmitted, in any form or by any other means, electronic, mechanical, photocopying or otherwise, without the prior permission of Harcourt Publishers Limited, 24–28 Oval Road, London NW1 7DX

First published 1998
Reprinted 1999

A catalogue record for this book is available from the British Library

ISBN 0 7020 2068 0

The
publisher's
policy is to use
**paper manufactured
from sustainable forests**

Typeset by Phoenix Photosetting, Chatham, Kent
Printed and bound by Bell and Bain Ltd., Glasgow

Contents

Contributors   ix

Introduction   xi

1.   **Ways of knowing in nursing and health care
     practice**   1
     Mike Nolan, Ulla Lundh

     Changing health care, changing knowledge   2
     Reality, knowing and method: some basic beliefs   4
     Ways of knowing: an overview   7
     Major contributors and their work   11
     Achieving a balance   16

2.   **The context of nursing and health care research**   23
     Susan Read

     Research in nursing before 1980   24
     Health services research before 1990   27
     The NHS R&D strategy   29
     The strategy for research in nursing   34
     NHS R&D from 1994   39
     Recent developments   42

3.   **Accessing sources of knowledge**   55
     Christine Hibbert, Patrick Crookes

     Successful literature searching   56
     Reading the literature   67
     Critically analyzing the literature   73

4.   Philosophical and theoretical underpinnings of research   **85**

Lorraine Ellis, Patrick Crookes

Philosophy and research   86
Paradigms in research   88
Theory and its relationship to research   95
Frames of reference in research   101

5.   Recognizing research processes in research-based literature   **116**

Ann Thomson

Factors influencing the choice of research design   116
Qualitative approaches   119
Quantitative approaches   123
Bridging the gap   129

6.   Evaluating methods for collecting data in published research   **139**

Nigel Mathers, Yu Chu Huang

Quantitative data collection methods   141
Validity and reliability in quantitative data collection   144
Sample size and quantitative methods   147
Sampling in qualitative research   150
Validity and reliability in qualitative data collection   151
Qualitative data collection methods   153

7.   Evaluating methods for analyzing data in published research   **162**

Nigel Mathers, Yu Chu Huang

Quantitative data analysis   162
Independent and dependent variables   168
Qualitative data analysis   173

8.   Populations and samples: identifying the boundaries of research   **181**

Christine Ingleton

Types of sample   182
Boundary setting in quantitative research   182
Sampling in the qualitative domain   189
Sampling for other reasons   193
What size of sample?   195
Sources of sampling bias   198
Critiquing the sample   199

9.   Critiquing ethical issues in published research   **204**
Liz Matthews, Angela Venables

The Four Principles plus Scope of Application approach   206
Autonomy   207
Beneficence and non-maleficence   214
Justice   218

10.   Reviewing and interpreting research: identifying implications for practice   **233**
Sue Davies

Types of review   234
Purposes of a literature review   236
A methodology for reviewing literature   238
Putting it all together   247
Putting reviews into practice   254

11.   Factors which may inhibit the utilization of research findings in practice – and some solutions   **259**
Ann McDonnell

Preliminary points   260
Do nurses use research?   263
Barriers to research utilization   264
Possible solutions   270

12.   Techniques and strategies for translating research findings into health care practice   **281**
Patrick Crookes

Background   282
Five factors crucial to the success of change management   286
Change agents   296
Change strategies and models of change   299

Glossary   311

Index   333

Contributors

Patrick Crookes BSc (Nursing) PhD RGN RNT CertEd
Senior Lecturer, Department of Nursing, University of Wollongong, NSW, Australia. Formerly Lecturer, School of Nursing and Midwifery, and Coordinator, BMedSci, Clinical Nursing and Midwifery, University of Sheffield, UK

Sue Davies BSc MSc RGN RHV
Lecturer in Nursing, Department of Gerontological and Continuing Care Nursing, University of Sheffield, UK

Lorraine B. Ellis BA (Hons) MSc RGN RNT
Lecturer in Nursing, Department of Acute and Critical Care Nursing, University of Sheffield, Sheffield, UK

Christine Hibbert RGN RNT Med
Nursing Lecturer, Department of Acute and Critical Care Nursing, University of Sheffield, Sheffield, UK

Yu Chu Huang BSc MMSc PhD RN
Head of Department, Der-Yu School of Nursing, Keelung, Taiwan, Republic of China

Christine Ingleton BA (Hons) MA PhD CertEd RGN RCNT
Lecturer, Department of Gerontological and Continuing Care Nursing, University of Sheffield, Sheffield, UK

Ulla S. E. Lundh BSc PhD RGN
Senior Lecturer, University College of Health Sciences, Jonköping, Sweden

Nigel Mathers BSc MD PhD DCH MRCGP
Director, Institute of General Practice and Primary Care, Community Sciences Centre, Northern General Hospital, Sheffield, UK

Elizabeth Matthews BSc (Hons) RGN
Lecturer in Nursing, Department of Acute and Critical Care Nursing, University of Sheffield, Sheffield, UK

Ann McDonnell BSc MSc RGN RNT
Lecturer in Nursing, Department of Acute and Critical Care Nursing, University of Sheffield, Sheffield, UK

Mike Nolan BEd MA MSc PhD RGN RMN
Professor of Gerontological Nursing, Director of Research, School of Nursing and Midwifery, University of Sheffield, Sheffield, UK

Susan M. Read PhD RGN RHV FWT
Senior Lecturer (Research), Department of Acute and Critical Care Nursing, University of Sheffield, Sheffield, UK

Ann M. Thomson BA MSc RGN RM MTD
Senior Lecturer in Midwifery, School of Nursing, Midwifery and Health Visiting, University of Manchester, Manchester, UK

Angela Venables BSc MA RGN RM CertEd
Senior Lecturer, Department of Acute and Critical Care Nursing, University of Sheffield, Sheffield, UK

Introduction

P. Crookes, S. Davies

Background to this book

In 1993, the Report of the Taskforce on the Strategy for Research in Nursing Midwifery and Health Visiting (DoH 1993) emphasized the need for research skills to be more widespread within these professions. The Taskforce were careful, however, to identify that such skills should not be developed via a proliferation of inadequately supervised, small-scale projects. Instead they took a wider perspective of the term 'research skills' to incorporate critical and analytical thinking. They also asserted that information literacy skills – accessing and evaluating literature (in this case research-based literature) were essential prerequisites for knowledge-based practice.

Shortly after the Taskforce Report was published, we found ourselves working together to develop a new research skills module for qualified nurses and midwives undertaking a 'top-up' degree at the University of Sheffield. Similar modules were being developed around the country as schools and colleges of nursing and health amalgamated with universities. We shared the views of the Taskforce about the need to widen the definition of 'research skills' since our experience of teaching nurses and midwives about research had led us to realize that many see it as of little relevance to their own practice. Many practitioners seem to view research as the concern of 'other people', not least because they associate the term 'research' with the need to actually carry out research themselves. As a result the utilization and implementation of research suffers from a lack of understanding, a lack of motivation and a lack of necessary skills.

We had both attempted to modify this view in our teaching by the use of a model – the 4 As of research skills (Awareness, Appreciation, Application and Ability). With this model we were able to differentiate between the skills of understanding available research reports and applying the findings in practice (necessary to all practitioners) and the skills to carry out research (necessary to a few). This philosophy provided the basis for the module Research Appreciation and Application. Our aim was to produce a programme which did not stop at the development of positive attitudes towards research and its role in clinical practice, but went on to facilitate the skills and knowledge required for the critical appraisal of research-based literature.

Our experience also told us that 'traditional' methods of teaching research do not typically lead to the development of the skills needed to appreciate and apply research. The content of courses and study days on research is often focused upon steps in the research process, on research methods and on writing research proposals, rather than on the identification and evaluation of the characteristics of research which have implications for the application of findings to practice. We feel it is more appropriate to focus *overtly* on the development of skills relevant to research utilization, including skills necessary to initiate and manage change. There are many barriers to research utilization in practice and the research-aware practitioner needs a full repertoire of skills and knowledge to help overcome these barriers.

As a result we developed a new approach to teaching research skills, one which focused on *overtly* developing skills in the critical appraisal of research reports and appropriate implementation of research findings. Our intention was to encourage, enable and motivate practitioners to:

■ access, read and understand research reports
■ apply research-based knowledge in the practice setting
■ influence colleagues on the use of research information
■ develop responsibility for their own professional development;

in other words, to accept research as a normal aspect of professional nursing and health care practice.

The module was also designed to promote the development of important generic skills (such as the use of information technology and writing systematic literature reviews) which could be applied in other contexts, as well as facilitating personal and professional development. In recognition of the findings of the Taskforce Report, we incorporated content which placed an emphasis on the context in which health care research is conducted, disseminated and utilized.

In developing the module, one of the first things we tried to do was identify a text which could support students (and us) through the course. Perusing the texts available at the time identified for us that the practice of equating research activity with 'doing' research has reached the point of ideology or dogma. Furthermore it is so pervasive that nursing research texts, which are largely north American in origin, cover material in such a way that the reader is taken through the processes of research by considering how to 'do it correctly', rather than by identifying important things to consider when evaluating a research report.

As a result, we decided to develop a text to reflect our own approach to teaching, not least to clearly and strongly assert that there are skills of research appreciation and application which are distinct from the skills necessary to undertake research. Furthermore we are keen to demonstrate that the skills of research appreciation and application are not inherently inferior to the skills necessary to 'do' research but that these skills complement each other in the context of modern health care.

Scope and purpose

This book is intended to prepare the reader to access, critically evaluate, synthesize and utilize research-based literature within professional health care practice. It is aimed at all health care professionals who need to develop skills in the appreciation and utilization of research. However, it should be of particular value to students undertaking educational programmes ranging from Diploma to Masters level, as these all require the development of skills in literature retrieval, analysis and review. We recognize that much of the material is drawn from a midwifery or nursing context, reflecting the backgrounds of the contributors. However, the book is intended to be relevant to all areas of professional health care practice and this reflects the importance of a multidisciplinary approach to research and research utilization.

How does this book differ from other books on research?

This text does *not* focus on how to do research. Instead it concentrates on the retrieval, analysis and application of existing research in order to identify and develop good practice. The traditional 'order' used in other texts based upon the stages of the research process has been avoided. Instead, we seek to *overtly* develop:

- an appreciation of the range of sources of knowledge which may inform nursing and health care practice
- an awareness of contemporary research and of the context within which health services' research and development takes place
- appreciation skills using an approach which examines the implications of features of project design and conduct for the critical evaluation of research reports and other research-based literature
- a recognition of the range of skills and insights relevant to the application of research findings and innovation within health care practice.

Throughout, the reader is encouraged to reflect upon the application of these skills within their own practice, and that of colleagues.

As you will see, the text is multi-authored to ensure that the content was written by people with particular expertise and insights. However, we have exercised our editorial influence in order to maintain overall coherence. As a result the chapters are presented in a similar style and contain a range of features including ongoing summary of content: reflective exercises, questions for possible discussion, and suggestions for further reading. These features are included with the dual intention of making the experience of reading the text as 'interactive' as possible, as well as emphasizing the 'so what?' of key issues covered.

The book is intended to be read in one of two ways, depending on readers' existing knowledge of research. The person new to research will benefit from reading the content as ordered in the text. Those with more knowledge and experience will also find this useful but may prefer to 'dip into' the text at particular points of interest. To make this easier, we now present the 12 chapters in overview.

Chapter 1 Ways of knowing in nursing and health care practice

There are a variety of ways of 'knowing' which may inform nursing and health care practice. Carper (1978), for example, distinguishes between empirical, aesthetic, moral and personal knowledge. Within this chapter, Mike Nolan and Ulla Lundh explore the concept of 'knowing' in detail, and encourage the reader to recognize the contribution that *all* types of knowledge can make to effective health care. A useful critique of the contributions of Patricia Benner and Donald Schön to current thinking about the ways in which nurses develop expertise is included in this chapter.

Chapter 2 The context of nursing and health care research

Sue Read begins with a brief historical overview of conditions and events which have led to the current emphasis on establishing the research base to nursing and health care practice. The contemporary context, including government policy and professional commentary within the last 5 years, is then explored in more detail, so as to inform the reader of the social and political context in which research is currently undertaken and applied. The aim is to alert practitioners to opportunities for utilizing research-based knowledge to inform and develop practice offered by national and local Research and Development strategies. Attention is also paid to the motivating forces which encourage individual researchers and research teams to undertake particular projects, as well as recognizing the effect that researcher motivation may have on findings and conclusions.

Chapter 3 Accessing sources of knowledge

As research activities become more central to nursing and health care practice, the range and volume of resources available to inform practice continues to increase rapidly. The ability to search the literature in a systematic and efficient way, is therefore, fundamental to the development of a research base to nursing and health care practice. In this chapter, Christine Hibbert and Patrick Crookes seek to enable the reader to identify and access research-based literature by suggesting ways of defining and refining topics for successful literature searching; considering different approaches to reading (e.g. skim reading, deep reading); presenting systems for recording and maintaining personal notes and references; and introducing the concept of critical analysis (we see the term regularly but what does it mean?). The chapter also contains an appendix presenting a range of databases and other sources of knowledge, which could be of use to health professionals.

Chapter 4 Philosophical and theoretical underpinnings of research

The aims of this chapter are to encourage the reader to appreciate the importance of recognizing the philosophical and theoretical perspectives which underpin research and to question and evaluate the theoretical and conceptual bases of individual research reports. To this end, Lorraine Ellis and Patrick Crookes highlight the major components of the relationship between research and theory – most importantly that research should be based upon and develop, theory and knowledge. The philosophical bases of three broad research paradigms – positivism, naturalism and critical theory are also explored, along with the processes of inductive and deductive reasoning. The roles of philosophy and reasoning within research processes are then described. Frames of reference (conceptual and theoretical frameworks) are discussed, and the contribution made by these frameworks to the development of research methodology and interpretation of findings is considered. In particular, the importance of identifying assumptions underpinning both the research questions and the research process for the study under evaluation is demonstrated.

Chapter 5 Recognizing research processes in research-based literature

Research design is a major factor to be considered when evaluating the appropriate application of research findings. For example, the findings of an ethnographic study are likely to have very different implications for practice, when compared with the findings of a large scale survey or randomized controlled trial. In this chapter, Ann Thomson describes the range of research designs commonly used in health care research generally, and in nursing and midwifery in particular and discusses the major strengths and limitations of each. The relationship between research design and level of knowledge (exploration, description and prediction) (DePoy and Gitlin 1993) is also examined.

Chapter 6 Evaluating methods for collecting data in published research

The value of a particular piece of research to nursing and health care practice is determined in large part by the rigour and credibility of its methodology. In turn, research rigour is related to the validity and reliability of all aspects of the research design. In this chapter, Nigel Mathers and Yu Chu Huang consider methodological rigour in relation to both qualitative and quantitative approaches to the collection of data. They also explore the issue of compatibility between procedures of data gathering and conclusions – an important aspect of evaluation when critically analyzing research papers. The significance of different methods for identifying a sample for study is also briefly considered.

Chapter 7 Evaluating methods for analyzing data in published research

In this chapter, Nigel Mathers and Yu Chu Huang shift their focus onto the evaluation of methods of analysis of both quantitative and qualitative data. Within the context of quantitative research, the reader is encouraged to consider whether a researcher has applied statistical tests appropriately, given the research design and nature of the data. Statistical tests which are commonly used in nursing and health care research are explained and the process of determining statistical significance is 'demystified'. Common approaches to the analysis of qualitative data are then explored. For both quantitative and qualitative data, the issue of compatibility of the analysis undertaken and the conclusions reached, is a key area of consideration and this is also discussed.

Chapter 8 Populations and samples: identifying the boundaries of research

The intention of this chapter is to make the critical reader of research more aware of the impact of sampling techniques on the implications of any research project. To do this, Christine Ingleton explores the range of sampling techniques commonly used in nursing and health care research. She then goes on to discuss the implications of using particular sampling techniques for extrapolating research findings to other populations and settings.

Chapter 9 Critiquing ethical issues in published research

A basic premise of this book is that nurses and other health care practitioners are expected to be involved in the evaluation and application of research findings. When reading and applying the findings of health care research there are a number of ethical principles to be considered. In this chapter, Liz Matthews and Angela Venables utilize the four principles and scope of application model of health care ethics to discuss ways of evaluating the ethical conduct of published research.

Chapter 10 Reviewing and interpreting research: identifying implications for practice

Identifying indicators for practice from research-based literature requires the synthesis of evidence from a number of projects investigating the same area. This may be complicated by the existence of apparently contradictory findings. In this chapter Sue Davies considers the purposes of a literature review and describes a number of tools and techniques which can help the reader to systematically review a body of literature in order to identify implications for practice, education and research. Approaches to structuring and writing a literature review are also presented.

Chapter 11 Factors which may inhibit the utilization of research findings in practice – and some solutions

A number of authors have identified that the utilization of research findings in nursing and health care practice is slow and is hampered by a wide range of factors. Ann McDonnell's chapter reviews the current literature in this field, and offers some possible solutions to perceived barriers.

Chapter 12 Techniques and strategies for translating research findings into health care practice

A range of methods and strategies have been identified as being effective in maximizing the success of innovation – namely 'models of change'. In this chapter, Patrick Crookes provides the reader with an overview of possible strategies for overcoming barriers to change and inertia within both individuals and organizations. This is an attempt to prepare practitioners wishing to apply the findings of research for the realities of the role of 'change agent'. The key argument of the chapter is that much of the innovation attempted in health care settings fails because people do not approach the management of change in a systematic and planned way. Criteria for the evaluation of previous innovation attempts are presented (those who ignore the mistakes of the past are destined to repeat them), as well as an overview of a number of models for planning change. The nursing context is used for much of the discussion, however, the principles discussed are relevant to any setting where change is being considered and planned.

We hope that this book will excite readers about the possibilities of using research-based knowledge to inform their practice. We have tried to demystify the terminology which can seem so off-putting for those new to reading research reports and hope that the book will enthuse readers to seek to expand their skills of research appreciation and application further. The satisfaction of being able to seek, find, and understand research-based literature which provides answers to our questions about practice is the ultimate reward.

References   Department of Health (1993) *Report of the Taskforce on the Strategy for Research in Nursing, Midwifery and Health Visiting*. London: DoH.

DePoy E and Gitlin L (1994) *Introduction to Research: Multiple Strategies for Health and Human Services*. St Louis, MO: Mosby.

1 Ways of knowing in nursing and health care practice

Mike Nolan, Ulla Lundh

'The essential nature of research lies in its intent to create new knowledge in whatever field' (Hockey 1996: 3)

Introduction

Although there are many definitions of research, the above short but important statement by Lisbeth Hockey, an early pioneer of nursing research in the UK, identifies one of its principal aims: to enhance our understanding by creating new knowledge. At first sight such an aim appears both reasonable and unproblematic. Unfortunately this is not the case. The question of what constitutes both research and knowledge is not straightforward and is a highly contested and hotly debated area. The main purpose of this book is to assist nurses and other practitioners to understand research and to play an active role in shaping debates about the value of research for their practice. However, as Hockey's quote suggests, research and knowledge, however defined, are inextricably linked and in order to appreciate the value of research it is also necessary to understand what is meant by knowledge. That is the purpose of this chapter.

It is not possible to provide definitive answers to these issues as there is no consensus on what constitutes 'knowledge'. However, there is broad agreement that there are differing types or forms of knowledge and that practitioners who work in disciplines such as nursing, teaching and social work draw on multiple sources and types of information to inform their practice. Whilst the emphasis within this book is primarily on scientific or theoretical knowledge, it is our hope that after reading this chapter you will have an understanding of different types of knowledge and will recognize the contribution that each has to make to improving practice.

In order to place our discussion in a suitable context we will begin with a brief consideration of the changing nature of health care, highlighting why it is important that all practitioners, and nurses in particular, draw on research-based evidence to inform their practice. Following this, attention is turned briefly to some philosophical considerations about the nature of knowledge. Although these issues will

See Chapters 2 and 4

be addressed in greater detail later in the book (see Chapters 2 and 4), it is necessary to introduce them here to give you a better appreciation of subsequent arguments. The remainder of this chapter will consider the differing types of knowledge commonly used in practice disciplines, stressing the potential value of each. The views of two major contributors to thinking in this area, Benner (Benner 1984, Benner *et al* 1996) and Schön (Schön 1987) are presented more fully and their relative merits identified. The literature in this area is extensive and it is not our aim to provide a complete account but rather to demonstrate the importance of adopting a critical and informed perspective. In concluding we will reiterate our belief that an eclectic and holistic approach to the use of knowledge is more appropriate than a narrow, discipline specific model. Essentially we will be arguing that there is a need to adopt a balanced stance which recognizes the important contribution of all types of knowledge, rather than a narrow, partisan position which prizes one form of knowing above another.

Key issues

- Factors influencing the emergence of research and development in the NHS
- The relationships between ontology, epistemology and methodology and the differing assumptions underpinning quantitative and qualitative research paradigms
- Types of knowledge including empirics, aesthetics, ethics, personal knowledge
- The place of 'intuitive' knowledge in practice disciplines
- Assumptions underpinning the work of Benner and Schön
- Arguments in favour of an eclectic knowledge base for practice

Changing health care, changing knowledge

Moody (1990) suggests that there has been an explosion in nursing knowledge over the last two decades, reflecting the scale and pace of change in the delivery of health care. Moreover, rather than slowing down, the pace of such change is increasing, fuelled by a number of factors such as:

- Advances in technology and treatment
- Demographic changes
- Increasing demands for health care
- The shift in focus and ideology towards primary care.

It is therefore now widely accepted that basic professional training provides only an initial platform of knowledge and skills and that it is essential that every practitioner updates themselves and keeps abreast of the latest developments. This is a prerequisite if 'knowledge-based decision-making' within the NHS (Secretary of State for Health 1996) is to be achieved. Furthermore, in recent years there has been an increasing realization that even medical practice must become far more research-based than is currently the case. For example, in 1991 Michael Peckham (then Director of Research and Development for the NHS) stated:

'Strongly held views based on belief rather than sound information still exert too much influence in health care'

(DoH 1991: Preface)

In order to address this perceived deficit the government of the day launched a strategy for research and development (R&D) in the NHS (DoH 1991). The primary objective of this strategy was to ensure that all those working in the Health Service used research to inform their day-to-day decision making.

In April 1992, a taskforce to consider the implications of the NHS R&D strategy for nursing, midwifery and health visiting was established. The terms of reference for this group were broad and included not only the scope and objectives of research in nursing, midwifery and health visiting, and how this activity should interface with other health-related research, but also the following issues:

■ Identifying research priorities
■ Mechanisms for taking research forward in clinical, managerial and educational environments
■ Training and recognition of research skills
■ Structures and incentives to ensure the dissemination of research findings
■ The role of the nursing, midwifery and health visiting professions in interdisciplinary work with other professions.

The Taskforce made a number of recommendations which are discussed more fully later (see Chapter 2). Central to their arguments was the belief that, whilst not all nurses should engage in research, it is essential for every practitioner to 'develop a capacity for critical thought' and that 'basic research literacy is an essential prerequisite for knowledge-led practice' (DoH 1993).

It is just such research literacy that this book is intended to stimulate and develop. Since this taskforce reported, the emphasis on R&D in the Health Service has increased, as has the expectation that all practitioners will develop their own knowledge base (Secretary of State for Health 1996). When used in this context, the term knowledge usually refers to 'scientific' or 'theoretical' knowledge. Yet – somewhat paradoxically – calls for the wider application of such theoretical knowledge are occurring simultaneously with trends in many practice disciplines, especially nursing, to place greater emphasis on practical or experiential knowledge. In order to understand the potential tensions and contradictions in nursing's move towards the intuitive rather than the rational side of care, it is necessary to refer briefly to more fundamental questions about the nature of knowledge. This is important as definitions of knowledge can only be appreciated when they are related to a more general set of beliefs about the world in which we live.

Reality, knowing and method: some basic beliefs

Different approaches to research and the generation of knowledge depend largely on the 'paradigm' that is adopted. According to Denzin and Lincoln (1994) a paradigm is a set of basic beliefs that guide action by providing a world view shaping the way we interpret and understand our environment. A paradigm is underpinned by a number of first principles or 'ultimates' (Denzin and Lincoln 1994) which can never be proven to be true but have to be accepted as being correct. Clearly it is not possible to believe in more than one paradigm, as each is based on differing beliefs about the nature of the world. Varying research methods reflect differing paradigms and

See Chapters 2 and 4

these will be explored in greater detail in subsequent chapters. For our present purpose it is sufficient to know that each paradigm attempts to provide answers to at least three sets of questions. Guba and Lincoln (1989) see these as being ontological, epistemological and methodological questions.

The most abstract of these is the ontological question, concerned with the nature of reality itself. The central issue is whether reality is perceived as something which is fixed and external or whether reality is shaped and influenced by how people interpret and interact with their world. The epistemological question asks 'what is knowledge?' and seeks to understand the relationship between researchers on the one hand and the subjects of research on the other. Methodological questions are the least abstract and are concerned with the methods and approaches that can be used to generate knowledge. It will readily be seen that although discrete, these questions are nonetheless related in a hierarchical fashion, so that answers to the ontological question influence the answers to the epistemological question, which in turn largely determines the methodological approaches that it is considered appropriate to use.

See Chapters 4, 5, 7 and 8

Such issues will be considered in more detail later in this book.

In this chapter we are interested primarily in epistemological questions – those seeking to establish the nature of knowledge. Debates in this area are complex and, as already highlighted, there is ultimately no way of proving them either right or wrong. Although important, the finer points of such arguments are of more interest to philosophers than to practitioners or researchers. We will therefore deal with them in a manner that some would consider to be superficial. This is inevitable in a book of this nature. The situation is further complicated by the fact that in qualitative research there are currently a number of differing paradigms each providing a different emphasis. Denzin and Lincoln (1994), for example, consider that in the last 60 years or so, five differing paradigms (they term them 'moments') of qualitative research have emerged and still co-exist. We will not be able to explore these approaches to qualitative research here and readers who are interested in a more detailed account are advised to consult the original text.

Here we will paint a deliberately broad picture highlighting the two issues which seem to us to be the most important. The first reflects the traditional debate about the difference between quantitative and qualitative research. The second is a product of more recent concerns about the role and value of scientific knowledge itself and the emerging argument that research should not simply aim to produce knowledge but that it should also actively seek to change and improve the world. From such a perspective research is seen to have a more overtly political and emancipatory agenda – as evidenced in approaches such as participatory action research, feminist research and ethnic research. Although such issues may appear rather academic at this point, an appreciation of them is essential to a better understanding of many of the current debates in the nursing literature.

Many readers will already have some familiarity with the long-standing quantitative/qualitative debate which, although it has raged for several decades, is still a preoccupation of many researchers and practitioners. Unfortunately arguments are frequently taken to extremes, with people adopting fixed and somewhat inflexible positions. The basis of such disagreements can be traced to the ontological assumptions underpinning qualitative and quantitative research.

The early development of science focused largely on the physical world involving disciplines such as mathematics, physics and chemistry. Indeed, mathematics is still seen as the 'queen' of sciences (Guba and Lincoln 1994). These disciplines rely heavily – almost exclusively – on quantification, in order to explain the world in terms of equations, statistics and laws. The success of the physical sciences in helping us to understand the world has led to the view that the methods they adopted are the only way to conduct good research. This became widely known as 'the positivist paradigm', which is based on the belief that there is an external reality and that the world is governed by universal laws or laws of nature, which apply at all times and in all places. Because knowledge consists of such laws, researchers can be totally objective and their own beliefs are not considered to influence the results of their research. Within the positivist paradigm, the best way to conduct research is to control and manipulate events, ideally in a laboratory setting.

Whilst such an approach seems reasonable in exploring the physical world, its application to the social world is seen by many as fundamentally flawed. It is argued that people are free agents, not governed by external laws but capable of taking independent decisions. An opposing set of beliefs, 'the qualitative paradigm', therefore emerged. Broadly speaking, those adhering to a qualitative paradigm believe that the social world is not fixed and external, but varies with time and place, and that human behaviour is not dictated by universal laws, but by the shared meanings people hold. As a result, it is not possible for researchers to be objective and value-free. Given these two premises, it is considered inappropriate for researchers to manipulate and control people and events as this alters the way they behave. Qualitative researchers therefore have a commitment to naturalism – studying people in their natural environment. This provides the broad methodological approach within the qualitative paradigm.

It can be seen that in terms of what constitutes knowledge there is considerable divergence between the qualitative and quantitative paradigms. However, despite such obvious differences both these paradigms have recently been criticized by those who believe that they place too much emphasis and importance on the role of the researcher. For example, although qualitative researchers recognize the importance of studying people in a natural setting and acknowledge that their own values can influence their results, ultimately it is still the researcher who takes the lead in deciding what is knowledge.

Critics of both qualitative and quantitative research argue that true power is still vested primarily with the researcher. They further believe that 'telling things as they are' and leaving them unchanged is not sufficient. The first set of arguments has been summarized by Elliot (1991) as follows:

> 'Whether the techniques generate psychometric measures, ethnographies or grounded theories does not matter. They are all symbolic of the power of the researcher to define valid knowledge'
>
> (Elliot 1991: 46)

This dissatisfaction with both qualitative and quantitative research has resulted in the emergence of much more radical and political interpretations of research underpinned by the need to empower people and assist them to change their situation. Such intentions are reflected within the critical theory paradigm discussed in detail in Chapter 4.

These shifts in ideology about the purpose of research reflect a more general move away from an uncritical acceptance of the value of traditional or scientific knowledge (theory) towards a greater emphasis on personal or experiential knowledge. This trend is mirrored in much of the recent nursing literature about intuitive, tacit or practical knowledge. Attention is now turned to these debates.

Summary

Empirical or research-based knowledge is not the only basis upon which decisions about health care should be made. However, the changing nature of health care, in part due to government pressure, highlights the imperative that nurses and other health professionals must be willing and able to draw on research-based evidence to inform their practice. The long-standing 'quantitative versus qualitative' debate and the perceived shortcomings of both these paradigms should not be allowed to obscure the value of empirical knowledge to contemporary health care workers.

Ways of knowing: an overview

As already indicated there are generally considered to be several different types of knowledge or 'ways of knowing'. This is complicated enough but as Eraut (1994) notes, the situation is not helped by the fact that differing terms are often used to describe essentially the same thing. Cohen and Manion (1985), for example, differentiate between experience, research and reasoning as ways of generating knowledge whereas Moody (1990) talks in terms of folklore, wisdom and scientific knowledge. Broadly speaking, several authors, by implication at least, distinguish the *source* of knowledge and how it is generated from the *type* of knowledge that results. For instance, Burns and Grove (1993) state that you can know a person, comprehend facts, acquire a skill or master a subject with the emphasis here being placed on different ways of knowing. They also suggest that nursing utilizes knowledge from many different sources such as:

- Tradition (custom and practice – 'it's always been done this way')
- Authority (based on expertise and power)
- Borrowing (from other disciplines such as medicine or sociology)
- Trial and error ('try it and see')
- Experience ('it worked for me')
- A role model or mentor (not dissimilar to authority).

Widening the debate somewhat, Meleis (1991) believes that there are also different types of 'knower' (Box 1.1). Here the emphasis shifts to characteristics of the individual with the assumption being that the way that nurses use knowledge is closely linked to their personality or the type of person they are.

For our present purpose we will focus mainly on different types of knowledge rather than on how knowledge is generated (although the two are clearly linked) or on the personal characteristics of individual practitioners. In the nursing literature the work of Carper (1978) is the most cited. Carper believed that nurses draw upon four different types of knowledge (see Box 1.2).

Box 1.1
Different types of knower

Silent knowers	accept the voice of authority and learn to be silent. May be skilled and knowledgeable but don't make their views known
Received knowers	accept the authority of others to generate knowledge, do not see the development of their own ideas as worthwhile
Subjective knowers	rely on personal experience as a source of knowledge
Procedural knowers	rely on rules, regulations and procedures
Constructed knowers	see knowledge as contextual and integrate/utilize different types of knowing depending on the context. Constantly redefine and reconstruct knowledge.

(After Meleis 1991)

Box 1.2
Different types of knowledge

Empirics	This is scientific nursing knowledge in the form of theories and models that can be tested against data gathered directly by studying the physical or social world. In other words such knowledge *and the way it is generated,* is publicly verifiable. The purpose of this type of knowledge is to describe, explain and eventually predict events. Empirical knowledge can be written down and learned as a set of ideas or principles constituting a 'body of knowledge'.
Aesthetics	This is often contrasted with empirics with aesthetics representing the artistic side of nursing. According to Chinn and Kramer (1991) aesthetics is nursing made visible through the actions, bearing, conduct and interaction of nurses with others (generally their patients). It involves engaging, interpreting and envisaging. To be engaged requires the direct involvement of self on an

Box 1.2 *(contd.)*

experiential rather than a cognitive level. It is about being rather than thinking. Interpretation is the process of making sense of and creating responses arising from interaction or engagement, whilst envisioning is about using knowledge to see or create new possibilities for change and growth. Aesthetics is not expressed in language but rather is experienced, although Chinn and Kramer argue that certain aspects such as empathetic listening or facial expressions can be communicated to others.

Ethics

Ethics is moral knowledge, a matter of what 'ought' to be, what is good or right. It involves having to make difficult decisions for which there are no prescriptive answers. Thus in contrast to scientific knowledge (empirics) ethics cannot be tested against reality as ethical decisions are underpinned by beliefs and values rather than facts.

Personal knowledge

This involves the inner experience of being self aware, the rationale being that in order to know others you have to know yourself first. Personal knowledge is seen as essential for the therapeutic use of self in nursing.

(After Carper 1978)

Chinn and Kramer (1991) contend that all the above types or 'patterns' of knowledge are required by nurses as each forms a distinct part of the whole. However, in most disciplines scientific knowledge is traditionally the most highly prized, since possession of a unique 'body of knowledge' is one of the main characteristics of a profession. Indeed the power of a profession lies primarily in its claim to have access to specialist knowledge; the more unique the knowledge and the less it is understandable to lay people, the greater the power (Eraut 1994). It is therefore not surprising that nursing, in its desire to compete with medicine, has placed great emphasis on scientific knowledge (Moody 1990, Chinn and Kramer 1991, Burns and Grove 1993, Meleis 1991, Rose and Parker 1994). This has also been the case in other disciplines aspiring to professional status such as teaching (Eraut 1994) and social work (Thompson 1995).

However, over the past decade or so, many practitioners have become increasingly disenchanted with scientific knowledge and have sought instead to highlight the value of practical and experiential knowledge. Once again a myriad of terms have been used but the essential argument turns on the relationship between knowing about something (expressed as facts and theories), knowing how to do something (in a practical sense) and how both relate to experience and intuition (Reason 1994).

It is interesting to trace this shift in emphasis within the nursing literature which, in the 1970s and 1980s, placed great store in theoretical knowledge (Hardy 1994). However, over the years there has been a growing discontent with theory (Lewis 1988, Moore 1990, Kenny 1993, Robinson 1994) so that it is now often seen as irrelevant, and many practitioners consider it to be a 'side issue' (Levine 1995).

Kenny (1993) rather prophetically suggested that the perceived failure of nursing theory would result in an increasing 'reification' of the experiential components of nursing. This is reflected in the growing calls to develop the intuitive aspects of nursing (Rose and Parker 1994) in the form of 'personal knowledge' (Sweeny 1994) or 'alternative theoretical frameworks' based on a tacit understanding (Lauder 1994) and 'informal' theories (Pryjmachuk 1996). This development is a facet of the basic tension apparent in most practice disciplines between propositional (theoretical) knowledge and practical (experiential) knowledge with Ryle (1949) coining the terms 'know that' and 'know how' to highlight this dichotomy.

These two types of knowledge should be complementary but unfortunately 'know that', as Kenny (1993) predicted, is becoming increasingly devalued, and 'know how' is currently seen by many as the way forward for nursing. There is therefore a growing tendency to 'undermine the rational in favour of the intuitive' (Bradshaw 1995), so that some feel that only practitioners can develop legitimate theory (Tolley 1995). Thompson (1995) argues that although appealing, the myth of 'theoryless practice' must be resisted and an appropriate balance has to be achieved between propositional (what he terms 'formal') knowledge and practical (informal) knowledge. As Eraut (1994: 42) so cogently points out 'to recognize that uncodifiable practical knowledge exists need not imply that stored, written knowledge is irrelevant'.

Such a balance is not readily apparent in much of the current nursing literature. As Hardy (1994) noted, many nurses jumped on the 'theory bandwagon' in the 1970s and 1980s and many are jumping on the 'experiential' bandwagon at the moment. It is easy to see the appeal of experiential knowledge, which stands in stark contrast to many nursing theories and models which are highly abstract and difficult to understand. Such models tend to confuse things unnecessarily by giving new theoretical names to things that would otherwise be seen as self-evident (Lundh *et al* 1988). Abstract theories often fail to recognize the unique needs of patients and alienate many practitioners who find it difficult to see how theory can provide an adequate basis for their day-to-day care (Lenz *et al* 1995). Experiential and practical knowledge on the other hand appears to be far more relevant. However, uncritical acceptance of experiential knowledge should be avoided. In order to illustrate this point the work of two influential authors, Benner (Benner 1984, Benner *et al* 1996) and Schön (1987) is now considered.

Summary

The most commonly cited model of 'ways of knowing' is that of Carper (1978). It should be acknowledged that all forms of knowledge have a place in health care decision making. For many years 'empirical' knowledge has held an ascendancy over the others, not least because the possession of a unique body of knowledge is a prerequisite for an occupational group to call itself a 'profession'. There are now signs, particularly within nursing, that the pendulum is swinging towards the view that 'personal' and 'aesthetic' knowledge are equally important – typically under the aegis of terms such as 'intuition' and 'experiential knowledge'.

Major contributors and their work

Patricia Benner

There can be few authors in the last 15 years whose work has had more impact on the nursing profession than that of Benner and colleagues (Benner 1984, Benner and Wruebel 1989, Benner *et al* 1996). Building on the model of the Dreyfus brothers (Dreyfus and Dreyfus 1986), Benner presents an elegant model of clinical expertise which has captured the imagination of numerous practitioners. Its appeal lies both in its apparent simplicity and the extent to which clinical nurses can identify with many of the stages on the road to expertise.

Benner (1984) based her adaptation of the original Dreyfus and Dreyfus model on detailed critical incident interviews with 93 nurses. From this empirical work Benner identified a number of competencies and seven main domains of nursing which she considered had to be mastered before expertise is reached. The route to expertise is primarily through experience rather than a reliance on theoretical knowledge. In Benner's view the more skilled a practitioner becomes, the less important is the role of theory. The development of expertise is depicted as a continuum comprising five sequential stages:

- Novice
- Advanced beginner

- Competent
- Proficient
- Expert.

Not all individuals reach expertise and many do not progress beyond competence.

When in the novice stage practitioners have little experience and rely heavily on taught rules and procedures. As a consequence they are unable to make discretionary judgements and practise more or less in a rote-like manner. As an individual gains more experience he or she is better able to see patterns or 'aspects' within a clinical situation, but in the advanced beginner phase such aspects are still treated separately and all are seen as being equally important. Decision making is largely focused on short-term goals. As competence is gained, the ability to set longer-term goals is enhanced and individuals are better able to deal with atypical or unusual situations. Proficiency is marked by a perception of situations as holistic, facilitating the setting of priorities in work. Eventually experts rely almost entirely on an intuitive grasp of situations and only turn to abstract reasoning in new or problematic situations. This progression has been described in the following way:

> 'The pathway to competence is characterised mainly by the ability to recognise features of practical situations and to discriminate between them, to carry out routine procedures under pressure and to plan ahead ... whereas proficiency marks the onset of quite a different approach to the job: normal behaviour is not just routine but semi-automatic; situations are apprehended more deeply and the abnormal is quickly spotted and given attention ... progression from proficiency to expertise finally happens when the decision-making as well as situational understanding becomes instinctive rather than analytic; and this requires significantly more experience'
>
> (Eraut 1994: 125–126)

More recently Benner *et al* (1996) have engaged in further empirical testing of this model, placing a greater emphasis on its implications for clinical practice and education. They highlight the importance of nurses knowing a particular patient, arguing that knowledge is socially embedded and context-specific, being based primarily on the ability to distinguish between 'saliences, nuances and qualitative distinctions'. This recent publication is more concerned than previous works with how expert practitioners can share their knowledge in order to create 'pooled expertise' that can be used to develop skills in other nurses.

There is no doubt that Benner's work has been very influential and has been adopted wholeheartedly, but perhaps somewhat uncritically, by many nurses. However, the model is not without its critics. In a lucid argument, Eraut (1994) is critical of the extent to which both the Dreyfus brothers and Benner spend too much time identifying the weaknesses of opposing models and not enough in exposing the limitations of their own. He believes that advocates of the novice-to-expert approach have tended to idealize the concept of intuitive practice and have ignored considerable research evidence, for example, in psychology, which stresses the fallibility of human judgement.

Moreover, virtually all of the empirical work undertaken by Benner has concentrated on acute and intensive care situations which call for rapid interpretation and decision making. The model has yet to be tested in care situations where the pace of work is slower, allowing greater time for active and purposeful contemplation. For example, the creation of a positive environment for the long-term care of older people should not be based primarily on intuition. It is more likely to be effective if it is underpinned by a sound theoretical rationale which recognizes individuality whilst appreciating the importance of group norms and expectations. The extent to which Benner's work can be applied successfully to the whole spectrum of nursing activity remains in the realms of speculation. Indeed Eraut (1994) considers that two important questions about the Dreyfus model remain unanswered:

> *'How serious is its neglect of the problem of expert fallibility? And what proportion of professional work does it cover? My own view is that it consistently underestimates the former and overestimates the latter'*

> (Eraut 1994: 128)

Such a critique does not mean that the work of Benner should be rejected but rather that it needs to be examined in greater detail. Often, however, there is a tendency to reify certain models and see them as inherently superior to alternative explanations. This is apparent in Benner's work and is also evident when the model of Schön (1987) is considered.

Donald Schön   If the Dreyfus model has had a significant impact on nursing, the work of Schön (1987) has achieved more widespread influence, affecting not only nursing but other disciplines such as teaching. Schön writes in a somewhat more accessible style than Benner and his use of metaphors to convey his ideas has instant appeal. He contrasts the world of 'technical rationality' (based on scientific knowledge) with the messy day-to-day world of real life practice. He argues that technical rationality is well suited to the 'hard high ground' where problems are easily identified and have clear-cut solutions, but believes that most practitioners occupy the 'swampy lowlands' where situations are often confused and problems are not clearly delineated.

Schön suggests that the most interesting and important problems occur in the swamps where the limitations of technical (scientific) knowledge are readily exposed. He questions the value and higher status accorded to theoretical knowledge and calls instead for an examination of the 'epistemology of practice'. Schön argues that we must recognize that the 'artistry' apparent in practical skills is an exercise of intelligence which is rigorous in its own terms. He believes that professional artistry is the type of competence that skilled practitioners demonstrate when they confront the 'unique, uncertain and conflicted situations of practice'.

As with Dreyfus and Benner, Schön stresses the value of tacit knowledge and understanding which allows us to know 'more than we can say'. He calls the normal, routine practice of a competent individual 'knowing-in-action', which is based on observable skilled performance, an explanation for which cannot usually be given. In other words, most practitioners perform tasks without being able to explain why. Normally in unproblematic situations, knowing-in-action is a spontaneous process that does not require conscious thought.

Occasionally surprise or unexpected events occur which require a rapid response and this, according to Schön, results in a process of 'reflection-in-action' in order to try and identify the cause of the unexpected failure. In such cases very skilled individuals can modify their performance in the middle of an action so that deficits are rectified instantly. Although Schön uses examples such as the gifted tennis player, he believes that expert practitioners are also capable of displaying such 'artistry', especially in uncertain situations where solutions may have to be developed, tested and refined almost immediately. He presents his model as a constructivist view of practice in which practitioners are constantly remaking or reconstructing their artistry as new events unfold.

Once again Schön has found advocates in many professional disciplines but his model is not without its critics. As with his critique of the Dreyfus thesis, Eraut (1994) poses some telling questions about the general applicability of 'reflection-in-action'. He highlights the fact that, as in Benner's work, Schön's focus is on the unpredictable aspects of practice which require fairly immediate action. As such Eraut believes that Schön's ideas, to the extent that they are applicable at all, relate only to a small section of the work of most practitioners.

> '. . . he is principally concerned with developing an epistemology of professional creativity, rather than a complete epistemology of professional practice'

(Eraut 1994: 143)

Furthermore, although Schön's use of metaphor is useful in presenting the basic philosophy underlying his model, Eraut is critical of the fact that there is little *but* metaphor in much of Schön's writing. Consequently the central feature of artistry, reflection-in-action, is, according to Eraut, rather vague, poorly defined and overgeneralized.

Another potential weakness of the whole notion of professional artistry is its failure to account adequately for the dimension of time. Some practical problems do not call for an immediate solution and Eraut argues that many activities, such as those common in engineering – building the Channel Tunnel for example – cannot be solved on the basis of intuition but call instead for strategic thinking. This requires the ability to weigh several different potential solutions in order to select the most effective. Professionals frequently face multiple and competing demands and Schön offers no adequate explanation as to how these are prioritized.

Within the context of the present health service Schön's work also suffers from two other major limitations. These relate to the need to account for multiprofessional and multiagency working and to incorporate the increasing expectation that patients (clients) and carers will play an active role in decisions about their care. Neither of these activities can be achieved by using intuitive action, reflective or otherwise, as there has to be a more overt, shared and readily observable set of interactions and perhaps outcomes. Eraut (1994) contends that in such circumstances there has to be conscious reflection, a willingness to learn from others and an openness to new ideas. He therefore argues that deliberation and metacognition are *also* hallmarks of professional expertise.

The emergence of 'several currently fashionable theories' of expertise over recent years has, according to Paley (1996), resulted in the use of sweeping generalizations, with people taking entrenched positions. Paley believes that many of the ensuing arguments have been 'juvenile' and have failed to address issues of central importance, such as the taken-for-granted assumption that professional expertise is inherently good. This, he contends, can lead to a blinkered self-serving approach and to the uncritical acceptance of the value of intuitive knowledge. It is our belief that *all* forms of knowledge are potentially useful and that the truly expert practitioner will be able to synthesize differing approaches and select the one that is the most appropriate. This suggests the need for an eclectic approach to practice, rather than one which sees certain types of knowledge as inherently superior to others.

Summary   Together, Benner and Schön present apparently cogent and compelling arguments in favour of using practical and experiential knowledge to underpin expert clinical practice. However, uncritical acceptance of the ascendancy of experiential over empirical knowledge should be avoided, not least because these models have yet to be tested in a range of clinical settings with a range of client groups. Nor do they take account of the fact that many aspects of health care delivery require deliberation and planning before any action is taken. Expert practitioners synthesize knowledge of differing types before reaching a conclusion regarding action. The need for an eclectic approach to professional knowledge and decision making therefore appears unarguable.

Achieving a balance

As already noted, concerns about the relative contribution and value of different forms of knowledge or ways of knowing are not confined to nursing but are apparent in a range of practice disciplines such as teaching (Elliot 1991), social work (Thompson 1995) and physiotherapy (Higgs 1992). This highlights the value of an 'extended epistemology' (Lincoln and Guba 1985, Reason 1994) which recognizes the validity and usefulness of all types of knowledge. However, we believe, as do others (Eraut 1994, Closs 1994, Paley 1996), that recent debates within the nursing literature have neglected the value of theoretical knowledge, placing too much emphasis on the intuitive side of practice.

In an attempt to regain a sense of balance Closs (1994) suggests that it is time to end what she considers to be rather sterile arguments about the art versus the science of nursing and recognize instead that a combination of experience, intuition, empathy and scientific knowledge is required. Indeed, Closs sees such an eclectic approach as one of nursing's greatest strengths. Even the proponents of intuitive knowledge recognize that it is not possible to excel without drawing on some 'articuable scientific knowledge' (i.e. theory) (Dreyfus and Dreyfus 1996). Yet as Eraut (1994) notes, action is required if equilibrium is to be restored:

> *Thirty years ago professional expertise tended to be identified with propositional knowledge and a high theoretical content regardless of whether such knowledge ever got used in practice. Whereas most of the theories of expertise . . . appear to have assumed that expertise is based mainly on experience with further development of theoretical knowledge having almost ceased soon after qualification'*
>
> (Eraut 1994: 157)

Many authors believe that one of the reasons why theory has not been adopted widely by most practitioners is the failure of educators to assist practitioners in 'transforming' theory before its use (Higgs 1992, Eraut 1994, Paul and Heaslip 1995, Thompson 1995). The simple learning of facts and theories is not sufficient in a practice discipline (Higgs 1992, Eraut 1994, Paul and Heaslip 1995) as the context of application is also of prime importance. Theoretical knowledge represents a useful set of guidelines for practice rather than a blueprint to be followed in a robot-like manner, and to be useful, theory has to be interpreted according to the demands of a given practical situation (Johns 1995, Paul and Heaslip 1995).

Elaborating on this idea Paul and Heaslip (1995) suggest that facts and theories learned in a classroom situation should be viewed as *information* rather than *knowledge* and that information does not become knowledge until it has been 'transformed'. This involves a deliberate intellectual effort of 'figuring out and reasoning about the problems one encounters in practice'. Starting from a similar premise, but in the context of physiotherapy practice, Higgs (1992) believes that effective clinicians require both knowledge and clinical reasoning skills. Within her framework, knowledge comprises personal, experiential and practical components based on a 'deep understanding' of each aspect. This alone is not, however, sufficient. To provide good care, knowledge must be married with clinical reasoning, that is, the ability to recall knowledge and analyze, synthesize and evaluate it in relation to each unique situation. In this way knowledge is constantly elaborated on (or 'constructed' in Higgs' terms) as it is applied and tested in practice.

When individuals become very skilled at such 'transformations' Paul and Heaslip (1995) contend that processing remains at a subconscious level and gives the appearance of intuition. On this basis they argue that within a professional context intuition is best viewed as a form of highly developed intellectual endeavour. Some support for this position can be gained from the literature on professional expertise. For example, most of the 'evidence' which is provided in favour of intuition is based on 'exemplars' or detailed descriptions of clinical situations which represent examples of practice. Schön (1987) in particular relies heavily on these to illustrate his arguments. In explaining the process of reflection-in-action he describes in some detail a 'problem' he encountered when building a gate. We quote this at length here as it is important not only in highlighting the rationale underpinning Schön's theories but because there is also one particular sentence which, for us, may help to reconcile the link between propositional (theoretical) knowledge and practical knowledge.

'Recently, for example, I built a gate out of wooden pickets and strapping. I had made a drawing and figured out the dimensions I wanted, but I had not reckoned with the problem of keeping the structure square. As I began to nail the strapping to the pickets, I noticed a wobble. I knew the structure would become rigid when I nailed in a diagonal piece, but how could I be sure

it would be square? There came to mind a vague memory about diagonals: in a rectangle diagonals are equal. I took a yardstick, intending to measure the diagonals, but I found I could not use it without disturbing the structure. It occurred to me to use a piece of string. Then it became apparent that, in order to measure the diagonals, I needed a precise location at each corner. After several trials, I found I could locate the centre point at each corner by constructing diagonals there. I hammered in a nail at each of the four centre points and used the nails as anchors for the measurement string. It took several minutes to figure out how to adjust the structure so as to correct the errors I found by measuring. And then, when I had the diagonals equal, I nailed in a piece of strapping to freeze the structure.

Here, in an example that must have its analogues in the experiences of amateur carpenters the world over, my intuitive way of going about the task led me to a surprise (the discovery of the wobble), which I interpreted as a problem. In the midst of action, I invented procedures to solve the problem, discovered further unpleasant surprises, and made further corrective inventions, including the several minor ones necessary to carry out the idea of using string to measure the diagonals. We might call such a process "trial and error". But the trials are not randomly related to one another; reflection on each trial and its results sets the stage for the next trial. Such a pattern of inquiry is better described as a sequence of "moments" in a process of reflection-in-action'

(Schön 1987: 26–27)

The fundamental problem Schön faced here was 'how could I be sure that it (the gate) would be square'. In order to begin the problem-solving process Schön states 'there came to mind a vague memory about diagonals: in a rectangle diagonals are equal'. We would suggest that here is an example of theoretical knowledge underpinning what is advanced as an exemplar of 'reflection-in-action'. In other words Schön's insights were actually based on geometric theory (the 'vague memory about diagonals') rather than intuitive knowledge. We are not arguing that this necessarily undermines Schön's approach entirely, but it does at least provide a potential illustration of the interdependent and mutually reinforcing nature of various forms of knowing.

Summary

It should be acknowledged that the skilled practitioner combines experience, intuition, empathy and scientific knowledge to inform the care and treatment they provide. Indeed this can be seen as one of nursing's greatest strengths. The work of Schön himself provides evidence that expert practice is built upon *all* forms of knowledge, working together in an interdependent and mutually reinforcing manner. To facilitate the development of this ability amongst the wider profession, more effort needs to be applied to the transformation of facts and theories (information) into knowledge which can actually be used in practice. Incidentally, in terms of knowledge of research appreciation and application skills, this is *the* intention of this text.

Chapter conclusion

Whether intuition, tacit knowledge and experiential knowledge exist as independent and discrete ways of knowing, or whether they are the skilful and imperceptible blending of propositional knowledge with experience, we believe that all knowledge is potentially useful. The expert practitioner is the one who draws on the most appropriate knowledge for the situation in hand. Eraut (1994) provides a useful metaphor when he suggests that practical situations can be considered as either hot or cold (and presumably somewhere in between). 'Hot' situations call for rapid decision making; an example in nursing would be a life-threatening event where action is needed instantly. In such circumstances deliberate and conscious thought does not overtly drive a response. In 'cold' situations on the other hand there is much more time for deliberation, and the use of forward thinking to anticipate potential problems and rehearse solutions is essential. Concepts of expertise and knowledge must account for both hot and cold situations and the numerous 'lukewarm' events that lie in between. Only then will a genuine extended epistemology be apparent.

It has been the purpose of this chapter to highlight a number of issues surrounding knowledge, ways of knowing and their potential inter-relationships. The remainder of this book will consider the role of research, the fundamental purpose of which, as we noted at the start of this chapter, is to add to our understanding by producing new knowledge. The debates about knowledge rehearsed here reflect similar arguments about the value of differing types of research, usually in the guise of the qualitative/quantitative debate. Some years ago Swanson and Chenitz (1982) cited Rubin (1981) in the following way:

'Our quarrels about the value of hard versus soft data are irrelevant to the world and its problems and are unnecessary and distracting for us. Differing research methods need not compete we need only to understand that they tell us different sorts of things'

If we may be allowed to paraphrase this we will finish this chapter with just such a message.

'Our quarrels about the value of scientific (theoretical, proposi-tional, formal) versus intuitive (experiential, tacit, informal) knowledge are irrelevant to the world and its problems and unnecessary and distracting for us. Differing ways of knowing need not compete, we need only to understand that they tell us different sorts of things'

Exercise 1.1

Think of a recent work-related event in which you had to make an important decision in:

- A 'hot' (i.e. rapidly changing) situation
- A 'cold' (more slowly evolving) situation.

For each situation, identify the types and sources of knowledge that you needed to reach your decision. Compare and contrast the two events and reflect upon whether your decision could have been improved and/or altered if differing knowledge had been applied.

Exercise 1.2

Refer to the 'types of knower' identified by Meleis in Box 1.1. Identify a colleague who you think would fit into each category (including yourself). Is this typology adequate or are there other 'types of knower'? Which approach do you think results in the most effective practitioner and why?

Further reading

Benner P (1984) *From Novice to Expert: Excellence and Power in Clinical Nursing Practice.* Menlo Park, CA: Addison Wesley.

Carper BA (1978) Fundamental patterns of knowing in nursing. *Advances in Nursing Science* **1**(1): 13–23.

Closs J (1994) What's so awful about science? *Nurse Research* **2**(2): 161–175.

Eraut M (1994) *Developing Professional Knowledge and Competence.* London: The Falmer Press.

Higgs J (1992) Developing knowledge: a process of construction, mapping and review. *New Zealand Journal of Physiotherapy.* **20**: 23–30.

Paley J (1996) Intuition and expertise: comments on the Benner debate. *Journal of Advanced Nursing* **23**(4): 665–671.

Paul RW and Heaslip P (1995) Critical thinking and intuitive nursing practice. *Journal of Advanced Nursing* **22**(1): 40–47.

Schön D (1987) *Educating the Reflective Practitioner.* San Francisco, CA: Jossey-Bass.

References

Benner P (1984) *From Novice to Expert: Excellence and Power in Clinical Nursing Practice*. Menlo Park, CA: Addison Wesley.

Benner P and Wruebel J (1989) *The Primacy of Caring: Stress and Coping in Health and Illness*. Menlo Park, CA: Addison Wesley.

Benner P, Tanner CA and Chesla CA (1996) *Expertise in Nursing Practice: Caring, Clinical Judgement and Ethics*. New York: Springer.

Bradshaw A (1995) What are nurses doing to patients? A review of theories of nursing past and present. *Journal of Clinical Nursing* **4**: 81–92.

Burns N and Grove SK (1993) *The Practice of Nursing Research: Conduct, Critique and Utilization*, 2nd edn. Philadelphia, PA: WB Saunders.

Carper BA (1978) Fundamental patterns of knowing in nursing. *Advances in Nursing Science* **1**(1): 13–23.

Chinn PL and Kramer MK (1991) *Theory and Nursing: A Systematic Approach*. St Louis, MO: Mosby Year Book.

Closs J (1994) What's so awful about science? *Nurse Researcher* **2**(2): 161–175.

Cohen L and Manion L (1985) *Research Methods in Education*, 2nd edn. London: Routledge.

Denzin NK and Lincoln YS (eds) (1994) *A Handbook of Qualitative Research*. Thousand Oaks, CA: Mosby Year Book.

Department of Health (1991) *Research for Health: A Research and Development Strategy for the NHS*. London: DoH.

Department of Health (1993) *Report of the Taskforce on the Strategy for Research in Nursing, Midwifery and Health Visiting*. London: DoH.

Dreyfus HL and Dreyfus SE (1986) *Mind Over Machine: the Power of Human Intuition and Expertise in the Era of the Computer*. New York: The Free Press.

Dreyfus HL and Dreyfus SE (1996) The relationship of theory and practice in the acquisition of skill. In Benner P, Tanner CA and Chesla CA (eds) *Expertise in Nursing Practice: Caring, Clinical Judgement and Ethics*. New York: Springer pp29–47.

Elliot J (1991) *Action Research for Educational Change*. Milton Keynes: Open University Press.

Eraut M (1994) *Developing Professional Knowledge and Competence*. London: The Falmer Press.

Guba EG and Lincoln YS (1989) *Fourth Generation Evaluation*. Newbury Park, DC: Sage.

Guba EG and Lincoln YS (1994) Competing paradigms in qualitative research. In Denzin NK and Lincoln YS (eds) *Handbook of Qualitative Research*. Thousand Oaks, CA: Sage, pp105–117.

Hardy LK (1994) The implication of jumping on nursing bandwagons – the case of nursing models in Newfoundland hospitals. *Canadian Journal of Nursing Administration* **7**(1): 21–30.

Hockey L (1996) The nature and purpose of research. In Cormack DFS (ed) *The Research Process in Nursing*, 3rd edn. Oxford: Blackwell Science, 3–13.

Higgs J (1992) Developing knowledge: a process of construction, mapping and review. *New Zealand Journal of Physiotherapy* **20**: 23–30.

Johns C (1995) Framing learning through reflection within Carper's fundamental ways of knowing in nursing. *Journal of Advanced Nursing* **22**: 226–234.

Kenny T (1993) Nursing models fail in practice. *British Journal of Nursing* **2**(2): 133–136.

Lauder W (1994) An exploratory study of the alternative theoretical frameworks of student nurses. *Journal of Clinical Nursing* **3**: 185–191.

Lenz ER, Supre F, Gift AG, Pugh LC and Milligan RD (1995) Collaborative development of middle-range nursing theories: toward a theory of unpleasant symptoms. *Advances in Nursing Science* **17**(3): 1–13.

Levine ME (1995) The rhetoric of nursing theory. *Image* **27**(1): 11–14.

Lewis T (1988) Leaping the chasm between theory and practice. *Journal of Advanced Nursing* **13**: 345–351.

Lincoln YS and Guba EG (1985) *Naturalistic Inquiry*. Newbury Park, DC: Sage.

Lundh U, Söder M and Waerness K (1988) Nursing theories: a critical view. *Image* **20**(1): 36–40.

Meleis A (1991) *Theoretical Nursing: Developments and Progress*, 2nd edn. Philadelphia, PA: Lippincott.

Moody LE (1990) *Advancing Nursing Science*

Through Research, Vol 1. Newbury Park, DC: Sage.

Moore S (1990) Thoughts on the discipline of nursing as we approach the year 2000. *Journal of Advanced Nursing* **15**: 825–828.

Paley J (1996) Intuition and expertise: comments on the Benner debate. *Journal of Advanced Nursing* **23**: 665–671.

Paul RW and Heaslip P (1995) Critical thinking and intuitive nursing practice. *Journal of Advanced Nursing* **22**: 40-47.

Pryjmachuk S (1996) A nursing perspective on the inter-relationship between theory, research and practice. *Journal of Advanced Nursing* **23**: 679–684.

Reason P (ed) (1994) *Participation in Human Inquiry*. London: Sage.

Robinson JJA (1994) *Problems with paradigms in a caring profession*. In Smith J (ed) *Models, Theories and Concepts*. London: Blackwell Scientific, 8–20.

Rose P and Parker D (1994) Nursing: an integration of the art and science within the experi-ence of the practitioner. *Journal of Advanced Nursing* **20**: 1004–1010.

Rubin LB (1981) Sociological research: the subjective dimension: *Symbolic Interaction* **4**: 99.

Ryle G (1949) *The Concept of Mind*. London: Hutchinson.

Schön D (1987) *Educating the Reflective Practitioner*. San Francisco, CA: Jossey-Bass.

Secretary of State for Health (1996) *The National Health Service: A Service with Ambition*. London: HMSO.

Swanson JM and Chenitz WC (1982) Why qualitative research in nursing? *Nursing Outlook* **30**(4): 241–245.

Sweeny (1994) A concept analysis of personal knowledge: application to nursing education, *Journal of Advanced Nursing* **20**: 917–924.

Thompson N (1995) *Theory and Practice in Health and Social Welfare*. Buckingham: Open University Press.

Tolley KA (1995) Theory from practice for practice: is this a reality? *Journal of Advanced Nursing* **21**: 184–190.

2 The context of nursing and health care research

Susan Read

This chapter is based on the belief that an understanding of the context of nursing[1] and health care research is essential when seeking to develop skills in reading and applying research in practice. The chapter recounts some of the history associated with nursing and health care research, exploring how reliance on tradition and custom is no longer accepted as a foundation for patient care. Context, however, is not just history and background, but should also look towards the future. *Chambers Everyday Dictionary* (1975) says that, in a literary sense, context is the parts of a discourse that precede and follow the passage under consideration, which may fix that passage's meaning. Readers will see that research in nursing and health care has grown almost beyond recognition in the 40 or so years since the word 'research' was first used in connection with nursing and other non-medical activities in health care in the UK. So whilst there may be a fixed core for the term 'research', such as this definition by McLeod Clark and Hockey (1989):

> *'Research is an attempt to increase available knowledge by the discovery of new facts or relationships through systematic inquiry'*
> (MacLeod Clark and Hockey 1989: 4)

The way that the research is planned, funded, carried out and reported is very different now from 40 years ago. Even more different is the health service in which that research takes place and the educational preparation available for health care professionals. This chapter considers the climate for research within the NHS and in the universities where many researchers learn and practise their trade, and considers issues which may have to be faced as we look into the future.

Inevitably, exploring the context of research involves an examination of policies developed by both government and organizations in the professions. Policies are also affected by economic arguments and by changes in public attitudes and expectations. Although many contextual features apply throughout the UK, some variations in

[1] The term 'nursing' in this chapter encompasses the professions of nursing, midwifery and health visiting.

research policy and opportunities exist in the four UK countries, and this chapter attempts to recognize these differences. Readers will find that the focus of the chapter moves between the nursing profession, other health care professions and the wider context of the NHS and its research and development (R&D) policies.

The chapter concludes by examining, in the light of the developments described in it, whether the balance has altered irrevocably between academic research, conducted for its own sake, and research into health care delivery required to improve the efficiency and effectiveness of the NHS. The reasons why every nurse and health care professional needs the skills to interpret and apply research are made clear as the chapter progresses. The goal of improving care for patients belongs to us all, whether practitioners or researchers.

Key issues

- The development of research in nursing before 1980
- The development of health services research before 1980
- The time of change in the early 1990s for R&D in the NHS
- The 1993 *Strategy for Research in Nursing, Midwifery and Health Visiting* and the response from the therapy professions to it, and to *Research for Health*
- Further developments in NHS R&D from 1994 onwards
- The recent nursing policy and educational context, and developments in other UK countries and further afield
- The balance between pure and applied research within health services' R&D

Research in nursing before 1980

Early days

Florence Nightingale is popularly remembered as 'the lady with the lamp' in sometimes sentimental recollections of her influence on nursing. We forget that she was also 'the lady with the statistical tables'. Nightingale's *Notes on Hospitals* (1863) set out her guidelines for recording hospital statistics in order to highlight differences in length of stay and complication rates for the same surgical procedures in different hospitals. League tables are not such a recent innovation! However, Nightingale's successors in the profession did not seem keen to emulate her example, and through late Victorian times and the first half of the 20th century there is no record of nurses becoming involved in research in the UK.

Lelean and Clarke (1990) tell us that the first known publication of research by a nurse in the UK was in 1953, when the Royal College of Nursing (RCN) published a report by Skellern (1953) on the teaching and management of nurses at ward level. Norton (1992), herself one of the early pioneers of nursing research, explains how the focus of the published studies in the 1950s tended to be nurses themselves, rather than patients – for instance Goddard (1953), Skellern (1953), Dan Mason Nursing Research Committee (1956) and Menzies (1960). These early projects were influenced by the techniques of work study and occupational psychology. Very gradually the focus of research began to include patients, beginning with Norton *et al's* ground-breaking study of care of the elderly published in 1962, and continuing with Hockey's research in the field of district nursing (1966 and 1968). A retrospective volume of *Nursing Research Abstracts* covering the years 1968–1976, published in 1982 by the Department of Health and Social Security, contained 700 items, of which the greatest numbers were in the categories of manpower and staffing, and education.

In the mid-1950s, two fellowships were established to enable nurses to undertake higher degrees at Edinburgh University. The same university pioneered the first undergraduate degree courses for nurses a few years later. However, during the 1950s and early 1960s most people in the nursing professions, including educators, were unaware that research in nursing was a possibility, let alone a necessity.

The first sign of impending change came in 1963, when the then Ministry of Health appointed Miss Marjorie Simpson as its first nursing research officer. This appointment heralded the beginning of a number of government initiatives to encourage the development of research in the nursing professions, through educational support, funding for nursing research units and programmes and dissemination of research findings (Lelean and Clarke 1990).

In the 1960s there was a strengthening of interest in research amongst professional organizations for nurses, notably the Royal College of Nursing (RCN), which hosted and supported *The Study of Nursing Care* project from 1965 onwards (McFarlane 1992). The project was funded by the Department of Health and Social Security (DHSS, later DH). The Queen's Institute of District Nursing (QIDN) was amongst the early publishers of nursing research reports, carried out by their own research officer (Hockey 1966, 1968).

Research base

'Nursing should become a research-based profession'
(Briggs 1972: 108)

This quotation from the report of the Committee on Nursing (Briggs 1972) marks the entry into the wider consciousness of the nursing professions, of the idea that research is an important foundation for practice. Briggs (1972) continued:

'While, as in other professions, the active pursuit of serious research must be limited to a minority within the profession, and there are benefits to be gained from a co-ordination of what research is being carried out, a sense of the need for research

should become part of the mental equipment of every practising nurse or midwife ... Educational and financial provisions must be made in order that the nursing and midwifery professions shall become more research-based'

(Briggs 1972: 108)

In the 1970s, there was an expansion of nursing academic departments in the higher education sector, the increasing recognition of research in post-basic nursing courses and, in 1977, the first mention of research appreciation in the syllabus for preregistration nurse education (Hayward and Lelean 1982). Another milestone was passed when

'... the need for a central index of nursing research was identified first in 1974, when it became clear that nurses were starting to seek ready access to research based information to help them in their work'

(Friend 1982: ii)

The identification of this need led to the establishment of the *Index of Nursing Research* at the DHSS in 1975. Nurses were invited to send details of completed and ongoing research projects for inclusion in the register. Quarterly volumes of *Research Abstracts* were published from 1978 onwards, including a retrospective volume going back to 1968, and publication only ceased in 1995 when the establishment of multidisciplinary regional research registers was thought to make a separate nursing register system unnecessary.

So far, in describing the progress of research in the nursing professions through its early stages up to the 1980s, the role of the government health departments, universities, professional organizations and nurse education (pre- and postregistration) have been mentioned. But it must not be forgotten that developments were also taking place within the service side of the NHS, such as:

- The establishment of research liaison posts at regional level (Norton 1980)
- Joint clinical/research posts at ward or unit level (Ashworth and Castledine 1980, Pearson 1983)
- Publication of research-based policies and procedures tested by nurses at a postgraduate teaching hospital (Royal Marsden 1984).

However, despite the efforts of research-minded nurses in service areas, backed up by educators, professional and statutory bodies and government health departments, it has to be admitted that by the end of the 1980s there were still many areas of nursing practice and organization that largely depended on tradition rather than research-based knowledge (Hunt 1981, Hunt 1987, Walsh and Ford 1989). In addition, the introduction of whole systems of nursing care such as the 'nursing process' (Walton 1987) and the use of 'nursing models'

(Aggleton and Chalmers 1986, Kershaw and Salvage 1986, Pearson and Vaughan 1986) – although frequently described as research-based – has often been carried out in uncritical acceptance. Transplanting systems and ideologies from the USA demands fuller examination and testing than has been the case. Such wide-scale adoption often leads to surface level implementation, with huge increases in paperwork but little real change in staff attitudes (Read *et al* 1994).

Summary

Between the 1950s and the 1980s there were numerous developments in nursing research in the UK. Not unlike today, the early stimulus came from academia (particularly the University of Edinburgh), government (the Ministry of Health) and from professional organizations such as the RCN and the QIDN. In the 1970s research began to appear in nursing curricula, first for postregistration courses, then for preregistration courses. This was in an era when university education for nurses gained ground in both undergraduate and postgraduate studies. The NHS also began to develop research posts. In spite of this, much nursing practice was based on custom and tradition rather than research.

Exercise 2.1

What do you think are the major requirements for a research base to nursing practice?
(Find the article by Lelean and Clarke (1990) for the answers!)

Health services research before 1990

Whilst nursing research was developing between the late 1950s and the middle of the 1980s, health services research was also developing as a multidisciplinary activity, although in its infancy it was largely dominated by the medical profession. Health services research is defined by the Medical Research Council (MRC) as:

'. . . *the identification of the health care needs of communities, and the study of the provision, effectiveness and use of health services*'

The Sheffield Centre for Health and Related Research (SCHARR) suggests this more detailed definition of health services research:

'*The systematic process by which the direct and indirect effects of particular health care interventions are assessed. It is concerned with the costs and effectiveness of interventions in their widest senses, and the use of the information obtained on policy and decision making at national, local and clinical levels. The interventions may be for purposes of prevention, diagnosis, treatment or palliative care. The subject of study might embrace content or method of delivery or its organisation*'

(SCHARR 1995: 11)

The conduct of health services research involves collaboration between a number of disciplines. These include:

- Health professionals
- Health economists
- Statisticians
- Medical sociologists
- Epidemiologists
- Information scientists
- Operational researchers.

When compared with biomedical research, with which it often has to compete for funds, it is clear that health services research is very much at the 'applied' end of the research continuum, whilst much scientific, laboratory-based biomedical research is at the 'pure' end of that continuum. Health research and development is funded from a variety of sources:

- The pharmaceutical and medical equipment industries
- The government health departments in the four UK countries
- The research councils (mainly the Medical Research Council)
- Universities
- Charitable foundations such as the Nuffield Provincial Hospitals Trust, the King's Fund, and the Wellcome Trust.

Health services research has often been based in research units attached to academic departments of public health medicine (Clarke and Kurinczuk 1992) but more recently separate designated units have been developed.

In the period from the 1970s onwards there has been a great deal of turbulence in the public services – particularly in the NHS – as pressure rises from increased demand linked to an ageing population and technological advances, and resources are stretched more and more tightly. It is not surprising that the search for effectiveness and efficiency has resulted in several reorganizations of the NHS; what *is* surprising is that so little of the reorganization process has been either based on research findings, or subjected afterwards to rigorous evaluation (Hunter and Pollitt 1992).

One research-related effect of the implementation of management change was that following the Griffiths inquiry (1983) there was a growth in interest in consumer-related research and quality assurance in the NHS. This would have pleased one of the early pioneers in health services research, Winifred Raphael, who dedicated herself to finding out what patients thought of their care in hospital (Raphael 1974).

Since the 1970s the basic policy governing the commissioning of research by government departments has followed the recommendations of Lord Rothschild's review in 1971 (Cmnd 4814). This introduced the customer/contractor relationship into research, in which (in this case) the Department of Health, as customer, specifies research needs, which the contractor (the researcher) seeks to meet.

Despite the establishment of Research Liaison Groups within the DHSS in the 1970s, by the mid 1980s there were indicators that further action was needed (Nuffield Provincial Hospitals Trust 1985) in order to prioritize the need for health services research. In 1988 the House of Lords Select Committee on Science and Technology:

> '... *criticised the lack of coherent arrangements for the NHS to articulate its research needs and to ensure that the benefits of research are systematically and effectively transferred into service'*
>
> (House of Lords 1988: 48, Clarke and Kurinczuk 1992: 1675).

The next part of this chapter examines the government's response to this criticism.

Summary

Health services research (HSR) is a multidisciplinary activity. The MRC defines it as research which 'involves the identification of the health care needs of communities, and the study of the provision, effectiveness and use of health services'. Government departments commission research in accordance with policies which depict the government as customer and the research community as contractors to supply their needs. As a result HSR workers have to compete for funds alongside biomedical researchers with more impressive 'track records'. It should be recognized that by the end of the 1980s, the imperative that nursing and other areas of health should wherever possible be based in a sound research base, had been well and truly articulated by government.

Exercise 2.2

Think about two nursing interventions which you make use of regularly in your own practice. This could be anything which you use with patients and/or clients – a pre-operative teaching programme, aromatherapy, a particular type of wound dressing.

Think about your own rationale for using each intervention. Is it based upon research evidence? Do you know? How could you find out?

The NHS R&D Strategy

In 1990 the NHS Management Executive responded to the House of Lords Report (1988) on *Priorities in Medical Research* by appointing a Director of Research and Development (DRD) with a seat on the board of the NHS Executive. Professor Peckham's brief was to establish a national research and development strategy for the NHS in England. The first edition of the strategy was published in 1991 (Department of

Health 1991a) with the objective 'to ensure that the content and delivery of care in the NHS is based on high quality research relevant to improving the health of the nation'. *The Health of the Nation* policy document was published in the same year (DoH 1991b).

A central R&D committee (CRDC) was established in 1991 to advise the NHS Executive on priorities for R&D in the NHS. When first constituted, two of CRDC's 29 active members were nurses, 19 were from a medical or science background and six from NHS management. Later, in 1996, only one of its 24 members was a nurse.

The 1991 Strategy for NHS R&D explained that the regions were to have a crucial role. They were to set their own priorities and to direct, commission and manage research in their own R&D programmes. Regions were to provide a forum for dialogue between local researchers, research managers and purchasers and providers of health care. To enable them to undertake this role, each region was to appoint a regional director of R&D and an R&D committee, and to set up structures both for managing research and for assessing its quality. Mechanisms were also established for cross-regional coordination, and each of the Regional Office R&D Directorates were to manage one or more of the national priority programmes (e.g. research on cardiovascular disease and stroke, or on the primary/secondary care interface).

It is important to note that the R&D programme involves more than merely commissioning new research. It also provides the focus for new initiatives on:

- Implementing the findings of research
- Developing health service practitioners' skills in critical appraisal
- Increasing investment and interest in multidisciplinary health services research.

This aspect of the R&D programme has been taken forward through the implementation of the Research and Development (R&D) Information Systems Strategy (DoH 1992a). A key feature of this strategy is the national project register which may be consulted via the regional R&D offices. NHS staff can use this register to find out what recent research exists in their field. A big expansion in short courses on critical appraisal of research literature is also taking place, which will mean that nurses, amongst others, can have access to such courses and develop the skills to evaluate the usefulness of research reports. In 1994, the NHS Centre for Reviews and Dissemination (CRD) at the University of York was set up under a contract from the Department of Health. Its review work includes issues relevant to nursing. The UK Cochrane Collaboration reviews clinical trials in nursing amongst other subject areas, and is the third aspect of the Information Strategy for R&D.

The term 'health technology assessment' (HTA) may seem irrelevant to nurses. However, the terminology is somewhat misleading since HTA is defined as:

'. . . the variety of methods used by health professionals to promote health, to prevent and treat disease, and to foster improved rehabilitation and long term care'

(DoH 1992b: 4)

Using this definition, it becomes apparent that many nursing interventions can be classified as health technologies.

When new interventions are planned, they should be rigorously evaluated before being widely implemented, and existing interventions should also be tested for effectiveness. The CRDC Standing Group on HTA suggests that:

'The challenge is . . . to shift the whole focus in health care, so that patients, professionals and managers recognize the extent of uncertainty about the effects of health technologies, share in efforts to obtain it, and use the evidence routinely as a basis for making decisions'

(DoH 1992b: 9)

The 1992 report stresses the importance of outcome measurement, including health status, quality of life, patient acceptability and cost effectiveness. It suggests that any new health technology should be assessed for its impact on the organization, on legal and ethical issues, and on social life, as well as on the more obvious safety and health gain measures.

Some examples of nursing health technology assessment in which this author has been involved are a study of triage in an accident and emergency department (George, Read, Westlake *et al* 1992) and a study of nurse-led ear care in primary care (Fall, Read, Walters *et al* 1997). In each case patient outcomes and patient satisfaction were compared for groups of patients who did or did not receive the service in question. The ear care study also compared the cost implications, showing that the nurse-led service was cheaper but led to greater patient satisfaction.

In 1993 a more fully developed research strategy for the NHS was published (DoH 1993a). This builds on the earlier reports, and recommends a partnership between NHS staff and the research community so that researchers will understand the needs of the NHS and design more appropriate research projects, and users will understand the benefits of research and be enabled to articulate problems for future research more clearly.

The strategy sets out six objectives, of which the most relevant to nurses and other professions allied to medicine are:

■ To facilitate the development of a knowledge-based NHS and encourage an evaluative culture within it

■ To ensure that the benefits of research are systematically and effectively translated into practice.

Research for Health (DoH 1993a) puts 'flesh on the bones' of the 1991 strategy, explaining how national priorities are identified, co-ordinated and then acted upon, either centrally, or by delegation to the NHS regions. The report describes an integrated approach to R&D which builds on alliances with the higher education sector, the research councils, charitable funding bodies, industry, the European Union and other bodies, both governmental and non-governmental. Great attention is paid to the dissemination of research findings, putting research into practice and the achievement of clinical effec-tiveness, ensuring that R&D affects purchasing and contracting, and the need for increasing research capacity through education. Criteria are given against which proposals bidding for NHS R&D funding can be assessed (Box 2.1):

Box 2.1
Criteria for assessing proposals for NHS R&D funding

Is the proposed research:
■ Designed to provide new knowledge necessary to improve NHS performance in enhancing the nation's health?
■ Designed so the findings will be valuable, relevant and gener-alizable?
■ Following a clear, peer-reviewed and ethically approved pro-tocol?
■ Stating well-defined arrangements for project management?
■ Intending to publish findings so they are generally accessible and open to critical appraisal?

(DoH 1993a)

Tremendous energy was invested in this period from the appoint-ment of the Director of R&D for the NHS in 1990 until the publica-tion of *Research for Health* in 1993. What was needed was for the whole culture of the NHS to change. Following a meeting in Trent Region in 1993 of NHS managers and researchers, Szczepura and Cooke (1993) reported that:

'One of the main obstacles to effective use of existing research-based information is that many staff see research as an activity divorced from everyday working practice, and which has mini-mal financial impact'

(Szczepura and Cooke 1993: 27)

The meeting suggested ways in which managers and researchers could stimulate use of research-based information. These included:

■ Provision of incentives for staff using research to improve health care

■ Insistence that all new procedures must either have research evidence of their effectiveness, or be introduced as part of an evaluation

■ Introduction of simple changes in technology by staff with all other factors remaining the same, so that benefits can be clearly attributed to the technology change

■ Encouragement of critical appraisal of existing practice, and of research-based teaching by clinical educators

■ Increased involvement of managers in planning national, regional and local research programmes, especially HTA

■ Increased effort by researchers to demonstrate benefits of HTA to managers, by regular meetings and by publication in accessible journals.

Summary

The appointment in 1990 of the first NHS Director of Research and Development, Professor Peckham, marked the beginning of a new era for health services research in England. *Research for Health* (DoH 1991a) laid the foundations for both central and regional determination of research priorities and the development of a coherent programme for research, development, dissemination and education. The NHS R&D Information Systems Strategy was published in 1992 to support the implementation of *Research for Health*. *Assessing the Effects of Health Technologies* (DoH 1992b) clarified the range of outcome measurements and research designs which can be considered in health technology assessment and stressed the importance of evaluating all forms of care. *Research for Health* (DoH 1993a) built on the preceding publications in strengthening the R&D strategy for the NHS. It explained the alliances with other bodies concerned with research which contribute to an integrated approach to R&D. A number of measures to stimulate the use of research-based knowledge in the NHS were introduced.

Exercise 2.3

Find a copy of one of the policy documents discussed in this section. These reports should be available in your local health services or university library. Alternatively, your manager may have copies. Read through the report, making notes about any important implications for your own practice.

One useful way of getting to grips with the range of policy documents which relate to nursing and health care practice and research is to share the responsibility with a group of colleagues. Each person agrees to read one document and present a summary of the key issues to the rest of the group. It's amazing how what appears to be quite dull material can come to life when it is summarized and the important issues debated!

The strategy for research in nursing

In 1992 a Taskforce chaired by Professor Adrian Webb and comprising eminent members of the nursing and medical research community was appointed by the NHS R&D Director and the Chief Nursing Officer. Its terms of reference were to consider the scope and objectives of research for the nursing professions, and the interface with other areas of interdisciplinary health and health services research, all within the context of the NHS R&D Strategy and the Strategy for Nursing (DoH 1989a). Identification of research need, and structures for strengthening research programmes, education and dissemination were all to be considered.

Florence Nightingale's birthday, May 12 1993, 130 years after the publication of her *Notes on Hospitals*, was the launch date chosen by the Department of Health for the *Report of the Taskforce on the Strategy for Research in Nursing, Midwifery and Health Visiting* (DoH 1993b). The Taskforce defined two objectives which were the focus for their 37 recommendations:

- To promote more and better research into nursing
- To enhance the research skills of nursing staff so as to increase their involvement in research in their own fields, and in health services research generally.

The Taskforce used the terms 'nursing' and 'the nursing professions' to encompass the nursing, midwifery and health visiting professions (as does this chapter) for brevity, and to emphasize the need for a common framework for growth in the research endeavour. The Taskforce also referred consistently to 'research in nursing' rather than 'nursing research'. It defined research as:

> '... rigorous and systematic enquiry, conducted on a scale and using methods commensurate with the issue to be investigated, and designed to lead to generalizable contributions to knowledge'

(DoH 1993b: 6)

As a means to defining research in nursing, the Taskforce report listed topics on which such research might focus:

> '... nursing practices; nursing service and service delivery; the nursing professions and issues concerned with the workforce and its deployment; health promotion; complex procedures or

patterns of intervention; service systems within which nursing plays but a part along with other health care professions'

(DoH 1993b: 8)

Glenister (1994) suggests that research in nursing 'involves any activity that may have an impact on the delivery of nursing care'. The Taskforce report highlights the need for work on outcome measures for nursing.

'Investigation of the effectiveness and efficiency of clinical intervention is essential and requires considerable preparatory work to establish outcome measures. Organisational structures, diverse patterns of professional practice and patients' attitudes and satisfaction must be taken into account'

(DoH 1993b: 9)

While acknowledging that research of value already exists in nursing, both nationally and internationally, the Taskforce considered that the amount and range of such research was inadequate.

'It is insufficiently cumulative and . . . much of it is too small in scale and discontinuous in nature and in its funding base. Moreover it is not disseminated and utilised as effectively as it should be'

(DoH 1993b: 10)

The Taskforce rejected the plea to 'ringfence' nursing research and its resources, but made a strong case for better research education for nurses and more financial support for research into nursing issues. The Taskforce's recommendations focused particularly on integration of nursing issues and researchers into the new R&D structures, on investment in research education, on identification of enhanced sources of funding, and on improvement of mechanisms for dissemination of research and the development of research-based practice (Box 2.2).

The Taskforce expressed the hope that its report would be viewed as a coherent strategy to be implemented in its entirety, rather than as a shopping list from which just a few items would actually be 'taken off the shelf'. Since various recommendations were addressed to different audiences (e.g. the research councils, statutory bodies, higher education, professional organizations, charities) as well as to the Department of Health, it is inevitable that the hopes for wholesale implementation have not yet been fully realized. The author of this chapter was project officer to the implementation team so was well placed to assess the early impact (Read 1994). The recommended full evaluation has not yet been conducted, four years later. However, by the time of the conference held to mark the first anniversary of the launch of the Taskforce report (DoH 1995d) 24 of the report's 37 recommendations had been implemented and addressed.

Box 2.2
Key recommendations of the Strategy for Research in Nursing, Midwifery and Health Visiting (Department of Health)

Recommendations on structure and organization included:

■ Encouraging senior executives in the NHS to influence the management culture of the NHS, to increase the awareness of the importance of research especially to professional practice

■ Giving consideration to nursing research in R&D processes of prioritization and decision making
  – commissioning and funding
  – assembling databases
  – dissemination and development
  – NHS contracting between purchasers and providers

■ Creating a regional and national network for support of research in nursing, involving regions, the NHS and academic departments

Recommendations on education and training covered:

■ Expanding research training for nurses and other health service staff

■ Ensuring adequate content and quality of research training courses and supervision

■ Encouraging provision of funds (especially by the regions) for research and to allow employment of staff to cover absence

■ Providing a central information resource on research and research training

Recommendations on research funding covered:

■ Recognizing a nursing research element in centrally funded research programmes and in regionally funded responsive schemes

■ Encouraging provision of research advisory resources in regions, and awareness of the Research Development Group of MRC

■ Encouraging research council and private sector funding for a long-term programme of nursing research

■ Encouraging academic departments of nursing to make links with regional R&D networks, to contribute to research training expansion and to concentrate research in areas where they have potential for excellence

Box 2.2 (*contd.*)

Recommendations on improving research dissemination and utilization covered:

■ Integrating the Index of Nursing Research and the Midwifery Research Database into the NHS R&D Information Systems Strategy Register and publicizing the availability of these

■ Building a nursing dimension into the Research Review Commissioning Facility – the planned Centre for Reviews and Dissemination

■ Initiating a feasibility study of how best to undertake systematic overviews of the field of research in nursing

■ Ensuring that a dissemination strategy is adopted by RHA, SHA and purchaser research departments, and that research contracts include a requirement for dissemination

(Adapted from DoH 1993b)

Probably the biggest talking point when the report was issued was on the lack of 'ringfencing' of nursing research, and the insistence that it should be fully integrated into NHS R&D. This recommendation gave rise to a number of concerns. One of the Taskforce members, Professor Luker, had said in 1992:

> *'Research into nursing practice is an essential ingredient in any comprehensive research strategy. The challenge for nurses is to ensure that the nursing dimension in any multi-disciplinary project is clearly defined and is adequately funded'*
>
> (Luker 1992: 1152)

Referring to life in a multidisciplinary research unit, Hardey and Mulhall (1994) suggested that:

> *'The participation of researchers from many disciplines in creating and promoting innovations in the delivery of nursing care does not imply that nursing research should lose its identity within health services research (HSR). It is important that nursing should have a distinctive voice that can contribute to HSR in its own right . . .*
>
> *It is important to recognize that members of multidisciplinary groups must be able to maintain links with their own discipline and should not be the sole representative within the immediate working environment'*
>
> (Hardey and Mulhall 1994: 16)

Another concern about the integration of nursing research into NHS R&D, with its emphasis on multidisciplinary teams and funding for priority topics, was that the more conceptual and theory-related work proper to academic nursing departments would be squeezed out in the pressure to win contracts for applied research. This concern is raised again later in this chapter.

As project officer to the implementation team for the Taskforce report, the present author (Read 1994) observed that the Strategy for Research in Nursing had had an impact:

- Highlighting the need for nursing representation on decision-making bodies
- Drawing attention to nurses' need for research education
- Widening the horizons of funding bodies and committees
- Encouraging research-based practice.

More particularly, most of the then 14 NHS regions had begun to actively consider their response to the Strategy, and several regions were making noticeable progress because of the presence of a nurse in the regional R&D 'core team' (Read 1994). Now, looking back over the years since the Taskforce report was published, it is clear that change has taken place in some areas. More nurses are being funded for research education from regional funds, particularly for taught masters' courses in health services research, and nurses are winning more research contracts, particularly at national level in Department of Health commissioned research, and as team members in HTA bids. Vigilance is needed, however, to ensure that in the changes at regional office level (regions are now part of the NHS Executive) and in the frequent financial crises at local level, nurses do not lose their hard won gains in the research battlefield for funds and influence.

Soon after the publication of the Strategy for Research in Nursing, a therapy professions' research group was convened to produce a position statement and response to the nursing and NHS R&D strategies. The group's report was published in May 1994, making 15 recommendations (Box 2.3).

Summary

The Strategy for Research in Nursing had two objectives:

- To promote more and better research in nursing
- To enhance the research skills of nurses.

It defined research as being 'systematic inquiry, conducted on a scale and using methods commensurate with the issue to be investigated, and designed to lead to generalisable contributions to knowledge'.

The strategy focused on the integration of research in nursing into the new NHS R&D structures and the health services research community; improving research education and training; and increasing the funding opportunities for nurses wishing to undertake research. The recommendations are summarized in Box 2.2.

Box 2.3
Therapy Professions Research Recommendations: Inclusion in decision-making structures

These recommendations aimed to ensure better representation of therapists in national, regional and local R&D bodies, including ethics committees

Management support infrastructure
This recommendation aimed to encourage managers to place more value on therapists undertaking research

Education and training
These recommendations aimed to persuade the Department of Health, NHS Executive and research councils to increase the numbers of doctoral and postdoctoral fellowships available to therapy professionals

Career opportunities
These recommendations aimed to encourage the provision of more career opportunities for therapists to move between practice, research and academic settings at both junior, mid-career and senior levels without financial disadvantage

Methodologies
It was recommended that a mapping exercise should chart the range of methodologies in use in therapy research, to enhance existing research reviews

Dissemination and implementation
These recommendations aimed to fully integrate therapy research into the NHS R&D Information Systems Strategy components – the project registers, the Cochrane Collaboration and the CRD

(Adapted from Therapy Professions Research Group 1994)

Considerable progress has been made with Strategy implementation, although concerns have been raised about monitoring a distinctive nursing contribution affording priority to the development of nursing theory.

NHS R&D from 1994

Although the 1991 and 1993 editions of *Research for Health* were milestones for NHS R&D, they have since been overtaken by a number of other reports with implications for health services research. However, the basic principles of *Research for Health* remain central to the thinking of the NHS Executive.

In 1993 the report *Managing the New NHS: Functions and Responsibilities* (DoH 1993c) was published. This document set out the framework of change for Regional Health Authorities to be reduced in number (from 14 to 8) and to become a direct arm of the NHS Executive. Because of the vital part that Regional R&D Directorates play in the *Research for Health* strategy, a further report was issued late in 1994 entitled *Research and Development in the New NHS: Functions and Responsibilities* (DoH 1994a). The report states one overall aim of the NHS R&D strategy:

> *'to secure a knowledge-based health service in which clinical, managerial, and policy decisions are based on sound and pertinent information about research findings and scientific and technological advance. This provides the basis for maximising the effectiveness, efficiency and appropriateness of patient services'*
>
> (DoH 1994a: 1)

The report identified four areas of activity which would be instrumental to the achievement of that aim.

- Increase of the **knowledge base** – by prioritization of NHS R&D needs and by ensuring that those needs are met by supporting R&D funding and education
- Ensuring that **information** is available and accessible to NHS decision makers about existing research-based knowledge and about ongoing research
- Promoting the use of research-based knowledge in its **implementation** by decision makers and clinical staff
- Instilling into the NHS a **culture of evaluation, review and learning**, so that R&D becomes a regular ingredient of policy decisions.

The report clarifies the responsibilities in these four key areas for the different levels in the NHS:

- The NHS Executive's central R&D Directorate
- The regional offices
- The purchasing authorities
- The providers
- The research community.

Finally, the report sets all this in the context of the wider Department of Health with its responsibility not just for health care and the NHS, but also for social care and public health.

The functions and responsibilities paper was followed up in 1995 by *Research and Development: Towards an Evidence-based Health Service* (DoH 1995a), a dossier of separate short papers on every possible aspect of NHS R&D, on the Department of Health's centrally commissioned research programme, and on broader research issues. This dossier includes detailed information on how to contact the key people in the various programmes, and on NHS R&D publications. In this way the NHS Executive begins to meet its own target for improving information on R&D.

Probably the most important of the recent developments, however, is the chain of events following the issue of the report of yet another taskforce on R&D. Known as *The Culyer Report* after the taskforce's chair, the 1994 report is called *Supporting Research and Development in the NHS*. Although the report owes its main impact to the changes in R&D funding which it recommends, its content is actually broader than just financial matters. Culyer himself, in another forum (Culyer 1996) discusses some of the concerns reported to the R&D Taskforce:

- Uncoordinated support systems for R&D
- Conflict between the NHS internal market and R&D
- Poor quality control and accountability in R&D
- Inadequate support for community- and primary care-based R&D, and for non-medical health services research (including nursing and therapy research)
- Confusion about who funds what, where and when in R&D
- Shortage of key research skills for NHS R&D, particularly in health economics, statistics, nursing and therapy professions and community and primary care.

The main recommendations of the Culyer Report (1994) include:

- Creation of a new single-stream of R&D funding for the NHS, by merging the numerous previous sources which discriminated against so-called 'non-teaching hospitals' and against primary and community care
- Compilation of a detailed register of all research activities in every NHS trust, however funded. Costing could then be attempted for all these activities as part of the process of determining the level of funding for R&D for each institution
- Later in the research registration exercise an attempt would be made to measure the quality of the research and its outputs and effects.

Other aspects of the Culyer Report (1994) cover the creation of a national forum for NHS R&D to bring together the varying bodies (public, private, charitable, educational and professional) which support NHS R&D, and the adjustment of membership of the Central R&D Committee to be more representative of all constituents, particularly purchasers and providers. Culyer recommends particular attention to increasing funding for primary and community care research.

The Culyer Report was followed up (DoH 1995b) by an implementation plan, and a more detailed outline of the new funding system (DoH 1996). The implementation of the Culyer recommendations will continue over several years, but has already resulted in a tremendous flurry of activity at trust and regional office level. Some trusts, of course, already had R&D directors and research registers. For these, fulfilling the Culyer requirements simply required some fine tuning of existing systems. For others, major effort was required. Regional R&D directorates were responsible for guiding the trusts in their registration activities, and then receiving and analyzing the resulting information.

The importance for readers of this book is that involvement in any research activity within the NHS must be made known to the relevant officer in the trust – whether the reader is actually doing research, collaborating in it, or helping enrol patients or staff for it. In addition, staff in hospital or community where facilities for involvement in research have not been available may expect improvement in the next few years.

Summary

Research for Health (DoH 1993) continues to supply a strategy for NHS R&D. Subsequent reports stress the importance of a knowledge-based NHS within an evaluative culture. Changes in funding mechanisms for NHS R&D are in progress, based on the recommendations of the Culyer Report, and should lead to better support for non-medical health services research, especially in community and primary care settings.

Recent developments

The beginning of this chapter described the early days of research in nursing in the UK; until the mid 1980s this development probably affected relatively few clinical nurses or their managers. However, the issue of the UKCC's *Code of Professional Conduct* in 1984 (revised in 1992) included in nurses' accountability the responsibility for maintaining and improving professional knowledge and competence. In the year that the Code was issued, Baroness McFarlane said:

> *'Research is not a luxury for the academic, but a tool for developing nursing decisions, prescriptions and actions. Whether as clinicians, educators, managers or researchers, we have a responsibility; neglect of that responsibility could be classed as professional negligence'*
>
> (McFarlane 1984: xi)

Glenister (1994) also points out the link between the Code of Professional Conduct and nurses' need to be aware of research.

> *'All members of the nursing professions need an understanding of the research process and the ability and time to retrieve and assess research critically. This is essential if professional knowledge is to be improved and nursing is to be practised competently'*
>
> (Glenister 1994: 22)

Although research awareness was introduced into the preregistration nursing curriculum in the late 1970s, and implied in the UKCC's code in 1984, and although Briggs had stated as early as 1972 that nursing should be a research-based profession, it was the Department of Health's *Strategy for Nursing* (DoH 1989a) which really made it plain.

> *'The basic requirements of nursing practice . . . should be of the highest possible standard and safety and should be founded on up-to-date research and knowledge'*
>
> (DoH 1989a: 10)

The Strategy continues:

> *'. . . professional education will need to foster an awareness of and an ability to use research findings . . . Ensuring that the results of current research are effectively disseminated to all health care settings and promptly incorporated into standard treatments and procedures will be increasingly important'*
>
> (DoH 1989a: 15)

The Strategy closes with the setting of targets – 44 in all, divided between practice, manpower, education, leadership and management. In the practice section, two are specifically related to research. Target Seven is 'All clinical practice should be founded on up-to-date information and research findings; practitioners should be encouraged to identify the needs and opportunities for research presented by their work'. Target Eight is 'Academic faculties with departments of nursing should be encouraged to broaden their links with, and deepen their expertise, in research-based practice'.

In 1993, another policy document for nursing, *A Vision for the Future* was published by the DoH (1993d) to carry forward the 1989 Strategy, in the context of the NHS reforms (*Working for Patients*, DoH 1989b), care in the community (*Caring for People*, DoH 1989c), the *Patient's Charter* (DoH 1991c), *The Health of the Nation* (DoH 1991b), and the *Children Act* (DoH 1989d).

A Vision for the Future discusses the effect of these policy initiatives on the nursing professions, emphasising that nurses need to carry awareness of them into all aspects of their work. As well as policy awareness, the concepts of audit, accountability, clinical supervision, contracting for services and professional development are woven into *The Vision*, which is crystallized into 12 targets. These targets were to be monitored over the ensuing two years – further reports were issued in 1994 (DoH 1994b) and 1995 (DoH 1995c).

Two of the 12 targets were specifically research oriented. Target Eight said 'At the end of the first year (i.e. by 1994) professional leaders should be able to demonstrate the existence of local networks to disseminate good practice based on research'.

Target Nine said 'By the end of the year providers should be able to demonstrate at least three areas where clinical practice has changed as a result of research findings'.

As a monitoring exercise after one year, 427 trust chief nurses were sent a postal questionnaire (DoH 1994b) and 60% of them replied. Of these, 95% claimed that they had established networks to disseminate research-based practice, using a combination of meetings and paper communication, and 44% reported that a research coordinator or facilitator managed the dissemination process. Furthermore, 86% of respondents stated that clinical practice had changed in response to research findings, particularly in areas of tissue viability, pain management, advice on prevention of cot death, managing potential suicides and handling challenging behaviour.

The difference in the way the targets were specified and then measured in *Vision for the Future*, compared with the non-specific nature of the 1989 Strategy targets, demonstrates how research awareness had affected leaders of the profession. The importance of precision in defining outcomes in nursing and health care research received much attention between 1988 and 1994 (Bond and Thomas 1991, Brown and Grimes 1992, Heater *et al* 1988, Lang 1994, Marek 1989).

In a period when the nursing profession and the R&D community has been overwhelmed with new policy initiatives, one other nursing report has to be mentioned. This was based on a debate at Heathrow which took place in 1993 amongst senior nursing leaders and academics from the four UK countries, and is entitled *The Challenges for Nursing and Midwifery in the 21st Century* (DoH 1994c). After a stimulating range of possible scenarios of how health care might be delivered in the year 2010, the report attempts to describe what is constant in the role of the nurse. It then asks how much of that constant role can be justified in terms of clinical effectiveness, because increasingly purchasers will only pay for what is effective. The conclusion is that:

> '... *nurses, along with every other supplier of services across the health and social care sector, must ensure that wherever they can, they clarify what works, get this information to those who need it and reflect it in practice. Effectiveness will increasingly be the key to recognition. Research-based knowledge must underpin and inform nursing practice*'

> (DoH 1994c: 22)

The most recent concept to gain widespread acceptance in the NHS is evidence-based practice (EBP). This is defined by Sackett *et al* (1996) as:

> '... *the conscientious, explicit and judicious use of current best evidence in making decisions about the care of individual*

patients. The practice of EBP means integrating individual expertise with the best available external evidence from systematic research'

JET LIBRARY

(Sackett *et al* 1996: 71)

According to Russell (1996) the criteria which are applicable in evidence-based practice are:

- **Efficacy** – can the procedure generate 'health gain' under ideal conditions?
- **Effectiveness** – does the procedure generate 'health gain' in clinical practice?
- **Acceptability** – is the procedure acceptable to patients, carers, staff?
- **Efficiency** – does the procedure give good value for money?
- **Wider implications** – does the procedure affect other aspects of the NHS or society in general?

These are questions which may usefully be applied by nurses to many aspects of their practice.

The role of statutory and professional bodies

Therapy professions

The context of nursing and health care research must also include the attitudes and policies of the professional and statutory bodies for the nursing and therapy professions. The position statement on R&D in the therapy professions (Therapy Professions Research Group 1994) was produced by a group drawn mainly from membership of the three professional associations involved: the Chartered Society of Physiotherapists, the College of Occupational Therapists, and the College of Speech and Language Therapists. All these organizations strongly support research in their respective clinical areas, and in multidisciplinary ventures.

RCN

The Royal College of Nursing (RCN) has had a distinguished history in support of research in nursing. The *Study of Nursing Care Project* was the starting point for many nurse researchers who went on to establish their reputations in research. The Royal College covers all four UK countries, and so its annual Research Society conference draws members from a wide geographical area, and from all levels of seniority from students to professors and now deans of university schools of nursing.

The RCN established a permanent research standing committee in the early 1990s (Hancock 1993) to coordinate and shape the RCN's research role, which includes:

- Promoting a research culture
- Marketing and disseminating research findings

■ Educating nurses for higher degrees
■ Commissioning and undertaking research.

More recently the development of the RCN Institute, Oxford, based on the pre-existing National Institute for Nursing in Oxford, the RCN Institute of Advanced Nursing Education and the RCN's Daphne Heald Research Unit, has strengthened the research role of the RCN.

UKCC   As the statutory body for the regulation of the nursing professions in the four UK countries, the United Kingdom Central Council (UKCC) for Nursing, Midwifery and Health Visiting's primary concern is for standards of education, conduct and practice in the three nursing professions. Wherever research plays a part in that concern, the UKCC is fully involved, and encourages the growth of research-based practice in support of the improvement of professional standards. As well as being a consumer and encourager of research, the UKCC has recently become a commissioner of research.

ENB   The English National Board (ENB) for Nursing, Midwifery and Health Visiting's primary role is to advise on educational programmes for the three professions and to validate courses. However, research also has a high profile at the Board, which developed an R&D Strategy in 1990 (Le Var 1995), and began commissioning research before that, in 1986. The Board has a strong commitment to disseminating the research it commissions through very wide distribution of its *Research Highlights* series. It gave a very positive response to the 1993 *Report of the Taskforce on the Strategy for Research in Nursing, Midwifery and Health Visiting* (Le Var 1994).

Education   The educational world of nursing has undergone enormous changes in the past five years, and is a very important part of the context for nursing and health care research. The change from certificate to diploma level in preregistration education, the move from colleges of nursing to integration with higher education, and the huge expansion of numbers of nurses with first degrees, and increasingly studying for higher degrees, must all speed up the culture change in nursing so that research-based knowledge and practice become the goal of all, rather than of the few. However, to undertake a research assessment of the impact of educational change on the research culture of the nursing profession would be a major undertaking – a challenge perhaps for the newly formed Centre for Policy in Nursing Research, funded by the Nuffield Provincial Hospitals Trust and based at the London School of Hygiene and Tropical Medicine. The centre's aim is to develop a coordinated professional strategy for nursing research throughout the United Kingdom.

UK variations   The mention of the lack of a coordinated strategy for nursing research throughout the UK leads to a brief discussion of the variations in approach to research in nursing in the four UK countries. England has been very fully dealt with in this chapter, partly because of the rapidly developing R&D context for nursing here, of which the author has had personal experience, and partly because of the comparative numbers of nurses in the four countries. However, the activities of the UKCC and the RCN Research Society do provide a forum for nurses throughout the entire United Kingdom.

Scotland   Scotland published its own *Strategy for Nursing Research* back in 1991 (Scottish Office 1991). (Readers will remember that Edinburgh University was home to the first academic department of nursing in the UK and hosted a nursing research unit for over 25 years, funded by the Chief Scientist's Office.) The ingredients of the Scottish Strategy were similar in some respects to the later English Strategy, including research education, funding and dissemination in its priorities, and stressing research links at trust and practice level. However, there was not the same thrust to integrate nursing with health services research, presumably in part because the *NHS R&D Strategy for Scotland* was not published until 1993 (Scottish Office 1993), but arguably also because of the already strong identity of nursing research in Scotland.

However, a major recent development has been the beginning of the Nursing Research Initiative for Scotland (NRIS), whose director, Professor Jennifer Hunt, took up post late in 1994. After a period of fact-finding and preparation based at the Scottish Home and Health Department, the Initiative now has an academic base at Glasgow Caledonian University, and a clinical base at Glasgow's Victoria Infirmary. NRIS's remit is 'to improve the care and treatment of patients or clients through scientific study related to direct patient or client care'. It is intended that research funded by NRIS will encompass all health care settings and therefore be of an interdisciplinary nature. NRIS aims to develop a relevant and useful research programme, based on identified priority topics, involving nurses and other direct care staff as much as possible. It will make research reviews available in a variety of formats, and set up link centres in different parts of Scotland where research advice and information will be accessible to nurses and others. One early function of the new initiative has been to encourage nurses to participate in the exercise declaring research activity in response to the Culyer Report's Scottish implementation (Hunt 1996).

The Scottish National Board for Nursing, Midwifery and Health Visiting has a strong interest in research, both as a commissioner and a consumer; it has a full-time research officer, and a newly established R&D team. The team's main thrust will be to:

- Pose new research questions
- Promote developments in research activity by members of the nursing professions
- Encourage research-based education and practice.

Wales

Following the publication of *Sharpening the Focus: R&D Framework for NHS Wales* in 1992 (Welsh Office 1992), the All Wales Nursing, Midwifery and Health Visiting Research Group produced *A Strategy for the Development of Research in Nursing in Wales* (Welsh Office 1993) as a discussion document. This was followed by a shorter document in 1994, *A Framework for R&D for Nursing in Wales* (Welsh Office 1994). This set the following objectives:

- To facilitate more effective nursing research
- To enhance the research skills and experience of nurses
- To identify R&D priorities
- To develop opportunities for research education and training for nurses
- To identify methods for dissemination and implementation of research findings
- To develop research leaders.

A small group is currently meeting to take forward the Strategy, but are already involved in the clinical effectiveness initiative for Wales (Welsh Office 1995) and are linked with the new Centre for Practice Research at the University of Glamorgan, and with the Cochrane Collaboration.

The Welsh National Board (WNB) for Nursing, Midwifery and Health Visiting is also involved in helping nurses to become research aware and research active. Its main activity is encouraging the research components of all its validated courses, especially in making the module on Research Application and Methodology compulsory at Diploma level for nurses undertaking its framework for continuing education. It also supports four research training fellowships a year for nurse teachers.

Northern Ireland

The Department of Health and Social Services of the Northern Ireland Office published an action plan for nursing R&D in 1993. The plan's aims were:

- To establish effective mechanisms for identifying priorities for nursing R&D and to develop a research programme
- To secure funding for nursing R&D
- To encourage interdisciplinary research
- To disseminate research findings and encourage implementation.

The National Board for Nursing, Midwifery and Health Visiting for Northern Ireland (NBNI) is also actively involved in identifying research priorities, particularly for nurse education, encouraging interest in and education for research, and lobbying for increased funding for research in nursing in the Province (NBNI 1991, 1994). The Board holds an annual research conference and sponsors competitive research awards.

International context

Beyond the four UK countries there are a number of organisations or opportunities for nurses to discuss their respective research agenda in an international context.

WENR

The Workgroup of European Nurse Researchers (WENR) meets every year to collate reports from member countries on the progress of nursing research. WENR also holds an open conference every second year.

Council of Europe

The European Union has a standing committee of nurses (Pritchard 1994) and also funds large research programmes. The Council of Europe, following a meeting of health ministers of member states, established a Committee of Experts on Nursing Research in 1993 to make recommendations which would improve the position of research in nursing across all European countries.

ICN

The International Council of Nurses, made up of national nursing organisation representatives, holds a quadrennial congress where presentation of research papers is invited. In 1996, to commemorate International Nurses' Day, the ICN published a monograph *Better Health Through Nursing Research* (ICN 1996).

Summary

The need to ensure that nursing practice is based on up-to-date research wherever possible, is a requirement of the UKCC's *Code of Professional Conduct*. The report *A Vision for the Future* (DoH 1993d) attempted to review the implications of a series of policy initiatives for nursing practice and identified targets for research dissemination and implementation.

The concept of evidence-based practice is continuing to gain widespread acceptance within the NHS. The report of the 'Heathrow Debate' identified the need to demonstrate effectiveness as one of the key challenges for nursing and midwifery in the 21st century, while statutory and professional bodies such as the RCN, UKCC and ENB have all played an important role in promoting awareness of the need for a sound research base to nursing practice. Initiatives to promote research cultures in the other UK countries (Scotland, Wales and Northern Ireland), have paralleled developments in England. This has included changes in the organization of pre- and postregistration nurse education, which have resulted in a greater emphasis on the goal of research-based knowledge and practice.

Chapter conclusion

This chapter has charted the development of research in nursing in the UK from its beginnings in the 1950s which involved the use of work-study techniques. The growth of academic nursing departments in universities encouraged development in methodologies and expansion of subjects researched. However, integration of nursing research into NHS R&D has highlighted an already existing dilemma. As Hardey and Mulhall put it:

'Within the academic tradition, research is seen as contributing to a body of knowledge and thus may not have any declared usefulness. In contrast, a commercial R&D tradition that is gaining influence within the restructured health care system seeks pragmatic and measurable research outcomes ... The balance between "research for its own sake" and "customer-directed research" is hard to establish'

(Hardey and Mulhall 1994: 6)

With the integration of nursing research and the current funding crisis in higher education forcing even higher workloads on researchers and increasing the pressure for them to win research contracts, the opportunity to stop and think, and to synthesize ideas from different projects or different disciplines is often lost. The worry is that, as Culyer (1996) suggests:

'... it is unlikely that excellence in research can be built and sustained on applied research alone. It is essential for applied research to form part of a larger (and wider) institutional (or departmental) portfolio of work which includes theoretical research, fundamental research with no specific "customer" in mind outside the academic peer group and the more general work of parent disciplines'

(Culyer 1996: 42)

Culyer maintains that it is the mutual interaction of the pure and applied research streams that produce the most fruitful results in both fields. So, perhaps we should take stock, and try to redress the balance.

Exercise 2.4

Browse through the papers in a recent issue of an academic nursing/midwifery journal such as the *Journal of Advanced Nursing, Midwifery* or the *International Journal of Nursing Studies*. What proportion of the articles have direct implications for nursing practice? How do the remaining papers contribute to nursing knowledge?

Exercise 2.5   How easy is it to identify the funders of research from papers published in academic nursing journals? Compare nursing and medical journals in this respect. Do you notice any difference? If so, think about why this might be.

Further reading   Baker M and Kirk S (1996). *Research and Development for the NHS: Evidence, Evaluation and Effectiveness*. Oxford: Radcliffe Medical Press.

This recent text is useful. However, since the context for research and development within the NHS changes so rapidly, the most important thing is to keep up-to-date with current developments. One way of doing this is to read the 'news' items in professional and academic nursing and health care journals. Useful information is also provided by R&D offices within trusts and regional R&D offices. Find out if your local office produces a newsletter and put your name on their mailing list.

References

Aggleton P and Chalmers H (1986) *Nursing Models and the Nursing Process*. Basingstoke: Macmillan.

Ashworth P and Castledine G (1980) Joint service/education appointments in nursing. *Medical Teacher* **2**(6): 295–299.

Bond S and Thomas LH (1991) Issues in measuring outcomes of nursing. *Journal of Advanced Nursing* **16**: 1492–1502.

Briggs A [chair] (1972) *Report of the Committee on Nursing*. CMND 5115. London: HMSO.

Brown S and Grimes D (1992) *A Meta-analysis of Process of Care, Clinical Outcomes and Cost-Effectiveness of Nurses in Primary Care Roles*. Houston, TX: University of Texas for American Nurses Association.

Chambers (1975) *Everyday Dictionary*. Edinburgh: Chambers.

Clarke M and Kurinczuk JJ (1992) Health Services Research: a case of need or special pleading? *British Medical Journal* **304**: 1675-1676.

Culyer AJ (1996) Taking advantage of the new environment for research and development. In Baker M and Kirk S (1996). *Research and Development for the NHS: Evidence, Evaluation and Effectiveness*. Oxford: Radcliffe Medical Press.

Culyer AJ [chair] Taskforce on research and development in the NHS (1994) *Supporting Research and Development in the NHS*. London: HMSO.

Dan Mason Nursing Research Committee (1956) *The Work of Recently Qualified Nurses*. Dan Mason NRC, London.

Department of Health (1989a) *A Strategy for Nursing*. London: DoH.

Department of Health (1989b) *Working for Patients*. London: HMSO.

Department of Health (1989c) *Caring for People: Community Care in the Next Decade and Beyond*. London: HMSO.

Department of Health (1989d) *The Children Act*. London: HMSO.

Department of Health (1991a) *Research for Health: an R&D Strategy for the NHS*. London: HMSO.

Department of Health (1991b) *The Health of the Nation*. London: HMSO.

Department of Health (1991c) *The Patient's Charter*. London: DoH.

Department of Health for NHS ME Research and Development Directorate (1992a) *Report of the NHS R&D Information Systems Strategy Study*. London: DoH.

Department of Health Advisory Group on Health Technology Assessment (1992b) *Assessing the Effects of Health Technologies*. London: DoH.

Department of Health (1993a) *Research for Health*. London: HMSO.

Department of Health (1993b) *Report of the Taskforce on the Strategy for Research in Nursing, Midwifery and Health Visiting*. London: DoH.

Department of Health (1993c) *Managing the New NHS*. London: DoH.

Department of Health (1993d) *A Vision for the Future. The Nursing, Midwifery and Health Visiting Contribution to Health and Health Care*. London: DoH.

Department of Health (1994a) *Research and Development in the New NHS: Functions and Responsibilities*. London: DoH.

Department of Health (1994b) *Testing the Vision*. London: DoH.

Department of Health (1994c) *The Challenges for Nursing and Midwifery in the 21st Century (The Heathrow Debate)*. London: DoH.

Department of Health (1995a) *Research and Development: Towards an Evidence-based Health Service*. London: DoH.

Department of Health (1995b) *Supporting R&D in the NHS: Implementation Plan*. London: DoH.

Department of Health (1995c) *A Vision for the Future: Report of the Consultation Exercise*. London: DoH.

Department of Health (1995d) *The Nursing and Therapy Professions' Contribution to Health Services Research and Development*. Report of a conference. London: DoH.

Department of Health (1996) *The New Funding System for R&D in the NHS: an Outline*. London: DoH.

Department of Health and Social Security (1982) *Nursing Research Abstracts: Retrospective Volume 1968–1976*. Foreword by Dame Phyllis Friend, Chief Nursing Officer. London: DHSS.

Fall M, Read S, Walters S *et al* (1997) *An Evaluation of a Nurse-led Ear Care Service in Primary Care: Benefits and Cost Consequences*. British Journal of General Practice **47:** 699–703.

Friend P (1982) Foreword in *Nursing Research Abstracts 1968–76*. DHSS, London.

George S, Read S, Westlake L *et al* (1992) Evaluation of nurse triage in a British accident and emergency department. *British Medical Journal* **304**: 876–878.

Glenister H (1994) Undertaking research in nursing. In Hardey M and Mulhall A (eds) *Nursing Research: Theory and Practice*. London: Chapman & Hall.

Goddard H (1953) *The Work of Nurses in Hospital Wards*. London: Nuffield Provincial Hospitals Trust.

Griffiths R (1983) *NHS Management Inquiry*. London: DHSS.

Hancock C (1993) Promoting Nursing Research: the RCN's role. *Nurse Researcher* **1**(2): 72–80.

Hardey M and Mulhall A (1994) The theory and practice of research. In Hardey M and Mulhall A (eds) *Nursing Research: Theory and Practice*. London: Chapman & Hall.

Hayward J and Lelean S (1982) Nursing Research. In Allen P and Jolley M (eds) *Nursing, Midwifery and Health Visiting since 1900*. London: Faber and Faber.

Heater BS, Becker AM and Olson RK (1988) Nursing interventions and patient outcomes: a meta-analysis of studies. *Nursing Research* **37**(5): 303–307.

Hockey L (1966) *Feeling the Pulse*. London: Queen's Institute of District Nursing.

Hockey L (1968) *Care in the Balance*. London: Queen's Institute of District Nursing.

House of Lords Select Committee on Science and Technology (1988) *Priorities in Medical Research*, Vol 1. London: HMSO.

Hunt J (1981) Indicators for nursing practice: the use of research findings. *Journal of Advanced Nursing* **6**: 189–194.

Hunt J (1996) Funding R&D in Scotland. *Nursing Standard* **10**(22): 32.

Hunt M (1987) The process of translating research findings into nursing practice. *Journal of Advanced Nursing* **12**: 101–110.

Hunter D and Pollitt C (1992) Developments in health services research. *Journal of Public Health Medicine* **14**(2): 164–168.

International Council of Nurses (1996) *Better Health through Nursing Research*. Geneva: ICN.

Kershaw B and Salvage J (eds) (1986) *Models for Nursing*. Chichester: John Wiley.

Lang AF (1994) Guidelines, protocols and outcomes. *International Journal of Healthcare Quality and Assurance* **7**(5): 4–7.

Le Var R (1994) The ENB's implementation of the new strategy for research. *Nursing Times* **90**(22): 36–38.

Le Var R (1995) Evaluating R&D at the ENB. *Nursing Standard* **9**(47): 29–32.

Lelean S and Clarke M (1990) Research resource development in the UK. *International Journal of Nursing Studies* **27**(2): 123–138

Luker K (1992) Research and development in nursing [guest editorial]. *Journal of Advanced Nursing* **17**: 1151–1152.

Macleod Clark J and Hockey L (1989) *Further Research for Nursing*. London: Scutari Press.

Marek KD (1989) Outcome measurement in nursing. *Journal of Nursing Quality and Assurance* **4**(1): 1–9.

McFarlane Baroness J (1990) The study of nursing care. Winifred Raphael Memorial Lecture. Reprinted in Denton PF [editor] (1992) *They Speak for Themselves*. London: RCN.

McFarlane Baroness J (1984) Foreword in Cormack DFS (ed) The Research Process in Nursing. Oxford: Blackwell.

Menzies IEP (1960) *A Case Study in the Functioning of Social Systems as a Defence Against Anxiety*. London: Tavistock.

National Board for Nursing, Midwifery and Health Visiting for Northern Ireland (Research Group) (1991) *Research and the National Board: Future Strategy and Funding*. Belfast: NBNI.

National Board for Northern Ireland (1994) *Research Group: Terms of Reference*. Belfast: NBNI.

Nightingale F (1863) *Notes on Hospitals* (3rd edn). London: Longmans, Green & Co.

Northern Ireland Office: Department of Health and Social Security (1993) *Action Plan for Nursing R&D in Northern Ireland*. Belfast: DHSS for Northern Ireland.

Norton D (1980) Research at work in a region. *Nursing Times* **76**(22): 59–61.

Norton D (1987) Remember with advantages – research efforts gone before. Winifred Raphael Memorial Lecture. Reprinted in Denton PF (ed) (1992) *They Speak for Themselves*. London: RCN.

Norton D, McLaren R and Exton-Smith AN (1962) *An Investigation of Geriatric Nursing Problems in Hospital*. Edinburgh: Churchill Livingstone.

Nuffield Provincial Hospitals Trust (1985) *A Fresh Look at Policies for Health Service Research*. Occasional Paper no. 3. London: NPHT.

Pearson A (1983) *The Clinical Nursing Unit*. London: Heinemann.

Pearson A and Vaughan B (1986) *Nursing Models for Practice*. London: Heinemann.

Pritchard AP (1994) Beyond the stereotypes. *Nursing Standard* **8**(26): 18–20.

Raphael W (1974) *Survey of Patients' Opinions in Hospitals*. Project Paper no. 9. London: King's Fund.

Read SM, Broadbent J and George S (1994) Do formal controls always achieve control? *Health Services Management Research* **7**(1): 31–42.

Read SM (1994) The strategy for research in nursing in England: initial impact. *Nurse Researcher* **1**(3): 72–84.

Rothschild NMV (1971) *The Organization and Management of Government Research and Development (Rothschild Report)*. CMND 4814. London: HMSO.

Royal Marsden Hospital (1984) *Manual of Clinical Nursing Policies and Procedures*. London: Harper and Row.

Russell I (1996) *Research and Development in the NHS: Culyer and Beyond*. Paper at the National Conference for Directors of Nurse Education, Cambridge.

Sackett D, Rosenberg W, Muir Grey J et al (1996) Evidence-based medicine: what it is and what it isn't. *British Medical Journal* **312**: 71–72.

Scottish Office: Home and Health Department (1991) *Strategy for Nursing Research in Scotland*. Scottish Office, Edinburgh.

Scottish Office: Home and Health Department (1993) *R&D Strategy for the NHS in Scotland*. Scottish Office, Edinburgh.

Sheffield Centre for Health and Related Research (1995) SCHARR Strategic Plan 1995–1998. Sheffield: SCHARR.

Skellern E (1953) *Report on an Investigation Carried Out to Study and Make Recommendations on the Practical Application to Ward*

Administration of Modern Methods in the Instruction and Handling of Staff and Student Nurses. London: RCN.

Szczepura A and Cooke P (1993) Softly, softly. *Health Service Journal*, 29 July: 26–27.

Therapy Professions Research Group (1994) *Research and Development in Occupational Therapy, Physiotherapy and Speech and Language Therapy: a Position Statement.* London: DoH.

United Kingdom Central Council for Nursing, Midwifery and Health Visiting (1984, revised 1992) *Code of Professional Conduct.* London: UKCC.

Walsh M and Ford P (1989) Rituals in nursing. *Nursing Times* **85**(41): 26–35.

Walton I (1987) *The Nursing Process in Perspective.* Department of Social Policy and Social Work, York University.

Welsh Office (1992) *Sharpening the Focus: R&D Framework for NHS Wales.* Cardiff: Welsh Office.

Welsh Office (1994) A *Framework for R&D for Nursing in Wales.* Cardiff: Welsh Office.

Welsh Office (1995) *Towards Evidence-based Practice: a Clinical Effectiveness Initiative for Wales.* Cardiff: Welsh Office.

Welsh Office: All Wales Nursing, Midwifery and Health Visiting Research Group (1993) *A Strategy for the Development of Research in Nursing in Wales.* Cardiff: Welsh Office.

3 Accessing sources of knowledge

Christine Hibbert, Patrick Crookes

Introduction

The aim of this chapter is to examine the practicalities of literature searching and to introduce the idea of generic critical reading skills, which are applicable when reading both research and non-research-based literature. The chapter is divided into three sections. The first section is about searching for literature, defining and refining topics for consideration and reflecting upon ways of putting boundaries around search areas. Strategies for successful literature searching are outlined, along with the use of resources additional to the library, such as subject authorities and relevant organizations. The second part of the chapter commences with a discussion of speed reading techniques which can help you to quickly ascertain the relevance of books and articles, without necessarily having to read them in depth. Pointers for practising 'skim reading' of both texts and journal articles are presented. This section of the chapter ends with a discussion of various systems for recording and maintaining personal notes and references. Examples of a selection of reference storage systems are presented. The third part of the chapter introduces the idea of critical analysis. The meaning of this term is discussed and a distinction is made between 'critical analysis' and 'critique' which is perceived as a higher order skill and not expected of those new to research. A simple exercise is then used to enable you to practise making balanced decisions about written work and writing about such decisions.

At the end of the chapter there is a checklist of the databases (electronic and print) which are most relevant to health workers, along with a brief summary of their contents. References and suggested further reading are offered throughout the chapter and summarized at the end. This chapter articulates closely with Chapter 10. Whilst this chapter looks at accessing and evaluating literature at a basic level, Chapter 10 presents more advanced criteria for evaluating the rigour of research-based literature, before moving on to the processes of collating information (synthesis) from a variety of sources to produce systematic, critical literature reviews.

See Chapter 10,
Reviewing and
interpreting research

Key issues

> ■ Strategies for defining and refining topics to facilitate successful literature searching
> ■ Techniques to allow rapid evaluation of the usefulness of literature
> ■ Methods for developing skills in critical analysis

Successful literature searching

Starting to look for literature can seem a huge task. It can be frustrating, but if the search is fruitful, very satisfying and useful. This section of the chapter is intended to help you to maximize the chances of success in any searches you may undertake.

Why carry out a search in the first place? Polit and Hungler (1991) identify two reasons for undertaking literature searches and reviews:

■ To develop a picture of what is known – perhaps as a preparation for undertaking research
■ Searching and reviewing may result in 'a critical summary of the state of the art of a topic, which may be an end in itself'. The latter is the focus of Sue Davies' chapter later in this book, as she discusses the synthesis of a range of material, then explores the constituents of critical literature reviews. Many health professionals undertake literature searches to complete an element of a course, whilst others have a specific question or area that they wish to explore, either for interest or perhaps as part of their work. This text as a whole seeks to further develop the skills needed to do these things more successfully.

See Chapter 10, Reviewing and interpreting research

Where to start?

The first section of this chapter contains suggestions and hints from experienced searchers about using different approaches to searching. These apply to searching both for journal articles and books. The first myth to dispel about searching is that it must start in a library. Many initial discussions about the focus of a search take place with peers and teachers. Resources can be shared and – in the initial stages particularly – it is worth talking to as many relevant and interested people as possible. Ideas and information can come from the most surprizing sources and settings. Informal discussions with colleagues can be useful in helping to broaden or focus a topic area and may even yield specific articles and references. For example, if the topic area is pain relief, advice from colleagues may be that this is too broad and that to focus on pain assessment tools might be more appropriate. Someone may have undertaken courses where this was discussed and have reference lists associated with it, whilst others may have examined the topic in some depth and have specific research papers that they are willing to share. Meanwhile, supervisors and teachers often have a variety of resources, not necessarily associated with their specialist area, or they may know of others who may be able to help. Adequate discussion and consideration about the intended focus of a literature search should take place before even setting foot in a library.

Searching needs to be systematic

A second myth to dispel about searching the literature is that as many references as possible should be collected on the topic in question. Burnard (1993) calls this the 'broad brush approach' to literature searching. However, this usually results in the collection of masses of references which then have to be sifted through to identify the ones which are, or appear to be, most relevant. Such an approach can be costly in terms of time and photocopying, not least because it is not always possible to be sure of the usefulness or quality of an article without reading it in full. There are times when this approach is particularly useful, for example when the (re)searcher has limited knowledge about the topic area and wishes to ensure that they are at least familiar with the range of material which is available on a topic. It can also help to verify or refute a perception that very little is known or has been written about a particular topic.

Defining and refining the topic

If the broad brush approach is used, the best place to start is somewhere quiet, not necessarily a library. Time and space to concentrate are very important, as beginning a search is a creative exercise which may require a degree of lateral thinking. A blank piece of paper and a pen are essential, while a dictionary and a thesaurus are useful. A sensible starting point is to write a sentence which encompasses all the important points or concepts within your topic area. If the reason you are doing the search is to write an essay, then split the essay title up into its constituent parts. If the reason is to find out more about a topic, then think through exactly *what* it is you want to know more about. As previously suggested, refining your topic may be helped by discussing things with experts and/or colleagues.

Having defined the search area, the next task is to refine it. Start by writing down as many words as possible that mean the same as the concepts within the title or topic area identified. More than one word can be used, for example 'nursing care' instead of just 'care'. These are called key words or subject terms. Having done this, write down as many words as possible connected with the key words (the dictionary and thesaurus are again useful for this). These are called associated key words. Once the key words have been worked through and refined in this way, it does not matter how many words there are or how the page is organized. Some people find it easier to make lists because they prefer to work with words on paper; others find it easier to use spider diagrams, conceptual maps or 'mind maps'. Buzan (1981) discusses this at great length and makes many suggestions about how much easier planning is if such methods are used. Figure 3.1 shows an example of a spider diagram, whilst Figure 3.2 shows a linear key word presentation for the same topic area – pressure area care. As you can see the end product is essentially the same – it is purely a matter of choice.

Figure 3.1
A spider diagram or mind map of concepts related to 'pressure area care'

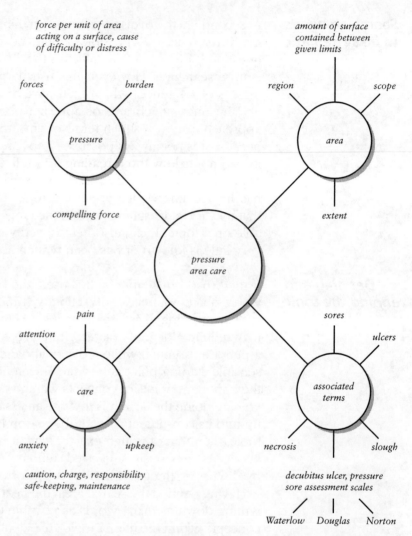

force per unit of area
acting on a surface, cause
of difficulty or distress

amount of surface
contained between
given limits

forces   burden   region   scope

pressure   area

compelling force   extent

pressure
area care

pain   sores

attention   ulcers

care   associated
                                    terms

anxiety   upkeep   necrosis   slough

caution, charge, responsibility
safe-keeping, maintenance

decubitus ulcer, pressure
sore assessment scales

Waterlow   Douglas   Norton

(After Buzan 1981)

Further refining of search terms

Once key words have been identified it is appropriate to turn to the indexes. Indexes are citations to journal articles, listed under subject headings and placed in alphabetical order. They may be either in a printed form or computer based (e.g. CD-ROM). These can be searched for references by simply entering keywords into the electronic databases or by hand searching printed indexes. This would be termed a 'free text' search of the index or database. Such a strategy may be the reason that some people fail to find as much material as they would like or perhaps expect, and may explain why many become disheartened and disillusioned. We suggest that you take an

Figure 3.2
*A linear presentation
of the same
brainstorming
exercise*

Key words or terms – pressure area care

Pressure: pressure, pressing, press, presses, force, forces, compulsion, compelling force, burden, cause of difficulty or distress

Area: area, region, scope, extent, amount of surface contained between given limits

Care: care, heedfulness, attention, caution, charge, responsibility, upkeep, maintenance, look after

Associated key words or terms
Sores, ulcers, necrosis, granulation, slough, decubitus ulcer, turning, pressure aids, mattress, pressure sore assessment tools, pressure sore assessment scales, Waterlow, Norton, Douglas

extra step to refine the key words you intend to search on within a particular index.

To do this you first need to identify which index you intend to access (see 'Which index?', page 61). Let's say that you intend to use the electronic database CINAHL (Cumulative Index of Nursing and Allied Health Literature). This database has a thesaurus within its programme, allowing you to check if the word(s) or term(s) you have identified actually appear in that database. An obvious issue is differences in spelling depending on where the index originates, e.g. 'oesophagus' (English) and 'esophagus' (American). On the other hand those who construct the index may not have categorized the term in the same way you do. For example, you may use the term 'pressure sores' while the index refers to these as 'decubitus ulcers', or you may use 'cancer' while the index lists such material under 'neoplasia'. The terms decubitus ulcers and neoplasia would therefore constitute 'subject headings' within that index. If you entered the term 'pressure sore' you would identify few (if any) references. However, if you entered 'decubitus ulcers' you would find far more references because you have used the correct subject heading *for that index.*

Each index has its own list of subject headings. Within CINAHL the online thesaurus fulfils this role and so refining your key words would involve applying the thesaurus option to each of them, to see if they appear in the database, or to suggest other terms which should be used in their place. If the online index you intend to use has no thesaurus facility *or* you are using a printed index, then the same process would apply, except that you would have to consult the printed 'subject heading index' (typically found in the reference section of libraries) for that particular index. It is important to recognize that because of the variation in subject headings between indexes, this process of refining and identifying terms needs to be repeated for each individual index. A successful search using key words refined from the CINAHL subject heading index *may not* be as successful when using the MEDLINE database. As a result, it is important that you record the indexes *and* the search terms you use for any search you undertake.

Exercise 3.1   Either choose a topic area relevant to your practice or use the heading 'management of acute pain', then brainstorm and list key words and present either as a mind map or a linear list. Next time you go to the library, locate and consult the subject heading index for an electronic database relevant to your discipline and refine your key words into the subject headings used by that database. Then search the index using those terms and note the results. You may find it interesting to do another search using your 'un-refined' terms to see just how many potentially useful references you might have missed.

In summary, it is important to appreciate that you need to put time and effort into the literature searching process *before* you are ready to peruse written or electronic indexes for references. Important and useful data can be missed, simply because inadequate preparation has gone into developing the search strategy. To draw an analogy with another systematic approach to problem-solving – medical diagnosis by doctors – inadequate preparation in developing a search strategy and moving straight to indexes is akin to a doctor deciding to operate on a patient with abdominal pain without first carrying out a detailed history and examination and reaching a diagnosis.

Refining a search is an ongoing process

Key words generated in this way enable you to search systematically through a print or an electronic index. However, the process does not necessarily end with looking for the terms in the print index or feeding them into the search field of the electronic database and then recording the results. To be most successful you need to be prepared to revise the search terms or use combinations of them. This is particularly true of searching using electronic databases as they have facilities for widening or narrowing searches depending on results. To return to the example of pressure area care. Having searched the terms 'pressure' and 'nursing care' individually and found literally hundreds of references, you might then reasonably combine the results of the two using the 'and' option (i.e. references including the term pressure '*and*' nursing care) so as to narrow the search down to a more reasonable number. If, however, you had found only a few references, you might have used the '*or*' option (pressure '*or*' nursing care references). If you find too many or only a few references, the search terms themselves may also need modifying, though this should not be the case if the above refining process has been carried out. There may also be some merit in examining the citations you get a little further. Rather than merely reading the reference and the abstract, you will find that somewhere in the citation is a list of other subject headings related to the topic area concerned. Extending the original search to include these terms *may* elicit further useful material. There are a number of these more advanced searching techniques. Our advice is to practise those we have discussed and then build upon them by consulting with library staff and undertaking training courses available at your library.

Which index?   A number of printed and electronic indexes are available. An index is a list of references organized under subject and author headings. An electronic index usually organizes references using a number of such 'fields', for example the related subject headings identified earlier. Some indexes even provide a short summary or abstract of the article, so that decisions can be made about whether or not they will be useful to the search at this point. This is very helpful as it can minimize time wasted retrieving items which appear to be relevant from their title, yet are of little value when the content is considered. Time can also be spent searching through the library catalogue system or the relevant section of the library to find books on the subject of interest.

With many indexes available, a number of other factors need to be considered when choosing which to search. Perhaps most obvious are that the index should be readily available to you and contains relevant material. With time and experience you will find that you come to prefer certain indexes more than others. The titles of indexes do not always indicate what they contain and, for this reason, Andrew Booth from SCHARR Information Resources at The University of Sheffield has produced a guide to the most commonly used nursing indexes (see Table 3.2, page 78).

It is not only important to consider the scope of the literature indexed, but also the coverage in terms of years. For example, CINAHL and MEDLINE do not index and review all nursing and health-related journals, even some that are quite well known to practitioners. Some indexes are only available for recent years, while others have extensive retrospective coverage. In your search strategy it is therefore worth including some indication of the years which you feel will be useful, as well as checking which journals are included in the indexes available to you. Decisions of this sort may be informed by the topic in question. For example 'shared governance', 'named nursing' and 'day-case surgery' are relatively recent phenomena so a search covering the last five or six years would probably identify the most relevant material. In time, you will become increasingly familiar with the index(es) which relate to material which is most relevant and useful to you.

Literature searching can be time consuming

At this point another myth should be dispelled. It is not usually possible to 'nip into the library at lunch time' to do a 'quick search'. Searching thoroughly usually takes some time. Time spent in the library should be allocated to three distinct tasks:

- Searching the indexes
- Finding the journal(s) or book(s)
- Photocopying the article(s).

First, allow time for searching in the indexes (electronic and print) for relevant references. Having found the references it will be necessary to find the specific journal on the shelves and check that the relevant item is included or order it from another library. Herein lies one of the biggest frustrations, particularly of using electronic indexes – they invariably identify numerous references to articles which appear very useful, but which are very difficult or expensive to access. Even if the journal title is held in the library, the particular issue or article you need may not be on the shelves. If books are identified as having possible use, then they should be quickly checked for their relevance (see exercise, page 68) and borrowed using the appropriate system. Finally, allow time to photocopy specific articles using the library facilities. Queues can form at busy times and so additional time may be necessary to use the photocopier or see the librarian. In view of the above, the processes of literature searching, collecting and reviewing, invariably takes more time than initially planned for.

Time is also a consideration because it is very easy to become sidetracked by looking at other interesting topic areas. Whilst searching on a particular topic, you need to be single-minded and focused to keep the process up to speed. The key word plan should help with this. It is also recommended that you keep a record of the key words used, the searches that have been carried out and the outcome(s) achieved, otherwise you will find yourself going over the same ground again and again. Using a systematic recording system reduces the likelihood of repeating searches and wasting time. This is especially useful if the searches are carried out on a part-time basis and over a longer period of time. If you are concerned that you will forget about material which *might* be useful at some later date, than keep a separate list for such references. A simple example of a search strategy record for the topic of 'shared governance' is presented as Table 3.1. It is useful to note that electronic databases will allow you to print out a copy of the strategy you use, for your records.

Incremental searching

Burnard (1993) also identifies the **incremental** approach to literature searching. This involves initially finding one or two pieces of literature on the chosen topic area, which may be chapters in books as

Table 3.1
A search strategy record for using CINAHL

No	Records	Search requirement
# 1	1468	Shared
# 2	577	Governance
# 3	479	Shared Governance
# 4	377	# 3 and (PY > 1990)

(PY = Publication year; > 1990 = after 1990).

See page 56, *Where to start?*

well as articles (though it is worth remembering that books quickly become dated), and then following up the references listed at the end of the piece. It is a strategy which is particularly useful when examining a topic on which little has been written, or when working in a very specialist or narrow field of study. An ideal place to start is with seminal texts on the subject. Which texts can be considered seminal is information which can be usefully sought from experts in the field, as discussed earlier. Literature retrieved from this exercise can then, in turn, be examined for further references to see if there are any which might prove useful. Searching for literature in this way can be as detailed as necessary. In practice this depends on what the aim of the search is. If it is merely to find out a little more about a topic then a few articles may suffice. However, if the intention is to find out what is known, then the search would continue to a point where little or no new information was being identified by ongoing searches.

There are problems associated with incremental literature searching. Perhaps the most obvious is that it can be very time consuming, particularly as reference lists are not always as accurate or detailed as they should be. There is nothing the searcher can do about this, other than be prepared for the time that will have to be spent 'chasing' references. The benefits of developing good working relationships with library staff should be reiterated here, as there are a number of techniques and short cuts (e.g. citation indexes, page 64) which can help in tracking down such material quickly.

Other problems include the fact that important pieces of work can be missed since they have not been cited by a particular author (who may not have been systematic in their search!). There is also the possibility of introducing a cultural bias, because authors tend to cite work from their own country. Some writers tend to use sources from their own reprint collections which means that they may omit more recent material. All of these problems can be limited by continuing the incremental searching process through as many references as possible, until it becomes apparent that no new writers, references or material are being identified. Properly done, the process can be seen as self-limiting, the end having been reached at this point of 'saturation'. Obviously other factors – most notably time, may curtail the search before this point is reached. The important thing is to recognize that such a search *may* be limited in terms of both scope and depth (one can not be sure as saturation will not have been reached). Furthermore, if the outcome of the search is a written review, then this potential limitation should be shared with the reader (see Chapter 10).

Citation indexes

Is incremental searching cheating? The simple answer to this is 'no'. It is a well-recognized method of searching the literature. In fact the *citation indexes* found in most libraries are actually lists of references presented by authors at the end of their articles. The best known nursing citation index is produced by the American Journal of Nursing and presented in its International Nursing Index (see Table 3.2 for more details). Such indexes are useful in several ways when searching for literature, including:

- Verifying journal citations inadequately cited elsewhere
- Following the progress of a theory or topic through publications
- Checking what other works an author has produced
- Getting some idea of who is writing in a particular field and perhaps who is being cited the most.

Exercise 3.2

Use the references at the end of this chapter to identify a book that you think might be useful for learning more about study skills. Write down the reference in full and during your next library visit, try to find it. Then make a decision about whether it is currently relevant to you. It may be useful to scan it to see if it is readable and easily understandable by picking pages at random and reading short abstracts. If the answer to the above questions is 'yes', then borrow it and read it in more detail.

Exercise 3.3

Find an article in a current journal on an area of interest to you, then check the references at the end and identify two that look useful. Note the journal titles and find out whether they are readily available in the library(ies) to which you have access. Write down the references in full and during your next library visit, try to find them. Again make a decision about whether the articles are currently relevant to you. Also scan them to see if they are readable and easily understandable. If the answer to the above questions is 'yes', then read the article in detail and perhaps copy it, if it is going to be of use to you in the future.

Techniques for improving 'scanning' are discussed in 'Reading the literature' (page 67).

Integrated approach

There is a third approach which is used frequently by experienced searchers. This is a combination of the two approaches discussed so far which we call the **integrated approach** to literature searching. When following this approach, the first thing is to find a good review article on the topic in question and follow the incremental approach already discussed. Again, the advice and counsel of someone knowledgeable in the field will be invaluable. Note that the suggestion is to find a *review* article, not a research article. This is because reviews are designed to do just that – to provide an overview of what has been written about a particular issue or topic. The references listed in the review (which will probably include empirical *and* review literature) can then be examined in more detail and useful material collected. Following this and whilst awaiting any papers which have had to be ordered from elsewhere, the broad brush approach can then be used to identify whether there are any omissions in the citations accrued from the incremental search.

Once the articles and books are retrieved these can also be incrementally cross checked for further references. Additional material can then be requested while the original sources are being read and analyzed. In this way, the time available can be used most effectively. It is important to reiterate here a point made earlier, that is, the need to keep a record of the search strategy followed and its results.

Other sources of information

Local sources

Using one or a combination of these approaches is possible in any professional library context independent of the topic area. The size of the library is immaterial. However, there are other sources of information. Searching for additional material outside the library should begin at a local level. Friends and colleagues often prove useful in this instance, as do clinical specialists within the various disciplines in practice settings. There are many other local sources of information, for example:

- Specialist departments (e.g. intensive care unit or coronary care unit)
- Health promotion units
- Voluntary organizations (e.g. The British Heart Foundation and the Stroke Association)
- Citizens Advice Bureau.

A telephone directory is a useful tool for identifying and locating such groups in your locality.

National sources

In Britain there are a number of national organizations willing to search for references, provided that they have a specific set of key words. Some require payment for this service, but the turnaround time from request to a list of available references delivered to the door can be very speedy. One example of this service is the English National Board for Nurses, Midwives and Health Visitors (ENB) which holds a database of mainly British sources to assist nurses. This service can provide a list of references based on the key words given to a home address in approximately 36 hours. The British Reference Library holds many journals and books and will provide an international service. However, a search for a specific article for an individual is very expensive and it is recommended that one of the professional libraries with whom they hold contractual arrangements should request the items. The Royal College of Nursing and the King's Fund also have extensive library resources. Many professional libraries will offer this or similar facilities. In the 'real world' therefore, a searcher needs to make a decision about the required depth of the search, as this will determine the need and practicality for using these invaluable but sometimes expensive resources.

World Wide Web

Access to the World Wide Web via Internet facilities is becoming increasingly available in many resource centres. This opens up access to a whole new dimension of world wide information. Using such facilities successfully can, however, be rather time consuming, particularly if you have not had a formal introduction to at least the rudiments of the system. It is very easy to spend several hours 'surfing the net' with little or no useful material to show for it at the end of the day. The various search engines and web site directories are helpful, but as with electronic databases perhaps the best advice is to get some training in their use before you waste a lot of time and are perhaps 'switched off' to the technology because of early failure. Most libraries equipped with such facilities will provide training programmes.

A final point to be made here is that the results of systematic reviews of evidence-based medical and nursing literature are increasingly available via traditional means (reports and circulars such as Oxford Health Authorities' *Bandolier* publication) and via the Internet (e.g. The Cochrane Collaboration Database and various Internet discussion groups).

Summary

Plan search strategies carefully. Get as much information as possible and define the search area as clearly as possible before you even access an index or database. Refine your search terms using thesauri and subject headings, remembering that subject headings vary from index to index. A combination of broad brush and incremental searching is often necessary. Recognize that a lot of information and advice can come from 'experts in the field'. These may be subject authorities, helpful library staff, or information specialists.

Once you start searching, keep records of the search steps followed and the resources examined. Try not to get sidetracked with material which looks interesting but is irrelevant to the task in hand. Remember that searching for references often takes more time than you originally thought. Expect to get frustrated as items are often missing or out on loan. Seek assistance from library staff, particularly about how to get the best from resources and training opportunities.

Reading the literature

Once literature has been obtained, the first step is to check it for relevance to the subject area and what you particularly want to know. With practice this can take very little time, provided that there are no distractions. This requires the skill of **skim reading**. This is an important skill because it means that you will not waste time reading material which is of little use to you. This section of the chapter is concerned with how to speed up the reading process and consists of suggestions about the usefulness of speed reading when trying to quickly evaluate the relevance of articles and books to a particular topic or line of research. There are also two exercises designed to help you to practise these skills of scanning and skimming.

Hector-Taylor and Bonsall (1994) suggest that there are three different levels of reading:

■ Scanning
■ Skimming
■ Deep study reading.

Whilst scanning and skimming literature help you to make decisions about whether it is relevant for your specific purpose, deep reading is required for understanding and considering the possible application of the literature to the 'real world'. The exercises below include the use of these strategies and highlight the fact that reading is an active process, that skills such as skim reading need to be seen as learned skills (rather than a natural ability) and finally that they have to be worked at, developed and practised. Deeper reading techniques are not discussed specifically here, since this text as a whole is designed to provide insight into research, and enable deeper reading of research-based literature.

'Skimming' a journal article

To check the relevance of a journal article it is worth reading the abstract. An abstract is a brief summary of the article and usually identifies what type of information is being presented. If there is no abstract then read the introduction and the conclusion. Reading these sections will give an indication of relevance to the subject area and to the paper's readability. The task is to check for relevance, not to read the document in its entirety or be diverted by interesting sections of it. There will be an opportunity for deeper reading at a later stage, if the piece is relevant. A decision can then be made about what type and what level of knowledge are reflected in the piece and thus whether it should be marked for further examination.

At this stage, the references should also be examined. Well-referenced pieces tend to carry more credibility. On the whole they should consist of up-to-date citations, unless classic pieces of research are cited. The references may also usefully contribute to further incremental searching.

The following exercise summarizes particular points to consider when skimming an article or book to decide whether to read it in more detail at a later time.

Exercise 3.4

Choose a recent journal article on a topic you are interested in and read the abstract or the introduction and conclusion. Look at the list of references but do not read any further. Try to answer the following questions.

- Is it currently relevant to you?
- What is the level of knowledge? (after DePoy and Gitlin 1994 – see Chapter 5)
- Does it look easy to read?
- Is it detailed or superficial?
- Is it well referenced?
- Are the references recent publications?
- Would you read the article in more detail if the opportunity arose?

'Skimming' a book

To check a book for relevance would seem initially to be a more difficult process. However, with a little practice it can take only a few minutes. In many ways, checking a book for relevance is a similar process to checking a journal article.

The first task is to look at the date the book was produced. Many books on specific subject areas quickly become dated. This is particularly the case for books which discuss clinical practice, which changes rapidly – though incrementally – all the time. Deciding whether a book should be considered current requires quite complex judgment, basically because you need some knowledge of the topic to know that the material has been superseded. If you do not have such knowledge, you should seek advice from specialists in the area, or possibly librarians, before continuing. If the book is considered current, the next task is to decide whether you think the author has credibility in the field. Points to consider in making this decision include relevant qualifications and any professional and academic positions held. Both of these will give some indication of their standing as an authority in the field about which they are writing.

Having decided that the author(s) appear credible, read the contents page(s). The chapter headings should give an overall picture of the book. Following this, read the introduction (sometimes called a preface) as in this section authors tend to give an overview of the reasons for writing the text and what they hope(d) to achieve by writing it. They often expand on chapter headings and how various aspects of the text tie together. It is recommended that you use this section to make a judgment on a book, rather than using the comments on the dust jacket which is invariably advertising material. Finally the references should be checked. There are usually two places to search for these. In edited books, references are often placed at the end of each chapter (as in this book). In other books they are placed after the text, before the main index. The reason for checking the references is the same as with a journal article – in case they are useful as primary sources and to make sure that they are concurrent with the publication date of the book. They should also be sufficient in number to suggest that a range of material has been considered.

Exercise 3.5   Choose a book and time yourself while you check the publication date, contents pages, introduction/preface and the references, then answer the following questions.

- Is it relevant to the work you are currently doing?
- Is the book relevant in terms of publication date?
- Does the author appear to be a credible authority on the subject in question?
- Which chapter(s) would you look at first?
- Were the intentions of the book stated at the beginning of the introduction or preface?
- Were there ample references and did any look interesting?
- Would you examine this book more closely if given the opportunity?
- How long did it take you to do this exercise?

The key to success with skim reading is practice. We therefore recommend that you repeat these exercises until you are satisfied that the answers to the above questions can be found quickly, for any article or book you choose to peruse. It is important to develop the confidence to feel that you will not miss useful information by checking books and journals in this way. From our experience we have noted that in high standard scholarly work, key issues are clearly identified at the start of any piece of writing, before being discussed in detail in the body of the work. Approach the task confidently.

Deep reading is also a skill that should be developed and practised. This is explored in some detail in Sue Davies' Chapter 10, where more advanced skills of critical analysis are discussed.

Summary

Skim reading skills are important because they help avoid wasting time reading material which is of little relevance to the task in hand. The key to success with skim reading is practice. Work through the exercises provided to help you structure this practice.

Making records and keeping notes

Having searched for and found appropriate literature, the next step is to consider how to organize and record the material (references for articles/books and notes). Bell (1993) and Northedge (1993) offer some very useful suggestions about using card indexes and boxes. Basically these systems involve making a record of each reference on a computer card. As most academic writing in the health and behavioural sciences uses the Harvard (author–date) system of referencing, it is sensible to record on card or computer information according to this system. Each card should include details of the author, date, title, publisher and source. For a journal article, the journal and page numbers should also be recorded. Additional information about where the piece of literature is kept can also be quite useful, especially if it is a book which has to be returned to the library. Finally, brief notes about the particular piece may prove useful, especially when using a computer card file, as this will assist in the retrieval of information. With increasing knowledge of both research methodology and the topic under consideration, these notes may extend to discussions of the rigour of research, the theoretical bases of arguments used and any recommendations made. Sue Davies provides an excellent framework for structuring such notes in Chapter 10.

Most computer database applications will contain some form of card file recording system. Essentially these differ from manual recording in that instead of writing the information on a card, it is recorded on a computer screen. An example of an entry in a computer card file index is presented in Fig. 3.3.

There are advantages and disadvantages to using either system (card or computer). Both require that you adopt a systematic approach to collating information and that it is an ongoing process. Both methods are quite time consuming at first, but time spent early on will save many hours of hunting for previously read documents and references in the future. Computer card files do have an advantage in that they often have a key word (text search) facility for searching through the collected references for a particular topic area. Card indexes need to be quite elaborately colour coded to achieve similar results.

There are a number of more advanced bibliographic software packages (e.g. EndNote and ProCite) which offer more than merely a computer screen version of a card. More detailed information of interest from references can be detailed under headings (also known as 'fields') such as 'themes', 'boundaries' and 'methods'. Key word searching is also available. Such packages can not only store

Figure 3.3
*Example of an entry
in a computer card
file index*

Dodd F (1996) Under pressure. *British Journal of Theatre Nursing*
6 (9): 33–35.

- Report of a study about pressure area care in the operating theatre
- Identifies that a thorough literature search has been undertaken, no details of this
- No methodological discussion, no theoretical or conceptual framework
- Study identifies detailed methods but no information about number of participants, ethical framework or length of time it took. Only seems to have been carried out in one area
- Detailed discussion about changes in practice as a result of this study
- Does identify that the report has been edited for publication, could possibly contact author for further information.

Held in HOME LIBRARY

references, but can also place them within text in a word-processed document *and* generate a reference list at the end. Developing such a database from the outset of any project or essay can save much of the time and effort which normally goes into the generation of reference lists. Fig. 3.4 shows an example of a more detailed reference entry, typical of EndNote.

Computers can be expensive, they are prone to break down and are not always portable – though all three aspects are rapidly changing. Using a paper system means that spare cards can be completed in the library and used wherever study takes place. Unfortunately, once the paper card system increases in size, it can be tedious to search for specific topic areas and increasingly loses its portability. Perhaps a combination of the two is best, where information is initially collated on cards then entered on the computer when accessible.

The importance of recognizing that systematically reading and recording useful references are essential aspects of the process of searching for and analyzing literature, cannot be emphasized enough. However, as with recording search strategies and their outcomes, they are often steps that are missed or dealt with in a haphazard manner because they are time consuming, laborious and appear to delay getting on with the 'real work'. Yet, when properly set up and maintained, they provide a useful and ongoing resource. As a potential 'life-long' learner, we encourage you to consider these suggestions for developing your own information database.

Figure 3.4
An example of an entry in a bibliographic software package

Author	Turner P
Year	1993
Title	Activity nursing and the changes in the quality of life of elderly patients: a semi-quantitative study
Source	Journal of Advanced Nursing
Volume	18
Issue	11
Pages	1727–1733
Publisher	
Place	
Summary	Activity nursing results in changes in cognitive functioning and quality of life
Themes	Therapeutic care Activity nursing
Boundaries	One hospital 23 patients 26 relatives 25 staff
Methods	Mental test score Holden communication scale Self-completion questionnaires to relatives and staff
Findings	Improvements in life satisfaction following introduction of individualized activity programmes. Relatives and staff were positive
Recommendation	More resources for activity nursing
Critique	No control group Not clear to what extent activities were taking place prior to baseline measurement Questions potentially leading Best seen as a useful exploratory study

Summary

A system for recording references and literature is an important feature of any strategy for collecting and storing information. Paper card files are portable and reliable but retrieving topic information from them can be a slow process. Computer card files facilitate quick topic retrieval, but they are less portable and not always available. The Harvard system is usually required for academic writing so it is worth recording references in this style. Computer-based bibliographic packages are useful as they not only retain reference material but also aid in the laborious task of writing reference lists. A combination of paper notes and computer files is perhaps the best way forward.

Critically analyzing the literature

This final section of the chapter focuses on the analysis of material retrieved from literature searches. This book as a whole is designed to facilitate insight into research processes, to allow readers to make reasoned decisions about the credibility (or otherwise) of research reports. However, at this point we wish to make general points about the processes of being critical and analytical, which can be exercized by anyone when reading or writing scholarly work. More detailed knowledge can then be brought to bear as it is assimilated.

It is difficult to articulate the difference between description, analysis and critical analysis. These terms invariably appear in the learning objectives for academic courses, but what do they mean? Description entails giving a narrative account of something, a statement of how something is, rather than what it could or should be. The word 'analyze' is defined as: 'to divide into component parts or elements; examine minutely; make a detailed description and criticism of' (Penguin Concise English Dictionary 1991).

In any analysis of a piece or a body of literature, there will always be an element of description to identify for the reader what the work is about. However, excessive description means that the reader would be better reading the original than your précis of it. Unfortunately, many people new to the art of scholarly or 'academic' writing have a tendency towards description rather than analysis.

What is critical analysis?

To be critical often implies that fault must be found with whatever is being reviewed. However, *The Penguin Concise English Dictionary* (1991) defines a critic as a 'professional reviewer of books'. It also states that to be critical means 'expressing sound judgment' and goes on to define criticism as being 'the art or process of judging merits of artistic or literary work; analysis or review of this work'. It can be seen from these definitions that being critical in its true sense involves making decisions about the worth or value of a piece of literature or other art. Furthermore, by referring to 'merits', the definition indicates that in being critical, a person should consider both the good and bad points of the work in question. This is perhaps a departure from the popular use of the term 'to criticize', with its typically negative connotations.

If we put this together with 'analyze', the term to 'critically analyze' a piece of literature can be seen to encompass breaking it down in some way (perhaps along the lines of ideas presented, or the research process) and examining it in detail, both in terms of its parts and how they fit together. It also includes an imperative to make decisions about the work – about what is good and bad about it; whether on balance it has merit; and whether it is of use to the reader. As no piece of literature is all good or all bad, it follows that having 'critically analyzed' it, a reader will end up with a balanced view of the material presented and will have reached decisions about its value.

It is perhaps worth noting at this point that there is a difference between critical analysis and **critique**. To critique a piece of literature is a high order skill requiring advanced knowledge of research ethics and methodologies. One would not expect those new to research to be able to work at this level. Try this next exercise, based on the kind of news presented on the health pages of some popular women's journals, to see if you can come up with a critical analysis of the following hypothetical paragraph. You are encouraged to think in terms of what the item is about (description) and its merits (positive and negative).

Exercise 3.6

> *Portable monitors designed to help protect asthmatics from ozone and pollution in the atmosphere may be placing people with chest complaints in danger. These monitors bleep according to the levels of ozone in the atmosphere and are meant to warn asthmatics when to take extra precautions. However, the monitors fail to bleep in the presence of lower levels of ozone and tobacco smoke – levels which, according to research, may still cause severe problems in susceptible people, says Doctor Marion Lewis-Day of Saint Patrick's College, Crookes University. Users could be at risk of severe breathing difficulties if they do not take adequate precautions based on this monitor's warning bleeps.*

Take a blank piece of paper and write a sentence describing what the paragraph is about. There are any number of variations in this sentence but the key is to narrow it down so that the description is as short as possible. Next, draw a line down the middle of the paper and write two headings 'positive' and 'negative', one at the top of each half. Read the paragraph again, identifying what you think are the 'merits' (including positives *and* negatives) of the piece. Write your thoughts under the appropriate heading.

The next task is to construct some sentences. In each sentence put in the positive and the negative comments. Remember to avoid unsubstantiated, overly argumentative or provocative statements. Words like 'must', 'should' and 'will' should be replaced with words like 'might', 'perhaps', 'suggest' and 'maybe'. An example of an unsubstantiated statement would be 'nurses do not understand research'. This could be replaced by 'the literature suggests that many nurses do not understand research'.

When describing a piece of literature, a good word to use at the start is 'this'. For example, you could say: 'This paragraph is about the problems associated with using portable monitors to detect pollution in the atmosphere'. In analyzing it most people find it easier to find fault with the literature but you are encouraged to try to reach a balanced decision. For every negative point that you make, try to think of a positive as well. In some cases you may find that the negative is the same as the positive – being brief and to the point can lead to a lack of detail, but also provide emphasis. Below is an example of the kind of things you might write.

POSITIVE	NEGATIVE
■ It raises awareness	■ It could be scare-mongering
■ It is short	■ There is not enough information
■ It is easy to read	■ There is not enough detail
■ A named scientist supports it	■ The named scientist might not be an expert in asthma
■ It says which institution she comes from	■ The university is not well known
■ It identifies that research has been carried out	■ There is no information about the scope and depth of the research
■ It gives a warning to asthma sufferers	■ It could be misleading because it initially sounds like these monitors are a good idea

Examples of the kind of sentences you could construct about the article are as follows:

'This paragraph is short. However, there is not enough information to make a decision about whether it is valuable. It is also easy to read but unfortunately there does not appear to be enough detail. Although this information is supported by a named doctor, there is no information about her area of speciality or area of practice. The university is named, however it does not seem to be a recognized institution. In addition, whilst there is acknowledgment that research has been carried out, there does not appear to be any information in the article about its methodology'

By using the key words in the initial analysis, it is quite easy to construct the sentences and already there is nearly as much written in the analysis as in the original article. Another point is that if all the sentences start with a positive and end with a negative it can become quite tedious, therefore it is worth considering varying the format. For example, 'It could be said that this information is misleading to asthma sufferers but at least it raises awareness about this issue'. The final step is to use the last sentence to leave the reader of the analysis with a lasting impression of your overall decision. If you think that overall, it was a good piece, it is worth considering ending with a positive comment. If, on the other hand, you think that it was a poor piece overall, you should consider ending with a negative comment.

You might like to consider using this exercise as a basic structure for making notes from material you read. As you learn more about research, this structure will naturally become more complex – as suggested by the criteria for evaluating research and non-research-based literature presented in Sue Davies' chapter (Chapter 10). The techniques demonstrated for attempting to ensure balanced analysis are also relevant when writing literature reviews – an issue also returned to in Sue's chapter 10.

Summary

Critical analysis of research literature involves judging the merits of the research and coming to a balanced decision about it. It is *not* merely the identification of what the researcher did wrong. No literature is all good or all bad. Therefore, when taking notes or when writing yourself, try to retain a balanced view. In particular avoid unsubstantiated statements as they can detract from the argument being presented. Finally, critiquing research is a very high order cognitive skill. It requires knowledge of the conceptual, methodological and ethical components of research. This book is intended to help you move towards this goal.

Chapter conclusion

In this chapter we have examined skills and knowledge which will enable you to be more effective in finding literature about any subject you have an interest in, and from there to make fairly quick decisions about its quality and relevance to you. To do this we described strategies for making index searching (paper and electronic) more effective – essentially by encouraging you to be systematic and perhaps putting a little more effort into preparing a search strategy before examining databases. Next, we described approaches to reading the literature discovered as a result of such searches. We particularly concentrated on techniques you can use to enable you to make quick decisions about the content – and therefore relevance – of texts and articles you find. This is important because, invariably, literature searching unearths far more information than you can actually use. Any mechanism which helps you to sort out 'need to know' from 'nice to know', without having to read it all in depth is very useful, not least because of the time it saves. We closed this section by making suggestions for ways of recording the results of your literature searches, either on paper or using computer software. Finally we discussed the issue of critical analysis of literature.

Being able to critically analyze and to demonstrate this ability in scholarly writing is an important skill, not least because it is typically required in diploma and degree level studies (and higher), as well as by credible professional journals. Critical analysis of research is also a basic require-ment of the clinician who wishes to be actively involved in evidence-based practice. However, it should be acknowl-edged that these 'generic' aspects of critical analysis need to be combined with an insight into research methodology, if you are intending to critically analyze scholarly (i.e. research and/or theoretically-based) literature. Furthermore, this book as a whole seeks to inform you, the reader, about key aspects of this knowledge base. Fairly advanced criteria for evaluating research and theoretically-based literature are pre-sented by Sue Davies in Chapter 10.

References

Bell J (1993) *Doing Your Research Project*. Milton Keynes: Open University Press.

Burnard P (1993) Facilities for searching the liter-ature and storing references. *Nurse Researcher* **1**(1): 56–63.

Buzan T (1981) *Make the Most of Your Mind*. London: Pan Books.

Carper BA (1978) Fundamental patterns of know-ing in nursing. *Advances in Nursing Science* **1**(1): 13–23.

Hector-Taylor M and Bonsall M (1994) *Successful Study: A Practical Way to Get a Good Degree*. Sheffield: The Hallamshire Press.

Northedge A (1993) *The Good Study Guide*. Milton Keynes: Open University Press.

Penguin Concise Oxford English Dictionary (1991) London: Penguin Books.

Polit DF and Hungler BP (1991) *Nursing Research: Principles and Methods,* 4th edn. Philadelphia, PA: Lippincott.

Table 3.2 Databases and information sources of use to health professionals (Compiled by Andrew Booth, Director of Information Resources, School of Health and Related Research, University of Sheffield)

Database name and dates	Coverage	Features	Access
AJN International Nursing Index 1982–	Produced by the American Journal of Nursing. Covers the international nursing literature including non-English materials.	Uses the Medical Subject Headings (MeSH) employed by MEDLINE. An invaluable feature is a citation index covering references used by the current year's authors which provides access to older materials.	Printed version, annual volume with three instalments a year
Applied Social Science Index and Abstracts (ASSIA) – 1987	Strong emphasis on the applied aspects of the social sciences. Particularly useful for materials on the social, political, economic and cultural context of health care.	Coverage: 40% UK, 45% USA, 15% rest of the world. Short informative summaries, full references and index terms. Approximately 550 world wide English language journals and newspapers are routinely scanned. About 80% are abstracted from cover to cover, 20% selectively.	CD-ROM Online via Knight Rider (Datastar/Dialog)
CRD Databases NHS Centre for Reviews and Dissemination (CRD) 1994–	Contains three databases covering systematic reviews and economic evaluations. Particularly useful for clinical effectiveness or cost effectiveness of treatments, especially those that are relatively recent.	Detailed summaries of published reviews in Health of the Nation topic areas, topics from the Effective Health Care Bulletins, pressure sores, cataracts, diabetes, and health promotion as well as health technology assessment. • Economic evaluations of health care • Full-text reviews either undertaken by CRD or produced by other organizations.	Available via the JANet network. Also included as part of the Cochrane Database of Systematic Reviews (see below)

Cochrane Database of Systematic Reviews Current	Contains reviews, bibliographies and details of Cochrane Collaboration activities and contacts. Useful for clinical effectiveness materials. Particularly strong in pregnancy and childbirth and stroke but other topics are being added all the time.	Full text of reviews organized by medical subject headings (MeSH). Also contains reference lists for existing systematic reviews, reviews assessed for quality by the NHS Centre for Reviews and Dissemination (CRD) and reviews on the database of the International Network of Agencies for Health Technology Assessment (INAHTA), together with methodological articles.	CD-ROM
Cochrane Pregnancy & Childbirth Database Current	Contains reviews, bibliographies and the full text of *Guide to Effective Care in Pregnancy and Childbirth*. Of great value to midwives and any staff involved in aspects of antenatal and perinatal care.	Includes critical comment on reviews including implications for care. Also contains a register of over 7500 controlled trials and a listing of articles on how to do a review. *Summary Effectiveness Tables* inform on whether an intervention is likely to be of benefit or harm.	CD-ROM
Cumulative Index of Nursing and Allied Health Literature (CINAHL) 1982–	Covers all aspects of nursing and allied health disciplines such as health education, occupational therapy, physiotherapy, emergency services and social services in health care.	Good coverage of therapy literature. Also includes some nursing theses (US) and provides citations at end of review articles. Strong American bias.	CD-ROM, online and printed versions
CRIB (Current Research in Britain) Current	National register of current academic research projects being carried out in the UK. Includes biological sciences, physical sciences, social sciences and humanities.	Location and description of research and research personnel, information on sponsoring bodies and references to both published and unpublished papers.	CD-ROM and printed versions

Table 3.2 (contd.)

Database name and dates	Coverage	Features	Access
DHSS–DATA 1983–	Covers health service and hospital administration, including health services facilities, equipment and supplies, public health, primary care; occupational diseases, social policy, social services for children, families, the handicapped and older people. Contains records formerly in *Nursing Research Abstracts*.	Articles from about 2000 mainly English language journals together with records of books, reports, pamphlets, administrative circulars and other official publications. Includes full details of DoH or DSS publications plus how to obtain them. Approximately 40% of the records carry abstracts and about 12 000 records are added each year.	Online via Knight-Rider (Datastar/Dialog). A CD-ROM is planned
EMBASE 1984–	Clinical medicine and medical research. Produced by Excerpta Medica. Superior to MEDLINE for European journal coverage.	Journal articles from about 3500 titles, only an overlap of 35% with MEDLINE coverage. Particular strength of this database is drug information and related areas. It *does not* cover nursing.	Available via the BIDS service on JANet network. Also online
English National Board for Nursing, Midwifery and Health Visiting Health Care Database Varies	Full range of issues relating to the nursing, midwifery and health visiting professions.	Journal articles, research reports, audio-visual materials and open learning packages.	Available via the English National Board
ERIC Most recent 4 years on CD-ROM. Online is more extensive	US database covering the journal and research literature in the field of education. Sponsored by the US Department of Education. Useful for nurse education and continuing education issues. Also for information on changing professionals' behaviour and practice.	*Resources in Education* (RIE), covers the document literature, and *Current Index to Journals in Education* (CIJE), covers over 775 periodicals. The database also includes the full text of ERIC Digest records – one- to two-page full-text records, which provide an overview of information on a given topic and supply references with more detailed information.	CD-ROM. Also online and printed versions

Health Education Authority Varies	Health promotion and disease prevention. With a UK focus. Particular strengths are AIDS and HIV prevention, ethnic health issues and dental health promotion.	In addition to journal articles and books used in the HEA bibliographies this Catalogue of the Health Promotion Information Centre (HPIC) also includes videos and health education training materials.	Access through the HPIC staff
HEALTHPLAN 1981–	Non-clinical aspects of health care delivery, including all aspects of administration and planning of health care facilities, financial management, licensure and accreditation, personnel management, staffing, planning, quality assurance and related topics.	Includes approximately 432 000 citations supplied by the US National Library of Medicine and the American Hospital Association. It also includes journal citations from the *Hospital Literature Index*.	CD-ROM and online. No exact printed equivalent
Health Management Information System (HELMIS) 1984–	Extensive bibliographic database on all aspects of health and social care management. Produced by the Information Resource Centre at the Nuffield Institute for Health, Leeds. Good UK focus.	Good coverage of general material on health outcomes, community care and comparative health systems.	Via JANet network for subscribers only
King's Fund 1984–	Coverage of health planning, management and social care including quality of care and administration. Covers books, reports and journal articles. Produced by the King's Fund.	Particularly strong on UK literature, carers, quality assurance and governmental and independent reports.	Searches can be requested from King's Fund Library. Plans to make available via Internet/ JANet

Table 3.2 (contd.)

Database name and dates	Coverage	Features	Access
MEDLINE 1966–	Citations and abstracts to world wide biomedical literature including research, clinical practice, administration, policy issues and health care services. Print equivalent: *Index Medicus, Index to Dental Literature, International Nursing Index.* Records held: 8 000 000 +, records added annually: 300 000 +	MEDLINE references articles from about 3400 journals published in 70 countries. MEDLINE also covers chapters and articles from selected monographs; author abstracts are available for about 60% of the citations since 1975. Searchable by subject headings found in the US National Library of Medicine's MeSH (Medical Subject Headings) thesaurus. Data is updated monthly with MeSH headings updated annually.	1966 to date available online. CD-ROM coverage varies according to local subscription
MIDIRS – Midwives Information and Resource Service	Midwifery, obstetrics and maternity care.	30 000 references to articles in popular and professional journals dealing with aspects of pregnancy, childbirth, preconceptual care, etc.	Searches done for a charge, contact MIDIRS
OSH–ROM 1960–	Brings together four complete bibliographic databases covering critical international occupational health and safety information. Useful for coverage of information concerning occupational health and safety, hazardous incidents, and the handling of dangerous materials.	Most useful component is HSELINE, from the Health and Safety Executive (UK). Four databases contain well over 300 000 citations taken from over 500 journals and 100 000 monographs and technical reports.	CD-ROM
Psycinfo/Psyclit 1967–1975	Coverage of psychology, clinical psychiatry, counselling, child development, child abuse, family therapy and psychoanalysis.	Some overlap with MEDLINE in psychology and clinical psychiatry.	Full database online. Also CD-ROM and printed versions

Research Activities and Projects Information Database (RAPID)	Covers health and health studies, research methods and welfare services. Useful for all non-clinical aspects of nursing research.	Information on Economic and Social Research Council (ESRC) research awards and publications. Publications include conference papers, non-refereed articles and some audio-visual materials.	Available via JANet network
RCN NURSE ROM Royal College of Nursing Database 1985–	Coverage of nursing, midwifery and health visiting. Journal articles and full text coverage of the *Nursing Standard*. Complements CINAHL by providing a UK focus but does not include allied health professions.	Consists of three databases: RCN Library's Journals containing 80 000 bibliographic records. Also includes a full list of journals held at the RCN Library; *Issues in Nursing and Health*, full text of recent position papers; and *Nursing Standard* text and images of 500 'clinical' articles (June 1992–December 1994)	Available on CD-ROM. Members may also contact the Royal College of Nursing Library
Science Citation Index and Social Science Citation Index 1983–	Coverage of scientific and social science literature. Health care topics are distributed between the two indexes depending on whether they are clinical subjects or examine organizational and social issues. Produced by the Institute for Scientific Information.	Provides references and abstracts to a great volume of the world's literature including European and Japanese journals. A major feature is the provision of cited references which can be searched across a period of years.	Available via the BIDS service on the JANet network
UK Clearing House on Health Outcomes Literature Database Varies	Coverage of health outcomes and their measurement. Produced by the UK Clearing House on Health Outcomes, Nuffield Institute for Health, University of Leeds.	Selective database covering general outcome issues and 'grey' literature.	Searches can be requested from the Outcomes Clearing House

Further reading

Buzan T (1991) *Speed Reading*. Newton Abbot: David and Charles.
Very detailed information about reading and planning, there is even information about the ambient temperature of a room. In-depth exercises also presented in a popular style.

Cuba L (1993) *A Short Guide to Writing About Social Science*, 2nd edn. New York: Harper Collins.
Good section on writing an essay (Form).

Freeman R (1991) *Mastering Study Skills*. Basingstoke: Macmillan Education.
A very basic guide for those who have limited experience of studying.

Freeman R and Meed J (1993) *How to Study Effectively*. Basingstoke: Macmillan Education.
A basic guide for the novice studier.

Parnell J and Kendrick K (1995) *Study Skills for Nurses: A Practical Guide*. New York: Churchill Livingstone.
Detailed information on reading activities and mind maps.

Redway K (1988) *Rapid Reading*. London: Pan Books.
A step-by-step approach to reading books, reports and journals.

Rowntree D (1988) *Learn How to Study: A Guide for Students of All Ages*. London: MacDonald Orbis.
Very detailed, worth reading though.

Williams K (1989) *Study Skills*. Basingstoke: Macmillan Education.
Good basic guide.

4 Philosophical and theoretical underpinnings of research

Lorraine Ellis, Patrick Crookes

Introduction

If there was a word more likely to engender a swift turning of the page, or a drift into the arms of Morpheus than 'research', then for many people it would be 'philosophy'. For others it would be 'theory'. Perhaps this is because these are terms that people don't perceive to have everyday relevance (Mike Nolan and Ullah Lundh point out in Chapter 1 (page 10) that 'know that' is currently seen as secondary to 'know how' in the minds of many nurses), or terms they don't really understand. However, they are terms which are of fundamental importance when considering research. In this chapter we cover these topics with the intention of explaining what they are and describing how a researcher's philosophical standpoint or 'world view' can impinge on the research they undertake and *how* they undertake it. This builds on material touched on in Chapter 1. We will then go on to discuss why any research study needs to relate to what is already known – or 'theory'. By developing an understanding of the philosophical bases of research paradigms and their associated methods, and by appreciating the relationship that *should* exist between theory and research, the critical reader of research will be well placed to evaluate research papers. You will be able to do so with regard to the appropriateness of the research design and research methods, the suitability of the research question, and the compatibility between the research methods, findings and conclusions.

We will first examine some of the assumptions and beliefs which underpin the traditional philosophical 'camps' of experimental-type (variously called quantitative, scientific or positivist) and naturalistic (qualitative or non-positivist) designs of research, then briefly compare these with a third research philosophy – critical theory. We will then re-visit the idea first raised in Chapter 1 (page 5), that no research philosophy or 'paradigm' (an example or model used as a standard) should be viewed necessarily as having the ascendancy over another, but rather that researchers should choose methods which reflect the level of knowledge on the topic in question and which will meaningfully add to that knowledge base.

From this starting point we will consider theory – what it is and how it can be generated or tested – including a brief explanation of inductive and deductive reasoning. This will lead on to a discussion of the relationships which (should) exist between theory and research. This is important because, as indicated already, being able to judge whether the right questions have been asked by a researcher is an important aspect of critically reading research reports.

Finally we will discuss how researchers use frames of reference, in an attempt to share their 'world view' with the critical reader and indicate how they perceive their research builds upon what is already known. This will include the identification of key points to consider when evaluating the conceptual bases of research studies. The most important thing to consider when reading research is whether or not it builds upon the existing body of knowledge, which in most cases will be indicated via links which can be drawn between the literature review and the research design. However, there are some researchers who attempt to clearly and overtly iden-tify the theoretical bases of their research. They do so through the presentation of a frame of reference. The final section of this chapter therefore concentrates on 'frames of reference in research'.

Key issues

- The relationship between philosophy and research design
- Paradigms in research
- Processes linking theory and research: induction and deduc-tion
- Theories as mechanisms for explaining and predicting phe-nomena
- Conceptual and theoretical frameworks

Philosophy and research

The term 'philosophy' has many definitions, as a brief perusal of any comprehensive dictionary will illustrate. Invariably such definitions refer to the pursuit of wisdom, allude to the system of values by which one lives and acknowledge that general principles underlie all branches of study, fields of activity or approaches to solving practi-cal problems. Definitions suggest that philosophy can be seen to be about the generation and development of knowledge, including an indication of what we as human beings *need* to know. Furthermore, they emphasize that to adhere to a particular philosophy can require a person to follow particular rules of conduct. Christian philosophy, for example, encourages forgiveness and love of fellow man. Philosophy also helps make explicit the general principles and beliefs which underpin particular fields of activity or study. For example, the philosophy of many medical practitioners, commonly termed the 'medical model' (or paradigm) of care, is said to be characterized by a concentration on the diagnosis and treatment of symptoms, rather than the implications of disease and its treatment for the patient.

In the same way, the various philosophies underpinning research can be seen to attend to these issues, for example by helping researchers:

- Identify issues 'worthy' of study – what do we *need* to know?;
- Decide what it is *possible* to 'know' about such issues;
- Identify a *process* to follow to ensure that they can be seen to have been systematic and rigorous in their work (Carper 1978) 'external verification' – see Chapter 1 (page 8), including making a decision about the appropriate relationship between the researcher and the researched.

These underpinning philosophies help us to make decisions about the 'ontological', 'epistemological' and 'methodological' questions discussed by Mike Nolan and Ullah Lundh in Chapter 1 (page 4).

Research paradigms reflect value systems which impinge on research design, data collection methods and the nature of researcher involvement in the field of study. By examining the philosophical traditions of positivism, naturalism and critical theory and how those traditions manifest in the research process, you as a reader should be more able to discern and appreciate valid and valuable research.

The authors first came to examine the issue of research philosophy when required to facilitate an educational discussion on the 'qualitative versus quantitative debate'. After much reading and discussion we came to a view that this debate continues (it is discussed in some form in almost all research texts) for two reasons:

- It is very difficult to state the difference between the two in a simple way.
- Researchers and people who write about research tend to either implicitly adhere to the scientific research process, or seek to undermine this in an attempt to justify their subscription to the use of 'non-scientific' research methods. Thus their ability to entertain an alternative or incompatible view is compromized and the 'debate' often ends on a 'my beliefs are better than yours' footing, rather than an acceptance that in certain circumstances some designs are more useful than others.

This latter viewpoint is the one accepted by the authors of this text, the suggestion being that critical readers of research should seek to satisfy themselves that the research design of a study reflects the nature of the research question(s). For example, if we are concerned with the issue of pain, can we ever truly appreciate another person's pain? (the naturalistic researcher's concern). On the other hand, can we produce useful and meaningful recommendations for the relief of pain without carrying out trials to see which forms of analgesia are most effective? (the aim of the 'scientist').

Some researchers and authors may not make their philosophical viewpoint explicit. This may either be because they see it as unnecessary, unquestionable, or because they are simply unaware of it. The following discussion is intended to indicate key points of similarity and difference between the two traditional research philosophies, along with a consideration of a third research paradigm – critical theory. The intention is to help the critical reader to consider the philosophical underpinnings of research studies they read. Detailed discussions of the limitations of each paradigm are not presented, not least because this has been eloquently done before. These references are offered as suggested readings in the text.

Paradigms in research

The Positivist paradigm

This can be seen as representing the traditional 'scientific' view of research and underpins what is commonly known as experimental research. As with any paradigm or world view, the positivist paradigm (also called quantitative and scientific, amongst other things) represents a particular way of viewing the world – in this case the world of research and knowledge, what can be known, and how such knowledge should be discovered and verified. The researcher operating in this paradigm believes that anything that is worth knowing can be known objectively (i.e. measured or quantified and typically represented numerically) and verified by independent observers. The positivist perceives that the object of research or study can only be truly understood by reducing it into parts and examining them in detail. Relationships between the parts considered important by the researcher can then be identified by repeated observation and measurement, leading finally to a point where it is considered reasonable to make predictions, based upon mathematical verification of the 'facts' (statistics). Positivism is based on the tenet that valid knowledge can only be discovered when the researcher occupies a position of detached observer (in other words unbiased and value-free). This is considered possible if certain 'universally' accepted research techniques or processes (essentially researcher as non-participant) are followed and reflect the stages of 'the' research process alluded to in most research texts. DePoy and Gitlin (1994) eloquently outline this approach as:

'... [having accepted] a theory or set of principles as holding true. Specific areas of inquiry (sic) are defined and hypotheses, or expected outcomes of an inquiry, are posed and tested ... data are then collected and mathematically analysed to support or refute hypotheses. Through incremental deductive reasoning ... "reality" can become predictable'

(DePoy and Gitlin 1994: 17)

A practical example of this approach to knowledge development would be an attempt by a 'researcher' to learn about the workings of a car engine by systematically dismantling and rebuilding it. Working in this paradigm he or she would seek to establish the *relationship(s)* between the component parts, e.g. cylinders, valves and pistons. The logical and structural principles that inform the relationship(s), such as combustion and emission, would also be discovered and through the collection and analysis of data, a theory would be tested which would allow us to *predict* phenomena from that which is already known. In this case perhaps a way for improving the performance of this and other car engines in the future could be established.

Table 4.1, adapted from Leininger (1985), summarizes key characteristics of the positivist research paradigm or world view. It also presents comparisons of this paradigm with the naturalistic and critical theory paradigms which will be discussed shortly.

Leininger (1985) could be said to be one of the authors who seek to undermine positivism to validate their use of naturalistic or 'non-scientific' research methods. Nevertheless, she presents an excellent exposition of the philosophical underpinnings of both quantitative and qualitative research paradigms, along with her views of the strengths and weaknesses of the two approaches with regard to research and knowledge development. You are recommended to read this text to supplement the necessarily basic discussion in this book. Table 4.1 summarizes these comparisons.

The Naturalistic paradigm

The naturalistic paradigm also has several different labels including qualitative, interpretive and phenomenological research, and non-positivism. It has also been termed 'holistic'. As with positivism, the naturalistic paradigm reflects a particular school of thought on the nature of knowledge, including: what we need to know; what can actually *be* known; and how best to find out or generate that knowledge. Meaningful parallels end at this point.

Unlike positivists, researchers in the naturalistic paradigm operate from the fundamental belief that humans need to know far more about themselves and the world in which they live, than can be 'measured' objectively. It is for this reason that it is considered by some to be 'un-scientific'. The kind of knowledge that is considered valid and useful therefore differs between the two paradigms. To

Table 4.1 *A Contrast of quantitative, qualitative and critical theory paradigms*

Domains	Quantitative methods	Qualitative method	Critical theory (action research)
Definitional focus	*Quantity:* Measurement focus of a thing, object or subject (how much)	*Quality:* Nature, essence, meaning and attributes (what it is and characteristics)	*Quality:* Meaning, perspectives and appreciation of issues
Orientation	Reductionist and deductive	Open discovery and inductive	Inductive, reflections on the phenomena of interest
Data sought	Measurable/quantifiable/numerical	Seek interpretive (subjective) and objective data. Emphasizes subject's personal interpretation of events	Context-specific, emphasizes subject's personal interpretation of events Pluralistic emphasis
Relation to people being studied	Detached observation, generally non-involvement, non-participation	Frequently direct involvement and participation with people. Close relationship between knower (researcher) and known (participant)	Role integral to the research setting, close involvement with participants, emphasizes collaboration and democracy
Research goal	Hypothesis testing/emphasizes cause and effect/prediction	Development of understandings and meanings of what one sees, hears, experiences and discovers. Access participants' experiences of *their* reality	Planning and taking action to change practice, introduce change to conditions to improve a situation. Problem resolution
Reliability indicators	Repeated measures, generalizability to other cases, reproducibility	Recurrent themes, patterns, lifestyles and behaviours	Patterns of behaviour
Domains of analysis	Predetermined, prejudgments and an *a priori* position taken, non-dynamic, fixed and planned research design	Can reformulate and expand focus of study as one proceeds, no predetermined *a priori* judgments	*A priori* position taken, dynamic and flexible, participants involved in the process of analysis, dialectic critique

(Adapted from Leininger 1985)

expand, positivism is based on the assumption that there is one truth and that this truth can be established objectively, i.e. *measured* in some way in a value-free manner. Naturalistic philosophy, however, reflects a belief that the meaning of human experience is affected by the interpretation placed on it by individuals, based on such things as previous experience and personal beliefs, and that therefore those who have experiences are the most knowledgeable about them. As a result, this philosophy allows for the fact that in certain circumstances there may be any number of 'realities' or truths regarding a particular research question, not least because the 'answers' are generated *post facto* from data derived from those who have had an experience – rather than being determined in advance by a researcher.

There is also an explicit acceptance within the naturalistic research paradigm that the role of researcher can never be one of neutrality or being value free, as is expected of the 'scientific' researcher. This is not least because the mere act of choosing to research something indicates that a value has been placed on it. Also, whilst the researcher may seek to be objective and detached they cannot control whether the research subject(s) view them as neutral and value free. It is because of the necessity of acquainting themselves with the research area and the subjects within it, that naturalistic researchers actually see merit in being 'subjective' and participating in the research context, to tune in to what people are saying and doing *within the natural context*.

Those coming from a naturalistic perspective also believe that, because positivist research methods require that the object of study be reduced into its constituent parts for closer examination, preferably in controlled and replicable conditions, then such approaches must be found wanting when attempting to explore and explain complex issues such as human motivation and behaviour. In other words, qualitative researchers believe that human experience and an individual's reactions to that experience are so complex that it is only possible to understand them by considering them holistically and in the 'real-life' setting, *not* by examining those aspects viewed as being of particular importance or relevance by researchers. This has been termed the 'gestalt' perspective, where the assembled parts are considered to accumulate to form a reality bigger or more complex than the sum of the individual parts would indicate.

The goal of a naturalistic approach to research is therefore to interpret, as fully as possible, the totality of whatever is being studied from the research subject's viewpoint (Leininger 1985, Meerabeau 1992). Research-based in the naturalistic paradigm is generally described as being diametrically opposed to reductionist positivism, as essentially it underlines the need to consider everything in its entirety, on the basis that in the social sciences everything influences everything else.

To explain this further, the researcher operating in a naturalistic paradigm might be interested in the concept of homeostasis from the point of view of the individual's *experiences* of blood pressure control and fluid balance. The researcher would be interested in the ways in which the quality of human life is affected by hypertension and fluid restrictions. Naturalistic inquiry seeks to capture the reality of these issues through the perceptions of those experiencing a raised blood pressure and restrictions in drinking fluid. The inter-relatedness of altered physiology (reality or the known), and the *experience* of altered physiology (the knower) underpins the research throughout. The researcher would not only be interested in predicting phenomena but also in *describing* and *exploring* the ways in which hypertension and a restricted fluid intake affect the lifestyle of research participants. The researcher attempts to tell it as it is, the 'is' being the participants' perspective. This is sometimes referred to as the 'emic' perspective. The different characteristics and emphases of the positivist (quantitative) and the naturalistic (qualitative) para-digms are contained in Table 4.1.

Like positivism, naturalistic inquiry has strengths and limitations. Qualitative research often produces large volumes of textual data which the researcher must analyze (Leininger 1985). For example, describing and exploring the participants' experiences of fluid restrictions and how this affects their quality of life would involve the researcher in encouraging participants to talk about themselves, per-haps using semistructured or unstructured interviews with several open-ended questions. The potential variety of responses makes handling the data difficult and introduces the possibility of bias in its interpretation. Conversely, this open and very flexible approach is a real strength of naturalistic inquiry, as it allows the researcher to explore the *complexities* and therefore the *completeness* (holism) of human experience. For example, the effects of a restricted fluid intake on the lifestyle and self-image of someone for whom drinking is a social occasion can only be effectively examined within a quali-tative research design. In these terms naturalistic inquiry lends itself to researching new, obscure and uncharted areas (Leininger 1985) leading to the generation of new theories.

Critical theory

Critical theory or critical social theory is an alternative research para-digm which reflects yet another particular world view. It is similar in many ways to the naturalistic paradigm in emphasizing the informant as knower; the creative nature of knowing; and a belief in the exis-tence of multiple realities. However, critical theory is distinct from positivism and naturalistic inquiry in two key respects: the purpose of the research *per se* and the role of the researcher in achieving that purpose.

Critical theorists aim to change the world by empowering the subject(s) of inquiry to enact social change. In this sense critical theory can be seen as a form of change management. Indeed Titchen (1993) makes the suggestion that critical theory reflects the philosophy of realism, as opposed to the 'objectivity' of 'science' and the idealism of naturalistic enquiry, neither of which appear to have an imperative for action to take place within their schema. Within this pragmatic paradigm the researcher's part in the research process is to act as a change agent (which may take many forms), the research itself being the vehicle through which change is enacted. Accordingly, the principal aim of this approach is to improve practical situations (Greenwood 1984, Hunt 1987, Wallace 1987, Carr 1989, Webb 1990, Elliot 1991). This is where the role of the researcher comes in. Underpinning the critical theory paradigm is a fundamental belief that when a power imbalance exists between one party and another, this has the effect of disempowering at least one of the parties.

Traditionally, in both quantitative and qualitative research, the role of researcher is one of outsider looking in. Webb (1990) refers to this as the 'smash and grab' approach to research, where researchers come into situations, grab data and then disappear again, without ever necessarily fully explaining what is going on to the 'subjects'. It is not uncommon for little or no personalized feedback to be given to them, though they may in due course read about themselves in a professional journal! In such circumstances it is not surprising that many subjects feel little or no ownership of the research and may fail to accept the findings or apply recommendations 'in practice'.

The researcher working within the critical theory paradigm – often termed an 'action researcher', seeks to avoid such problems by involving subjects throughout the research process (including identifying what needs to be researched) in such a way that the researched are also the researchers. There is also a tendency for the researcher to be an active participant in the clinical area in question so that they too are 'the researched'. In addressing the imbalance of power in these ways, it is considered that the clinicians involved in the research will develop and maintain a sense of ownership for the research findings and seek to apply them to their practice, whilst the researcher will be firmly grounded in 'reality' and so generate reasonable and realistic solutions to problems identified.

Action research does not therefore sit easily in either the qualitative or quantitative camp, not least because it stems from a different, more pragmatic philosophical standpoint than its more traditional siblings. However, building on Leininger's (1985) work, it is possible to highlight some of the characteristics of this philosophy and indicate some of the major differences between paradigms, as in Table 4.1.

As with other paradigms, critical theory has strengths and

limitations. A major strength of action research is its ability to empower subjects through participation (Hart 1995). However, as one might imagine, the success of this approach is heavily dependent on the accessibility of the research setting and the role of the researcher in what may be a politically sensitive area, as well as their communication and research skills. The researcher must take account, for example, of participants' traditional view of their role in the overall plan of care and in the decision-making process. Acting as an agent of change, the researcher must be sensitive to participants' agendas and consider the perceived impact of events, developing, where necessary, an ongoing strategy to enact change. Creativity is characteristic of this paradigm, with the action researcher acting as an imaginative diplomat introducing change. Unlike positivism the researcher forms an integral part of the research setting which, whilst crucial to the success of action research, poses questions of validity. The action researcher establishes validity by processes of self-validity, participant validity and peer validation (Titchen 1995). Whilst this process establishes the rigour of the research it is extremely time consuming and is therefore a disadvantage of researching within this paradigm. Nevertheless, checking out the multiple truths of reality across participants also serves to highlight differences in orientation and potential barriers to change. Titchen (1993) presents an excellent discussion of all three research paradigms. You are recommended to read this in addition to Leininger's work.

Implications for the reader of research

There should be no such thing as the 'quantitative versus qualitative' debate. This is not only because there is another paradigm to consider, but also because all three possess strengths and weaknesses which depend very much on how they are used – to paraphrase the point made in Chapter 1 (page 20), 'different research methods need not compete as what we need to understand is that they tell us different things. The real issue for a researcher should therefore be 'how can I best go about answering the research question?', rather than basing design selection on a view that some methods are more 'scientific' than others. It is for the reader to decide whether this is what the researcher actually did, which is possible because unlike other 'ways of knowing' empirical knowledge is 'publicly verifiable' (Carper 1978).

Another issue to consider is your own philosophical viewpoint. It may be that, wittingly or otherwise, you are of the view that some research methods, based on the various theoretical perspectives discussed, hold an ascendancy over others. If this discussion has made you reconsider that mind-set, then it has been useful.

Theory and its relationship to research

The meaning and characteristics of theory

Numerous definitions of theory can be found in research texts and in books on nursing theory. In fact, there seem to be as many definitions of theory as there are nurse theorists. It is hardly surprising that some definitions are as different as some are alike. For example, theory is defined as a set of concepts (Burns and Grove 1993, Polit and Hungler 1991), a set of constructs (Kerlinger 1973) and a set of related ideas (DePoy and Gitlin 1994). Despite such incongruities it is possible to discern commonalities among these definitions. Most authors refer to theory as an abstraction consisting of a set of inter-related components. Kerlinger (1973) suggests that theory is a set of constructs, definitions and propositions, while McKay (1969) defines nursing theory as logically inter-related sets of confirmed hypotheses. Taken together, such definitions suggest that theories *are representations of reality comprised of a combination of concepts and/or constructs that are in some way related*. The nature of these concepts and the relationships between them can be determined and verified through research.

The purpose of theory

Theory forms an inherent and arguably necessary component of professional practice and everyday life. Theories inform and guide how we think and how we behave though we may not be consciously aware of this. Theories may allow us to predict what might happen in a given set of circumstances (via deductive reasoning) or they may provide a means for us to interpret and explain reality (via inductive reasoning). Without theory we would be in the position of trying to comprehend what goes on every day as if everything was a new and novel experience, as well as being denied the opportunity to postulate what the effects of our actions will be. For the most part we are not aware of our use of theories, yet we use them constantly. For example, the theory of meteorology seeks to predict the likelihood of sunshine or rain, whilst the theory of probability allows us to decide whether or not it is wise to believe the weather forecast, based on the perception that it is often wrong!

The theory of meteorology is a theory of the physical sciences. Other theories belonging to this category include Einstein's theory of relativity and Newton's law of gravity. Theories generated or developed in the context of health services research are often associated with the human and social sciences. They include, for example, Becker's theory of health-seeking behaviour, or, the 'Health Belief Model' (Becker 1987), and Orem's theory of self-care – the 'Self Care Model' (Orem 1985). Whether a theory is of the physical or social sciences, the purpose is still to interpret and explain reality (Benoliel 1977) or to predict human experiences (DePoy and Gitlin 1994), and so provide information to guide everyday and professional life. This is none the less so in the world of research, and as such, theories perform similar functions within research projects.

Given our reliance on theory we need to have confidence in its approximation to reality. This requires that we are able to examine the premise(s) on which the theory is based. It is critical that we consider the underlying processes which may have led to the generation and/or testing of theory.

How research processes contribute to theory development

In general, researchers are concerned with finding meanings, explanations and solutions to problems, all of which involve generating and/or testing theory. Broadly speaking, theory development and testing involves two processes, known as induction and deduction. These processes can be described as ways of thinking or reasoning, by which one can come to a conclusion.

Induction and deduction are processes which reflect particular routes or patterns of enquiry. The researcher using deductive reasoning starts from the general (G) or whole, and moves in the direction of the specific (S), whilst the researcher using inductive reasoning travels from the specific (S) moving towards the general (G) or whole. Put differently, inductive reasoning starts at the micro level and evolves into the macro level, while deductive reasoning commences at the macro level developing into the micro level (Figure 4.1).

Figure 4.1
*Deductive and
inductive reasoning*

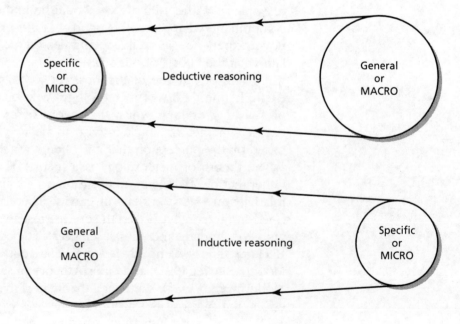

For example, someone using deductive reasoning might reason as follows:

All books on research are boring	(General)
This is a book on research	(Specific)
This book is boring	(Generalization)

Through this process the theorist/researcher has moved from the general to the specific, resulting in the generalization that this literary work is boring!

Conversely, a person following inductive lines of reasoning might reason as follows:

This is a very interesting book on research	(Specific)
There are several interesting books on research	(More general – less specific)
All books on research are interesting	(Generalization)

In this example the theorist/researcher has moved from the specific instance of what constitutes a 'good read' for them and generalized that information to apply to all other books on research.

In the context of health, deductive reasoning may involve the following:

All human beings experience loss	(General)
All adolescents are human beings	(More specific)
All adolescents experience loss	(Specific)

(adapted from Burns and Grove 1993)

In contrast someone using inductive reasoning could proceed as follows:

Jennifer had a mastectomy and felt a loss of self-esteem	(Specific)
Many women have a mastectomy	(General)
All women who have a mastectomy feel a loss of self-esteem	(Generalization)

In general, the inductive researcher begins with an individual case or cases, out of which general rules evolve, processes normally associated with the *generation of theory*. The reverse is true of the deductive researcher who begins with a belief or general principle which is then applied to a specific case, a process normally associated with *theory testing*. Research processes allow for such lines of thinking and argument to be tested and validated in some way, and then shared with the reader.

Inductive and deductive reasoning processes therefore have

varying parts to play in any research project. The degree to which they do so depends on the intention of the research itself, whether it is to explore, explain or allow predictions to be made. The following examples serve to explain this further.

Deductive reasoning and theory testing

Before engaging in the collection of data, the researcher using deductive reasoning starts with an accepted general truth or theory. For example, Wilson-Barnett (1978) studied the effect of informing patients about barium X-rays on their emotional reactions. Through a review of the literature Wilson-Barnett identified the existing level of knowledge or theory in relation to the effects of stress and anxiety. The theory was considered sufficiently substantive for the researcher to accept the general *truth* or theory that patients who are given detailed information procedures will report less anxiety than patients who are not informed. Using an experimental approach, an intervention group were provided with an explanation of forthcoming events and a control group were given no additional preparation. A self-report scale of emotions was used to compare the level of anxiety reported by the informed patients with those of patients (controls) who did not receive this information. In this way the researcher applied and tested the general theory of anxiety through the collection of empirical data to see whether the theory fitted. The theory was then modified accordingly.

Inductive reasoning and the generation of theory

In contrast, the inductive researcher starts from the specific individual experiences of research participants and seeks to generate theory in relation to topics about which little is known. For example, Mackenzie (1992) studied the experiences of district nurse students in the community. She adopted an ethnographic approach (see Chapter 5) (page 120) and collected data through interviews and observations of district nurses and district nurse students. The starting point for Mackenzie's research was the real-life experiences of the students. The researcher looked for explanations for the events, some of which fitted Knowles' (1984) theory of adult learning. The researcher developed generalizations and explanations of the observed phenomena, generated new theory and informed and built upon existing theory.

Summary

The thoughtful researcher therefore uses inductive or deductive reasoning depending on their approach to the problem or question under investigation, along with the existing body of knowledge. How these factors influence the researcher and how they think about the problem inform a number of things, including: the research design; the research methods; and, in due course, the body of theory (knowledge) produced. As a critical reader of research, you should observe for evidence of such processes throughout any research report.

What should *be the relationship between theory and research?*

Perhaps the most important point to be made about the relationship between theory and research is that research studies should build upon the existing body of knowledge. Ascertaining what is already known about a topic in order to identify a focus for new research constitutes vital early work in the process of any research project. Such insight ensures that the work is placed within a theoretical context and consequently that the research is informed by – and indeed adds to – the existing body of knowledge. This notion of research growing from and building upon what is already known is explained further by the following example of how you might go about researching something as commonplace as a garden.

Researching a garden

Suppose we asked you, a visitor from Mars, to research a garden. In the first instance you would presumably describe it: the size and shape of the ground covered; the presence of walls or fences; perhaps areas of light and shade, wet and dry. This could be followed by a description of the plants within the garden -- trees, shrubs, flowers, weeds and grass. Such descriptions would usefully include reference to sizes, shapes and colours of the plants. At this stage, however, you would be unable to name them owing to a lack of knowledge of earth vegetation. If you wished to pursue your interest further, you could consult experts or access books on earth flora, and from your initial descriptions begin to identify the various species of plant in the garden. This would be possible because the existing knowledge of earth flora is such that others have already examined and classified all the *known* plants growing on the planet. The plants have probably been photographed and presented in texts. As a result you would soon be in a position to differentiate between trees, shrubs, flowers and vegetables and probably name all the vegetation to be found in the garden under research. You would therefore be operating at the *exploratory* level of knowledge by attempting to describe, clarify and name objects (concepts) you have seen.

Ongoing observation of the garden would, however, indicate that you are not aware of all the information which could be useful to you, such as changes to the plants occurring through the seasons. You might also become aware from your observations that some plants tend to flourish in certain areas of the garden but not in others.

This could be seen as reflecting knowledge at the descriptive level, as having clarified the objects and issues involved (such as the various plants, light/shade, wet/dry conditions), you have begun to consider possible relationships between things like the rapid growth of certain plants in particular areas of the garden. However, you would not be sure of the *nature* of the relationships identified, that is, whether they are cause and effect relationships.

Suppose then, that you had noticed that there was a relationship between the strong growth of azaleas and the acidity of the soil, i.e. these plants appeared to flourish in such soils. It would be easy to jump to the conclusion that azaleas prefer acidic soils – but could it not also be the case that azaleas make the soils around them more acidic? For your knowledge to be at the level of *explanation or prediction* you would have to carry out some sort of trial to establish the true cause and effect of this apparent relationship. Having done so, you would be able to state with some certainty that azaleas do indeed prefer acidic soils and, as a result, be able to recommend certain sites for planting them – in other words, to make predictions.

Basing research on what is already known has other benefits:

■ Minimizing the chances of repeating the past mistakes of others and unnecessarily duplicating work
■ Informing decisions regarding research methodology such as what level of questioning is indicated? what level of data will be collected? and what methods of data analysis will be used?
■ Maximizing the chances that conclusions reached and any recommendations made will be realistic and based on the findings.

Identifying the relationship between what is known (theory) and empirical knowledge which is sought (research), is therefore an imperative for a researcher in the development of their research methodology. There is also a need to share the links between theory and research, as viewed by the researcher, with the research consumer. This can be seen to be an integral part of the discursively generated and publicly verifiable nature of empirical knowledge identified by Carper (1978) and discussed by Mike Nolan and Ulla Lundh in Chapter 1 (page 8).

Implications for the reader of research

We should recognize that theories are not merely abstract notions but useful mechanisms for explaining and predicting phenomena. They are representations of reality and as such they are as useful in 'real-life' as they are in research.

In research, theories are particularly useful because they offer a means of articulating to the reviewer of research (as well as clarifying for the researcher) just how the researcher believes a particular set of concepts or constructs are related, so allowing them to follow lines of argument and reasoning (inductive and/or deductive), as well as the evaluation of results (explanations and/or predictions) and any recommendations made.

The most important thing to consider when reading research is whether or not it builds upon the existing body of knowledge, which in most cases will be indicated via links which can be drawn between the literature review and the research design.

There are some researchers, however, who attempt to clearly and overtly identify the theoretical bases of their research. They do so by presenting a 'frame of reference'.

Frames of reference in research

See page 99

In this section we will examine frames of reference (conceptual and theoretical) and their role in research. We will then discuss points to consider when critically analyzing frameworks used in published research.

Earlier in this chapter, the importance of research studies being based upon what is already known – the existing body of knowledge – was discussed. Using the example of 'researching the garden', we suggested that ascertaining what is already known about a topic is work that should be undertaken very early on in the process of research.

Being able to clearly trace the researcher's thoughts, reasoning and decisions about all aspects of the research process throughout a research report conveys a sense of transparency to the work. Frames of reference can greatly enhance the ability of the researcher to share their thoughts and decision-making trails with the critical reader and hence facilitate transparency.

What is a frame of reference?

Burns and Grove (1993) suggest that frames of reference are abstract and logical structures of meaning which guide the development of a study and, in time, enable researchers to link their findings to existing knowledge. Moody (1990) takes this further by suggesting that by helping to guide the researcher in decisions about data collection and the interpretation of data, the researcher is more able to weave the facts into an orderly system, which in turn facilitates understanding in the reader. Frames of reference are therefore necessarily derived from the existing body of knowledge.

Frames of reference can also be seen as mechanisms by which researchers attempt to share abstract conceptualizations with others (Burns and Groves 1993). This may entail the clarification and description of concepts to be investigated in the study; suggestions about how the researcher perceives a group of concepts relate together; or both. All these attributes are important, as a theoretically

Figure 4.2
*Conceptual
framework to
suggest the factors
influencing quality of
care for older people
in continuing care
settings*

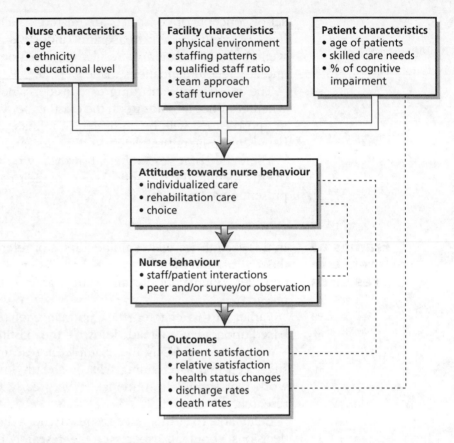

Nurse characteristics
• age
• ethnicity
• educational level

Facility characteristics
• physical environment
• staffing patterns
• qualified staff ratio
• team approach
• staff turnover

Patient characteristics
• age of patients
• skilled care needs
• % of cognitive
  impairment

Attitudes towards nurse behaviour
• individualized care
• rehabilitation care
• choice

Nurse behaviour
• staff/patient interactions
• peer and/or survey/or observation

Outcomes
• patient satisfaction
• relative satisfaction
• health status changes
• discharge rates
• death rates

(Adapted from Wright 1988)

sound, well-thought through and clearly presented frame of reference can act as a link between the researcher and the reader, affording a degree of insight into the thoughts, reasoning and conclusions of the researcher.

The conceptual framework presented in Figure 4.2 demonstrates the functions indicated above and clarifies the various concepts, such as relevant characteristics of nurses and patients. Possible relationships between the various concepts are also indicated. As a result the reader is in a position to make decisions about whether they concur with the concept definitions and lines of argument which the researcher is putting forward, in this case what factors lead to the presence of good quality, individualized nursing care of the aged in continuing care settings. Again this can be seen as an example of transparency within a research process, as the researcher's thinking is laid open to scutiny.

Frames of reference also guide researchers in the development of research methods and instruments, as exemplified in Box 4.1.

Box 4.1
Example of a conceptual framework informing the development of a research instrument

In a study of the educational needs of community nurses in relation to their teaching role with students of nursing, Thomson *et al* (1995) drew on a theory known as Bradshaw's taxonomy of social need to provide a framework for the study. The researchers designed a questionnaire to reflect the four different types of need identified within the taxonomy. Bradshaw's definitions of each type of need are shown below, together with examples of questions from the questionnaire, designed to reflect the different types.

Normative need: need identified by a governing body or profession, e.g. *What qualifications or courses are you required by your employers to have attended in order to be allocated responsibility for supervising students?*

Comparative need: need identified by comparing individuals/ organizations on the same attribute, e.g. *What arrangements for liaison exist between the educational centre from which the students come and the community placement areas?*

Felt need: need experienced/articulated by the individual, e.g. *What attributes/skills do you think community nurses and midwives need to help students to learn in community placements?* followed by
In your opinion which of your own attributes/skills require further development?

Expressed need: 'felt' need expressed as a request or demand, e.g. *In the past three years have you identified any courses that you wished to undertake to assist you with your role in helping students to learn?*

(Based upon Thomson et al 1995)

Where do frames of reference come from?

In some cases a researcher may utilize an existing frame of reference, for example, theories of nursing presented by Roper, Logan and Tierney (1996) or Dorothea Orem (1985). This can add credibility to a study as it should ensure a firm theoretical basis to the work and facilitate comparison of findings with existing knowledge. However, this is only the case if the frame of reference chosen is clearly related to the study in hand. It is not unusual, for example, to find reports of studies examining adult learners such as nurses, using theory derived from work on how children learn.

Alternatively, a frame of reference may be generated by the researcher and may be quite original, though concepts within it may have been identified and refined by other researchers. An example of this is the conceptual framework of *potential causal routes of*

Figure 4.3 *Potential causal routes of complicated grief reactions in nurses and midwives*

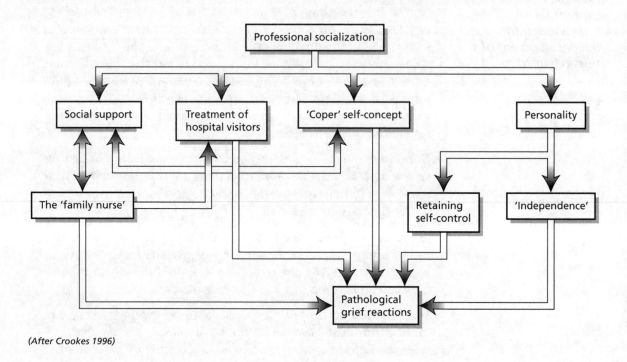

(After Crookes 1996)

complicated grief reactions in nurses and midwives (Figure 4.3) which Patrick Crookes developed for his study on personal bereavement and Registered General Nurses (Crookes 1996). In the exploratory aspect of this work, previously clarified concepts such as 'social support' and 'coping' were utilized, along with less well-defined concepts such as 'the family nurse' role, to facilitate sharing of ideas about ways in which being a nurse may potentially complicate personal bereavement.

An interesting point to be made here is that conceptual frameworks reflect the thought processes and world views of those who develop them. While both Roper *et al* and Orem's conceptual frameworks for nursing are based on the principle of promoting independence and 'self-care' in patients, the ways in which they articulate their ideas about how this can/should be applied to real life are very different. Theories (in this case in the form of conceptual frameworks) are only systematic versions of reality – not real life.

It is not uncommon to see a hybrid of the two approaches to the development of theory outlined above, with existing theory(ies) being incorporated within a new and perhaps wider application. An example of this is provided by McDonnell *et al* (1997) who utilized a number of theories related to health promotion and readiness to change (Prochaska and DiClemente 1983); and research utilization

(Funk *et al* 1991) in their study of research utilization by practice nurses in the area of cardiovascular disease and stroke prevention.

How are frames of reference usually presented?

The way in which a frame of reference is shared with the reader varies. It may be in the form of descriptive text (e.g. Roper *et al* 1996), a diagram (as in Figures 4.2 and 4.3), or a combination of the two. Using both has the benefit of providing a visual summary along with written details of concepts and relationships considered in the study and can facilitate a greater understanding in the reader. This is obviously an important function of a framework, as others apart from those directly involved in a study need to be able to comprehend the theoretical bases on which a study is founded. Frameworks provide terms of reference by which the methods of enquiry used, the study findings, their interpretation and any conclusions or recommendations made, can be considered by the research consumer – therefore, a well thought-out and presented framework adds to the transparency of the work for the reader.

In summary, 'frames of reference' or 'frameworks' occupy a pivotal position within the process of research, acting variously as:

- A guide to the researcher and the critical reader to demonstrate that the work is pitched at a level which reflects what is already known about a research topic
- A means of clarifying concepts by offering 'visual' representations of abstract propositions about the topic being researched, to make them more accessible to the research consumer
- A bridge between what is 'known' and what is elicited by the current study
- An aid to both the researcher and the critical reader when examining the decision trails throughout a study
- An indication of the processes followed by the researcher in developing rigorous research methods and instruments.

Frames of reference should be placed where perceived relationships between concepts, and decisions about method, are discussed. However, overt discussion of the theoretical underpinnings of research projects is often lacking in published research papers. Frames of reference may also be offered or discussed in other areas (e.g. when findings and their implications are considered), depending very much upon the nature/level of the study, i.e. whether it is at the exploratory, descriptive or predictive level (Brink and Wood 1988).

Relationships between levels of research and frames of reference

Frames of reference can be categorized as either conceptual or theoretical frameworks. A perusal of the research literature indicates that the terms are often used interchangeably, both by researchers and authors of research texts. Is it correct to do this? Are there any important differences between conceptual and theoretical frameworks?

Conceptual frameworks

Newman (1979) defines a conceptual framework as 'an organisation or matrix of concepts, that provides a focus for enquiry'. A conceptual framework is developed by linking concepts selected from theories, experience and/or other studies (Burns and Grove 1987) to form new and as yet untested propositions. They therefore reflect 'grand theories' (Moody 1990: 218) in that few of the concepts or relationships involved will have been formally tested. Their function is to act as a means by which hypotheses can be derived to be submitted to testing at a later date (to generate middle-range theory). For those interested in a more detailed discussion of levels of theory, Moody's (1990) text is recommended.

In essence, conceptual frameworks are more correctly used in exploratory research studies. These are studies which are undertaken with the intention of exploring and clarifying concepts and possible relationships between them. Exploratory studies are appropriate when the existing body of knowledge is such that there is little or no empirical literature on either the topic or the population under examination (Brink and Wood 1988). In turn, such studies may act as 'groundwork' for further investigation at the descriptive or predictive level, where the identification of relationships between concepts indicated by the exploratory work provides the focus.

An example is provided by Crookes' (1996) study. As a result of this exploratory work, based around the conceptual framework in Figure 4.3, a theoretical framework was developed which proposes ways in which societal expectations of nurses and midwives *could* lead to complicated grief reactions in some individuals (see Figure 4.4). In other words, *possible* relationships between being a nurse and a predisposition to complicated grief reactions are put forward. It is intended that this will form the basis of further research aimed at testing such propositions.

Theoretical frameworks

Nieswiandomy (1993: 834) suggests that theoretical frameworks provide a framework for studies 'based on propositional statements from a theory or theories' – in other words, studies in which the concepts or variables involved have been truly substantiated by previous research, and where the intention now is to test perceived relationships between them. At the descriptive level of research, this involves verification that relationships between variables do exist. To return to the garden analogy, this would relate to the identification of a relationship between leguminous plants (such as Brussels sprouts and green beans) and high

Figure 4.4 *Theoretical framework representing factors thought to predispose Registered General Nurses to complicated grief reactions.*

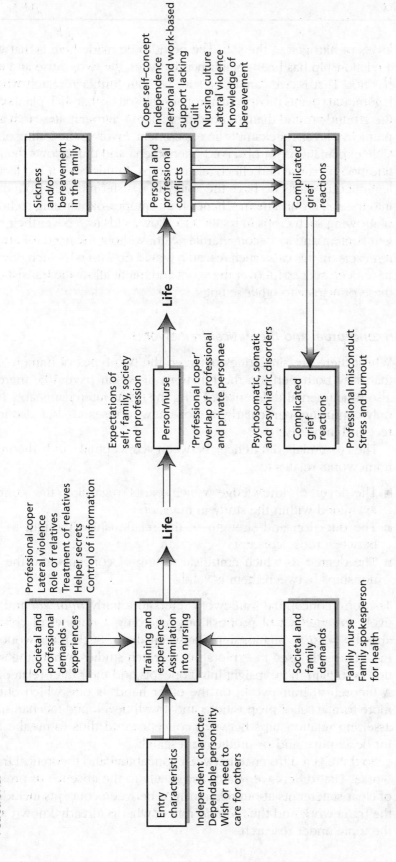

(Crookes 1996)

levels of nitrogen in the soil. The point to be made here is that while a relationship has been established between the two, cause and effect has not. That is, we cannot be sure without further research whether leguminous plants prosper in nitrogen-rich soil *or* that such plants cause the ground around them to become richer in nitrogen. Research at the predictive level, for example an experiment, involves the testing of possible explanations for observed phenomena and thus allows the identification of 'cause and effect' relationships. In this case, it is a fact that leguminous plants do have the ability to transfer nitrogen from the air into the soil around them – hence the centuries-old farming technique of growing such crops in rotation to allow fields to recover their nitrogen content and so become fertile again, without the need for artificial fertilizers. In this case, such research would *explain* why such practices have been successful over the years and might allow the translation of these principles to other settings.

The relationship between conceptual and theoretical frameworks

Whilst there are similarities between the two types of framework in that they both perform the functions listed on page 105, there are also fundamental differences. Using the terms interchangeably is not only confusing, particularly to those new to research, but also incorrect and imprecise.

The essential difference between conceptual and theoretical frameworks relates to:

- The level of knowledge which exists regarding the concepts examined within the study in question
- The direction and strength of the relationships thought to exist between those concepts
- The degree to which empirical testing of concepts and the relationships between them is valid.

The term conceptual framework refers to a fairly *informal* and relatively *untested* set of propositions regarding a number of concepts and the *possible* relationships between them. Such frameworks are most correctly used in exploratory research studies, where the intention is to gain more insight into concepts and their inter-relatedness. A theoretical framework, on the other hand, is one which offers a more formal set of propositions and a well-developed mechanism for asserting relationships between concepts, and thus forms the basis for descriptive and/or predictive research.

So there is a difference between conceptual and theoretical frameworks! That difference relates essentially to the absence or presence of clear statements about relationships between concepts included in the framework and thus *should* reflect what is already known about the topic under research.

Where are frameworks found? In a detailed research report, a framework (conceptual or theoretical) will typically be found in a chapter of its own, often sandwiched between the literature review and the methods section. This is apt, as an effective framework acts as a bridge between what has gone before (theory and/or existing knowledge) and what is to come (the prospective study). It may be in the form of a diagram, a description and/or discussion of relevant concepts, or both. However, frameworks may also be found later in research reports, for example in discussion or conclusion sections, when a product of the research has been the refinement of a conceptual framework or the development of a theoretical framework. This demonstrates that frameworks can have relevance in various parts of research studies, as a linkage between the conceptual and empirical aspects of a study and also as an endpoint, to demonstrate perceived relationships between concepts. Their effectiveness therefore must be measured against their stated intention within the work.

It is rare, however, for research consumers to have access to detailed reports. Usually they must rely on the brief overview papers published in professional journals. Historically, such papers have tended not to include overt discussion of – or even reference to – the conceptual underpinnings of the research (Polit and Hungler 1993) though this would appear to be changing within the 'quality' nursing journals. Absence may be as a result of the researcher not developing or using a frame of reference, or they may have failed to articulate it adequately for the reader (perhaps even for themselves). Whilst this does not nullify such work out of hand, its credibility and potential application to practice is inevitably brought into question. It may also mean that the report is much more difficult for the critical reader to 'appreciate', due to the effect on the transparency of the work.

Alternatively it may be the case that in brief reports, the theory underpinning the research is presented either under a specific heading such as 'frame of reference', or clearly discussed in the literature review section. Examples of these include Graydon (1994), who utilized Lazarus and Folkman's (1984) theory of stress and coping to help explore the quality of life of women following mastectomy, and defined this under the heading 'theoretical framework'. Before undertaking a study exploring the abilities of cancer nurses to provide psychological care to cancer patients in cancer care settings, Hanson (1994) explored three particular areas of the literature – stress theory and research; stress and its relationship with cancer; and psychological concepts pertaining to stress and persons with cancer. In this case the literature review structured around these areas presents pertinent theory to the reader and so clearly fulfils the remit of a framework discussed earlier, without overtly placing it under such a heading. It is the end and not the means that is therefore important when evaluating this aspect of a research report.

What to look for in the framework section of a study

Having discussed the function of frameworks and identified their importance in the research process, specific points to consider within research reports are offered here in brief.

- First and most obvious – is there a conceptual or theoretical framework? Is it made explicit?
- Has it been derived from – and with reference to – the existing body of knowledge?
- Is the framework appropriate for the study?
- Are the concepts clearly defined and understandable to the reader?
- Are relationships between the concepts clearly stated and understandable to the reader?
- Does the framework appear comprehensive?
- Is there an apparent linkage between 'theory', research methods and instrumentation, results, and conclusions/recommendations?

If the answer to these questions is 'yes', then the frame of reference has done its job. Concepts and perceived relationships between them have clearly been articulated for the reader, having been derived from the existing body of knowledge and leading to the use of research methods which clearly focus on the research question(s). The framework will also have been effective because it is important that a critical reader is able to discern clear links between the research findings and the existing body of knowledge. It is surprising how often researchers fail to discuss their research findings adequately in the light of data from other studies.

If a theoretical framework has been put forward and so propositional statements are to be 'tested', then further questions can be asked:

- Are appropriate definitions provided for the concepts that will be tested?
- Is the propositional statement(s) which guides the research question or hypothesis, clearly identifiable?
- Is the methodology chosen (questions/hypotheses; instruments; analyses; findings; conclusions) consistent with the theory?
- Does the theory provide an adequate framework within which to describe, discuss and interpret the findings?

Summary

In research, correctly used conceptual frameworks are typically associated with exploratory studies where existing theory is inapplicable or insufficient. They allow the researcher to clarify concepts and *possible* relationships between them for the reader and thus provide a bridge between what is 'known' and what is intended to be elicited by the study in hand, as discussed earlier. The point to remember is that if used correctly, the term 'conceptual framework' refers to a fairly *informal* and relatively *untested* set of propositions, regarding a number of concepts and the *possible* relationships between them.

The term 'theoretical framework', when correctly used, describes a rather more formal and well-developed mechanism for organising phenomena to be examined, than does a conceptual framework. The major difference is that a theoretical framework contains a set of propositions that assert relationships among the concepts. In descriptive research, such propositions can only indicate the existence of such relationships. On the other hand, predictive research seeks to substantiate cause and effect relationships and so verify or refute theory. Theoretical frameworks allow researchers to explain observations and make predictions about what is likely to happen in a given set of circumstances.

A theoretical framework may *sometimes* be a natural progression of a conceptual framework, as research based on a conceptual framework may lead to substantiation and clarification of concepts and indicate relationships between a number of them (Crookes 1996). A theory of how concepts inter-relate can then be developed, which is then articulated to the 'audience' as a theoretical framework.

The following exercise is designed to illustrate and reinforce points made in this text about frames of reference.

Box 4.2
Conceptual and theoretical frameworks: an exercise

Consider each of the following conceptual/theoretical frameworks together with the list of research questions below. Identify the framework(s) which could provide a useful basis for an exploration of each question.

Health belief model (Becker 1978) *Health-seeking behaviour is influenced by a person's perception of a threat posed by a health problem and the value associated with actions aimed at reducing the threat. The major components of the Health Belief Model include perceived susceptibility, perceived severity, perceived benefits and costs, motivation and enabling or modifying factors.*

Learned helplessness theory (Seligman 1976) *People tend to behave resignedly if their personal competency levels have been eroded and they feel that whatever behaviour they engage in, they cannot produce desired outcomes. Unless the environment is changed, apathy and depression are likely to result.*

Readiness to change model (Prochaska and Diclemente 1986) *When attempting to modify their own addictive behaviour, individuals move through a series of stages. The process begins with* **pre-contemplation** *(when the individual is not at all interested in changing their behaviour), through* **contemplation** *to* **preparing a change, making changes** *and finally* **maintaining**

change. Individuals who leap to action without adequate preparation or contemplation are a high risk for relapse.

Crisis theory (Aguilera and Messick 1980, Woolley 1990) *Crisis is defined as an upset or disequilibrium in a steady state occurring when usual problem-solving strategies are ineffective. When an individual experiences an emotionally hazardous situation and is unable to use previously learned coping behaviours effectively, or to reduce the stress using new problem-solving strategies, an emotional crisis may result. Immediately following a crisis event, prompt and skilful interventions are necessary to assist individuals towards maintaining or regaining emotional equilibrium.*

Orem's theory of self-care (Orem 1985) *Focuses upon each individual's ability to perform self-care. The need for nursing arises from self-care deficits, which occur when a person does not have the capacity for continuous self-care. Three categories of self-care requisites are proposed: universal requisites associated with physical life and the maintenance of human structure and functioning; developmental requisites associated with developmental processes at various stages of the life cycle; and health deviation requisites (arising as a result of an illness process or abnormality).*
The nurse's role may be wholly compensatory, partially compensatory or supportive–educative.

Maslow's theory of motivation (Maslow 1962, 1987) *Individuals strive for holistic growth through a hierarchy of values needs (which Maslow presented in pyramidal form). The base of the pyramid represents physiological and safety/security needs. These basic needs demand an individual's attention until satisfied. Only when these needs are met can attention be directed towards affiliation and self-esteem needs and eventually to self-actualization.*

Exercise 4.1   **Research questions**

■ To what extent do hospital inpatients wish to be involved in planning their own care?

■ What sort of interventions should practice nurses make in attempting to help people to stop smoking?

■ How can nurses ensure that their work with elderly patients on a rehabilitation ward is optimally therapeutic?

■ What factors affect compliance among young people with newly diagnosed diabetes?

■ What nursing actions are most effective in meeting the needs of suddenly bereaved family members in the A&E Department?

Exercise 4.2   Take time to think about your views on what knowledge is important and valid, and what isn't.

Exercise 4.3   Find a number of research articles on a topic which interests you. In the light of points discussed in this chapter identify the research paradigms which inform them. Having done that, decide whether the approaches chosen accurately reflect what the researcher(s) really wanted to know.

Using the same articles, identify whether the research undertaken builds upon existing theory (what is known) or not. If it does, how is this link articulated for the reader?

Chapter conclusion   In this chapter we have explained and compared three research philosophies: the positivist; the naturalistic; and critical theory paradigms. We did this to highlight the fact that each has its strengths and weaknesses in terms of informing research processes. As such, we have attempted to undermine the traditional 'quantitative versus qualitative' debate and move you, the critical reader of research, to a position of judging the approach taken by a researcher on the basis of how well it asks the relevant questions, rather than how well it adheres to a particular world view. Different research methods should not compete. What we need to understand is that they tell us different things.

We have also discussed 'theories', making the point that they are useful mechanisms for explaining and predicting phenomena – not merely abstractions with no real purpose. In research, theories are particularly useful because they offer a means of articulating just how the researcher believes a particular set of concepts or constructs are related together. We then presented arguments regarding the relationships which should exist between research and theory – particularly the point that research should stem from and build upon what is already known. The nature of theories and the processes of inductive and deductive reasoning were presented in support of these arguments, as was a classification of levels of knowledge ranging from exploration, through description, to explanation and prediction. The key point from this section is that research should build upon what is already known. It is up to the researcher to ensure that they do this and to demonstrate this clearly in the research report.

Finally we covered the issue of 'frames of reference' in research. This included explanations of what they are, their function within the research process, how they are generated and presented, and what to look for in the framework section of a study. The fact that clear explication of the theoretical underpinnings of any research project facilitates 'transparency' for the reader, was a point repeatedly returned to within the chapter.

We hope that after reading this chapter, you will feel more confident about evaluating the theoretical aspects of research reports you read in the future. This should be so because you will be better prepared to evaluate the appropriateness of the research design and research methods; the suitability of the research questions; and the compatibility between the research methods, findings and conclusions.

References

Aguilera D, Messick J (1980) *Crisis Intervention: Theory and Methodology*. London: Mosby.

Becker M (1978) The Health Belief Model and sick role behaviour. *Nursing Digest* **6**: 35–40.

Benoliel JQ (1977) the interaction between theory and research. *Nursing Outlook* **25**: 108–113. February.

Brink P and Wood M (1988) *Planning Nursing Research: From Question to Proposal*. Boston, MA: Jones Bartlett.

Burns N and Grove SK (1993) *The Practice of Nursing Research: Conduct, Critique and Utilisation*, 2nd edn. Philadelphia, PA: WB Saunders.

Carr W (1989) Action research: ten years on. *Curriculum Studies* **21**(1): 85–90.

Carper BA (1978) Fundamental patterns of knowing in nursing. *Advances in Nursing Science* **1**(3): 13–23.

Crookes PA (1996) *Personal bereavement in registered general nurses*. Unpublished PhD thesis, University of Hull, UK.

DePoy E and Gitlin LN (1994) *Introduction to Research: Multiple Strategies for Health and Human Services*. St Louis, MO: Mosby.

Elliott J (1991) *Action Research for Educational Change*. Milton Keynes: Open University Press.

Funk SG, Champagne MT, Wiese RT and Tonquist EM (1991) Barriers: the barriers to research utilisation scale. *Applied Nursing Research* **4**(1): 39–45.

Graydon J (1994) Women with breast cancer: their quality of life following a course of radiation therapy. *Journal of Advanced Nursing* **19**: 12–20.

Greenwood J (1984) Nursing research: a position paper. *Journal of Advanced Nursing* **9**: 77–82.

Hanson E (1994) An exploration of the taken for granted world of the cancer nurse in relation to stress and the person with cancer. *Journal of Advanced Nursing* **19**: 45–51.

Hart E (1995) Developing action research in nursing. *Nurse Researcher* **2**(3): 4–14.

Hunt M (1987) The process of translating research findings into nursing practice. *Journal of Advanced Nursing* **12**: 101–110.

Kerlinger FN (1973) *Foundations of Behavioural Research*, 2nd edn. New York: Holt, Rinehart & Winston.

Knowles (1984) *Androgogy in Action*. San Francisco, CA: Jossey Bass.

Lazarus RS and Folkmann S (1984) *Stress appraisal and coping*. New York: Springer.

Leininger MM (1985) *Qualitative Research Methods in Nursing*. Saunders.

McDonnell A, Davies S, Brown J and Shewan J (1997) *A detailed investigation of the implementation of research-based knowledge by practice nurses in the prevention of cardiovascular disease and stroke prevention*. Report to the NHS Executive, Northern and Yorkshire Region.

Mackenzie AE (1992) Learning from experience in the community: an ethnographic study of district nurse students. *Journal of Advanced Nursing* **17**: 682–691.

McKay R (1969) Theories, models and systems for nursing. *Nursing Research* **18**: 393–399.

Maslow AH (1987) *Motivation and Personality*. London: Harper and Row.

Meerabeau L (1992) Tacit nursing knowledge: an untapped resource or a methodological headache? *Journal of Advanced Nursing* **17**: 108–112.

Moody LE (1990) *Advancing Nursing Science Through Research*, Vol 1. Newbury Park, DC: Sage.

Newman (1979) Theory Development in Nursing, Philadelphia: Davis.

Nieswiandomy RM (1993) *Foundations of Nursing Research*, 2nd edn. Norwalk, Connecticut: Appleton and Lange.

Orem DE (1985) *Concepts of Practice*, 3rd edn. New York: McGraw-Hill.

Polit DF and Hungler BP (1991) *Nursing Research: Principles and Methods*. Philadelphia, PA: Lippincott.

Polit DF and Hungler BP (1993) *Essentials of Nursing Research – Methods, Appraisal and Utilisation*. Lippincott.

Prochaska JO and DiClemente CC (1986) *Towards a comprehensive model of change*. New York: Plenum.

Roper N, Logan WW and Tierney AJ (1996) *The Elements of Nursing: A Model For Nursing Based On a Model of Living*, 4th edn. Churchill Livingstone.

Selye H (1956) *The Stress of Life*. New York: McGraw-Hill.

Thomson A, Davies S, Shepherd B and Whittaker K (1995) An investigation into the changing educational needs of community nurses, midwives and health visitors in relation to the teaching, supervising and assessing of pre- and postregistration students. Report to the English National Board for Nursing, Midwifery and Health Visiting, University of Manchester.

Titchen A (1995) Issues of validity in action research. *Nurse Researcher*.

Titchen A, Binnie A (1993) Action research as a research strategy: finding our way through a philosophical and methodological maze. Changing Nursing Practice Through Action *Research Report No. 6, National Institute for Nursing*, Oxford.

Wallace M (1987) A historical review of action research: some implications for the education of teachers in their managerial role. *Journal of Education for Teaching* **13**(2): 97–110.

Webb C (1990) Partners in research. *Nursing Times* **86**(32): 40–44.

Wilson-Barnett J (1978) Patients' emotional responses to barium X-rays. *Journal of Advanced Nursing* **3**: 37–46.

Woolley N (1990) Crisis theory: a paradigm of effective intervention with families of critically ill people. *Journal of Advanced Nursing* **15**: 1402–1408.

Wright L (1988) A reconceptualization of the 'negative staff attitudes and poor care in nursing homes' assumptions. *Gerontologist* **28**(6): 813–820.

5 Recognizing research processes in research-based literature

Ann M. Thomson

Introduction

A research process, sometimes referred to as the research design, is the plan utilized to undertake a research study (Parahoo 1997). For midwives and nurses to fulfil the requirements of the *Code of Professional Conduct* (UKCC 1992) their care must be research-based wherever possible. However, individual practitioners need to be able to assess the value of a research report to their own individual practice. To do this the practitioner must understand the design of the research. This chapter has been written to meet that need.

Key issues

- Relationship between levels of knowledge and research design
- Qualitative designs (ethnography, grounded theory, ethology, ethnomethodology, phenomenology)
- Quantitative designs (experiment, survey)
- Designs which combine qualitative and quantitative approaches (historical research, action research, case study)

Factors influencing the choice of research design

Research design is 'usually a compromise reflecting ethical as well as scientific realities' (Gliksman 1993: 23) and the design used depends on the questions being asked. Evans (1979) suggests that:

> *'What kind of shoes you need depends on which route you're taking and what you're carrying'*

(Evans 1979: 82)

However, before deciding which route to take, and therefore whether sandals or boots are required, one also has to assess how well one can walk. For example, a newborn baby would not be given shoes as the baby cannot walk, whereas a hiker would want boots to give support around the ankles and provide protection in the terrain. Using this analogy the researcher in midwifery and nursing has to assess the level of knowledge on the topic under consideration as this will affect the level of design used to investigate the question (Brink and Wood 1989). Similarly, the critical reader of research needs to assess whether the research design was appropriate to the existing level of knowledge in relation to the topic being studied. This requires a consideration of the review of the literature providing the rationale for the study.

Brink and Wood (1989) and Depoy and Gitlin (1994) describe three levels of research design:

■ Exploration
■ Description
■ Prediction.

At the first level (exploration) there is very little knowledge about the topic under investigation, the researcher will be developing theory and will therefore require a research design which will allow exploration of the topic. At the second level (description) surveys are often used to describe features of sample groups and identify relationships between variables. Surveys can test findings from existing studies and can build on the work of level one studies. Level three studies (at the level of prediction) test theory, either in laboratory settings or in controlled trials. The relationships between the various types of research design are shown in Figure 5.1. The decisions on which type of design is appropriate can only be made after a critical review of the literature (LoBiondo-Wood 1994 and Chapters 3 and 10) and careful definition of the question to be answered. The research design includes a plan, structure and strategy for conducting the research (LoBiondo-Wood 1994).

The nature of the research questions will affect the decision on the approach used for the investigation. For example, Chamberlain (1996) and Davies (1996) found a paucity of

Figure 5.1
Relationships between research designs and level of questions

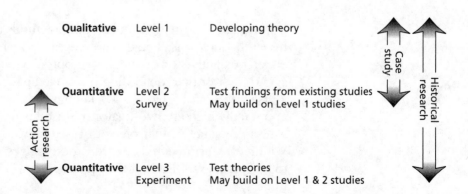

literature on the topic of how students learn to become mid-wives. These topics were therefore at the level of exploration and led both researchers to use a qualitative research design. Robinson *et al* (1983) wanted to analyze the role and responsi-bilities of the midwife in the late 1970s. There was existing lit-erature, and in order to investigate this level two topic they needed to obtain the views of a large number of people from a variety of professional backgrounds. For this reason they undertook a survey (Robinson *et al* 1983, Robinson 1985, 1989). Alexander (1996) was forced to reconsider the advice she was giving to pregnant women on the treatment of inverted and non-protractile nipples by the women she was advising. Alexander noted that the women did not relish the idea of wearing the shells which were routinely advised for these conditions. On reviewing the literature she was surprised to discover that despite the fact that shells had first been pro-moted 50 years ago (Waller 1946) and were recommended uni-versally to treat inverted and non-protractile nipples, there had been no controlled trials to evaluate the effectiveness of the treatment. This was a level three question at the level of pre-diction and she therefore conducted a randomized controlled trial (Alexander 1996).

Exercise 5.1   Select a research report from a copy of one of the academic nursing and midwifery journals (e.g. *Journal of Advanced Nursing*, *Midwifery*, *Journal of Clinical Nursing*). The paper should report an empirical research study, i.e. based on original data rather than a summary of other people's research. Read the literature review and identify the research question(s) which the study is addressing. Decide whether the questions are at level one, two or three.

Unfortunately, instead of developing methods appropriate to answer research questions, health care researchers have tended to adopt either qualitative or quantitative approaches and some researchers spend a lot of time defending one style against the other (Field and Morse 1985 and Chapter 4). Recognizing and understanding the approach which an investigator has used is not enough to be able to assess the value of that piece of research to our individual practice. Within each approach there are various stages and levels which have to be considered. Each of the approaches will now be considered in turn.

Summary

A number of factors influence the choice of research design within an empirical study. These include the nature of the research question(s) and the existing level of knowledge in relation to the topic under consideration. Design types can be broadly classified as qualitative or quantitative. Qualitative designs are more commonly used to answer level one questions whereas quantitative designs provide answers to level two and three questions. However, this is something of a generalization and qualitative approaches can also be used to test theory.

Qualitative approaches

Qualitative approaches to research have their origins in social anthropology and sociology, and develop theory inductively from the data (Field and Morse 1985 and Chapter 4). Qualitative approaches are typically used where very little is known about a topic and the researcher's intention is to construct theory (Morse and Field 1996) or where the researcher is trying to understand a phenomenon from the perspective of the actors in the situation (Brink and Wood 1989, Polit and Hungler 1991). In using this approach the researcher tries to assess the problem with an 'open mind' in order to consider all the possible options available. This is not easy as few researchers have blank minds and it is very difficult not to prejudge a situation or to forget existing assumptions. This style of research has been called 'soft', because it does not involve 'counting' or statistical analysis and has been suggested by some not to constitute science (Morse 1994a). However, failure to recognize the strengths of qualitative approaches means that we lose the contribution of exploration and theory generation in relation to a research problem which may later go on to be tested by a quantitative method. An excellent example of this is the study of selection of midwifery students where initially Phillips (1996) used a qualitative approach to identify key issues and then utilized a quantitative approach to seek findings which could be generalized to a wider population.

An important strength of qualitative research is that it is usually undertaken in a naturalistic setting (see Chapter 4, page 89) and so events reflect what would normally take place as far as possible. In qualitative research, the context is recognized to be part of the phenomenon (Morse and Field 1996) and careful description of the setting is essential to allow the critical reader to assess the relevance of the study for their own practice. This style of research is sometimes referred to as phenomenology. However, this terminology is somewhat misleading since phenomenology is a discrete qualitative approach in its own right (see below). In qualitative approaches, phenomena are investigated in depth, providing a considerable amount of 'rich' data from a relatively small number of respondents.

The aim of the researcher is to make explicit that knowledge or meaning which is known implicitly within a society (Morse and Field 1996). How scientists probe the implicit knowledge depends on the concerns about life experiences that they hold. Ethnography, ethnoscience and ethology have been generated in the anthropological tradition whilst the sociological tradition comprises ethnomethodology and analytical sociology (Field and Morse 1985). Phenomenology has its roots in philosophy (Polit and Hungler 1993). The following sections describe these approaches in more detail.

Ethnography

Like phenomenology, the term 'ethnography' is frequently used interchangeably with 'qualitative research style'. This is incorrect, as ethnography is just one of the approaches to undertaking a qualitative study. Ethnography is a generalized approach to developing concepts to understand behaviours from an 'emic' point of view (i.e. the view from within) (Field and Morse 1985, and Chapter 4). Its central tenet is that behaviour can only be understood in context and therefore during the analysis phase of a study the behaviour cannot be separated from its meaning and purpose (Boyle 1994). A further definition is provided by Leininger (1985) who suggests that ethnography is:

> '. . . the systematic process of observing, detailing, describing, documenting and analysing the lifeways or particular patterns of a culture (or subculture) in order to grasp the lifeways or patterns of the people in their familiar environment'
>
> (Leininger 1985: 35)

For example, in order to understand the nature of behaviour within the culture of the labour ward, and in particular at the 'shift handover' Hunt (1990):

■ Undertook observations and wrote field notes on them
■ Conducted interviews with key informants
■ Wrote notes on settings
■ Made reports of conversations
■ Collected 'off-duty' rotas, delivery records, request books, notices and letters.

In this way she was able to obtain information on the functioning and habits of those providing care and the situations in which the observed behaviours occurred. Mackenzie (1992) also used an ethnographic approach to explore the learning experiences of student district nurses undertaking community placements. Using a combination of observation and interviews she identified that one of the main influences on the nurses' behaviour was the need to 'fit in' with the social environment in which they were placed. Boyle (1994) describes the historical development of ethnography and states that there are different types of ethnography which are dependent upon the discipline of the investigator. Certainly, a review of the literature on ethnography suggests that different authors have interpreted the term in different ways (for example, Hammersley and Atkinson 1993, Rosenthal 1989, Leininger 1985).

Ethology

Ethology is the minute observation and description of non-verbal behaviour (Brink and Wood 1989). This approach originated in zoology in research on animal behaviour and has been modified in order to 'accurately record, describe and derive explanations for the behaviours' (Field and Morse 1985). Ethology was used, in particular, in research undertaken into the visual capabilities of preverbal babies (McGurk 1979). Whilst early work using this approach had to rely on repeated photographing of behaviour, current techniques use video recordings which are subsequently analyzed frame by frame. The advantage of using video recordings is that data collection is valid and because the video recordings can be replayed data analysis is usually reliable, especially as inter-rater reliability can be determined (Field and Morse 1985). However, there are ethical considerations in relation to who should have access to the video recordings and for how long after data collection they should be kept (see Chapter 9).

Ethnomethodology

Ethnomethodology has its roots in sociology and the purpose is to clarify understanding of everyday, taken-for-granted practices in society (Field and Morse 1985, Polit and Hungler 1993). Data collection methods include documentary analysis, audiovisual taped materials and participant observation. The focus of the research is to expose 'rule use' (Morse and Field 1996). To achieve this the ethnomethodologist often takes the opposite path from that of the ethnographer and instead of focusing on the common event examines unusual events which do not fit the normal pattern in order to identify the rules of everyday life. Mallett (1990) used an ethnomethodological approach to examine nurses' interactions with patients coming out of anaesthetic in the recovery room. This approach has also been used to explore interactions within medical consultations (Heath 1986).

Ethnomethodologists also differ from other qualitative researchers in that they sometimes undertake ethnomethodological experiments (Polit and Hungler 1993). During the experiments the researcher interferes or disrupts activities and violates the group's rules in order to observe the group members' responses to the dislocation.

Phenomenology

Phenomenology is the investigation of everyday experience from the perspective of those living the experience as it is considered that meaning can only be understood by those who experience it (DePoy and Gitlin 1994). The researcher's attention is directed towards participants' subjective perceptions of their own experiences with the aim of presenting these perceptions clearly and understanding their basic structure and meaning through a process of interpretation (Hallett 1995). Data are collected by interview which uses a biographical framework. The researcher strives to present the participants' views as accurately as possible and sometimes feeds back their interpretation to the participants to ensure that this is the case. The value of phenomenology to nursing lies in its ability to describe and clarify some of the most important issues for nursing practice from the perspective of service users.

Phenomenology has been used widely in research relevant to midwifery and nursing and health care. For example, two studies using this approach have been used to investigate women's experiences in childbirth. Berg *et al* (1996) tape recorded interviews with women to describe the experience of the encounter with the midwife during labour and delivery. Halldorsdottir and Karlsdottir (1996) also tape recorded interviews with women to explore the lived experience of childbearing. In a more general setting, Gaskill *et al* (1997) used phenomenological interviews to explore the phenomenon of isolation for patients cared for in reverse isolation for bone marrow transplant. Nay reports a phenomenological study to explore older people's experiences of relocation to a nursing home (Nay 1995).

Grounded theory

This is a form of analysis rather than a distinct qualitative approach (Field and Morse 1985). Its foundations are in the symbolic interactionist perspective (Chenitz and Swanson 1986) which asserts that meaning is socially constructed, negotiated and changes over time (Blumer 1962). Data collection continues until the researcher has enough data to have gained understanding of the particular situation and no further new information is being obtained (Morse 1994b). Not only does data collection continue until 'saturation' has been achieved (Walker *et al* 1995) but the researcher may return to the participants in order to ask them to verify the analysis (for example, Patterson 1995). Both inductive and deductive approaches to theory construction (see Chapter 4) are used as constructs and concepts are 'grounded' in the data and hypotheses are tested as they arise from the research (Field and Morse 1985). Data collection and analysis are undertaken concurrently and consideration of the analysis of the data will then affect the type of data collected in the future. At the same time data are constantly being re-analyzed to ensure that all possible explanations have been considered. For example, in her study of the similarities and differences in midwives' and women's views of motherhood, Laryea (1989) found that constant re-analysis of data showed that she had to be more specific when collecting data on how women were assisted to feed their babies. To examine the themes which had appeared in the initial analysis of their study of parents' experiences of care in a children's ward, Callery and Luker (1996) collected data and analyzed it concurrently. They continued with data collection until no new themes emerged.

Using existing data in qualitative research

Data do not have to be specifically generated for them to be used in a qualitative study. To assess the effect of atopic eczema upon a child and the rest of the family, Elliott and Luker (1997) used qualitative content analysis to analyze accounts written by mothers. The mothers had been asked to write these accounts for their first hospital appointment.

Summary

A wide range of qualitative approaches has been used in research of relevance to nursing and midwifery. The most commonly used approaches include ethnography, ethology, ethnomethodology, phenomenology and grounded theory, the latter being more accurately described as an approach to the analysis of qualitative data. To appreciate the value and relevance of a qualitative research study, it is important to recognize and understand the focus of the particular approach which has been used. For example, ethnography focuses on describing the behaviour of groups or cultures, whilst phenomenology stresses the significance of lived experience.

Exercise 5.2

Obtain a copy of one of the research reports referred to in this section. Read the report carefully, and try to answer the following questions:

- Is the investigation at the level of exploration, description or prediction?
- What was the research strategy or design used in the study?
- Was it appropriate for the existing level of knowledge?
- Was it appropriate to answer the research questions?
- How could nurses and/or other health care workers make use of the findings of the study?

Quantitative approaches

Burns and Grove (1995: 22) describe the quantitative approach to research as a 'formal, objective, systematic process for generating information about the world'. Its purpose is to describe and test

Experiments

The experimental approach originates from pure science, and is recognized in the field of health care as one method for assessing clinical interventions (Cochrane 1972). Experimental design incorporates an element of 'control': that is, the investigator is able to manipulate one or more variables in order to demonstrate a causal relationship (Cook and Campbell 1979; Greene 1979; Siegel and Castellan 1988). Controlling a situation in a laboratory using chemicals, or even animals which have been bred for the purpose, is relatively easy. However, controlling a situation involving people, who are all different, is more difficult. The difficulty arises from attempting to control for intervening variables without compromising internal and external validity (Cochrane 1979, Chalmers 1989). Internal validity refers to the exclusion of factors in the study design to give confidence that the findings reflect the relationship between the variables being investigated (Parahoo 1997). To assess the internal validity of an experiment the reader should assess whether flaws in the study design might have biased the study results. Are there uncontrolled factors which may have confounded the findings and caused changes in the variables in which the researcher is interested (Brennan and Croft 1994)? External validity is the extent to which the findings can be generalized beyond the immediate sample or setting and is largely dependent on how the sample was selected.

There are various levels of experimental design. These range from studies attempting to assess the impact of an event, 'before-and-after' studies, and the use of historical controls in assessing the efficacy of a new treatment, to randomized controlled trials (RCT) where the researcher attempts to manipulate the treatment under investigation and control for all extraneous variables.

The rigour of the research design will affect the confidence with which the findings of the study can be accepted, and therefore their value to practice. The most rigorous type of experiment (the RCT) involves the random allocation of participants to the treatment(s) (intervention group) or non-treatment (control group). They have no control over which arm of the trial they are in, and neither they nor their health care provider know which treatment they are receiving. This measure is undertaken to reduce the effect on outcome of a person knowing that they are taking part in a study, or the placebo effect. This type of study is known as the double-blind, placebo controlled trial and is used frequently to test drugs. In order to reduce potential bias even further the person undertaking the statistical analysis is unaware which of the groups is the treatment or control group. However, it is not always possible to use this very tight method of control in a study. For example when comparing restricted and liberal use of episiotomy, Sleep *et al* (1984) had to tell the midwives which group the women they were delivering were in, otherwise the midwives would not have known which treatment to use. In her pilot study of an RCT of pushing techniques in the second stage of labour, Thomson (1990, 1993) had to tell both the women and the midwives which group the women were in, because the midwives had to know which pushing technique to tell the women to use and obviously the women knew which technique they were using. There was no other way of undertaking these two studies.

When undertaking an experiment of the effects of a self-demand infant feeding regimen when compared with that of the traditional, fixed schedule, Illingworth and Stone (1952) recognized that an RCT would not be feasible. This is because women within one geographical area – the ward – would be using different treatments for both the feeding regimens and there was the potential for contamination of the two treatments as the women could have discussed this with each other. However, comparing treatments in two different geographical areas affects the rigour of a study because both the subjects and the care providers can affect the outcome of the treatments. The subjects may not be comparable, and the carers may be extra enthusiastic about the application of the treatment, particularly if they know they are using the experimental treatment. The latter is known as the 'Hawthorne effect' (Roethlisberger and Dickson 1939). As a safeguard, Illingworth and Stone (1952) designed a 'cross over' study whereby the ward areas were allocated to use the experimental or control treatment and then after three months 'crossed over' to use the opposite treatment for the next three months. In this way the researchers were trying to control for the possible effects of the characteristics of the subjects and health care providers.

Luker (1980) also used a cross over design in her RCT of focused health visiting to older women living alone. The concept of random allocation to treatment group is difficult to understand and may be more so for older people. Luker felt that it was possible that either women would decline to participate because they did not understand the concept or – worse – they would agree to take part without fully understanding the implications. She therefore undertook the randomization process before approaching the women to recruit them to the study. On visiting the women she was able to tell them that they would initially be in either the treatment or control group and would then 'cross over' into the other arm of the study. While this is a less rigorous way of undertaking the study (since knowing which group they were in may have affected the women's willingness to take part), Luker was able to give the women an explanation

See Chapter 9, *Critiquing ethical issues in published research*

of the study at a level that they could understand. It was therefore likely that they were able to give informed consent to participate (see Chapter 9).

A straight RCT with a control group and one experimental treatment may not always answer the question of which treatment is best, particularly if a combination of treatments may be appropriate. In this situation a factorial design may be more appropriate (Cochrane and Cox 1957) as it allows an opportunity for the comparison of two or more variables and provides scope for complexity in analysis (DePoy and Gitlin 1994). This type of design has been used to assess the efficacy of different cord treatments in newborn babies (Mugford *et al* 1986) and in assessing whether Woolwich Shells or Hoffman's stretching exercises are of any value in the treatment of inverted or non-protractile nipples (MAIN Trial Collaborative Group 1994).

The design of a randomized controlled trial is shown in Figure 5.2.

Figure 5.2 *Randomized controlled trial – flow chart*

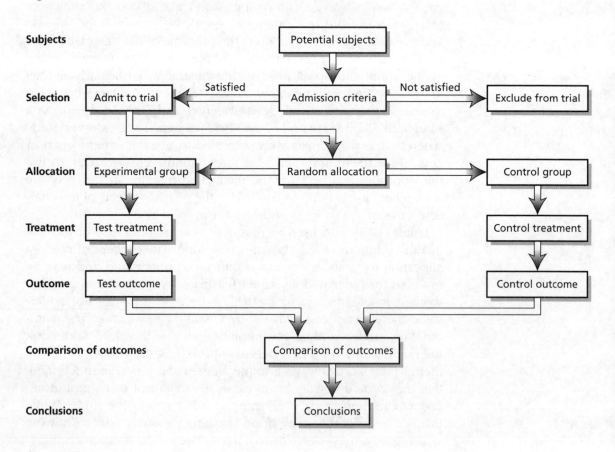

(Grant 1983)

Surveys   In opening their book *Survey Methods in Social Investigation* Moser and Kalton (1971) imply that it is impossible to define the term 'survey'. This is because the range of types of survey is so vast that any definition would be so general that the purpose would be defeated. Some authors go so far as to use the negative definition of 'non-experimental' when referring to a survey (Treece and Treece 1986, LoBiondo-Wood and Haber 1994). Types of surveys include the classic poverty studies (e.g. Booth 1889–1902, Rowntree 1941, 1986), Gallup Polls, market research, the General Household surveys, studies of transport use or local facilities and studies undertaken on matters to do with health and welfare.

The earliest known surveys were censuses involving all members of a population or group, and it is believed that the first known census affected the birthplace of Christ and the second was the Doomsday survey. Because both were undertaken by invading powers for tax purposes censuses were not very popular! Whilst there had been attempts as far back as 1690 to undertake a census in the UK the current series of censuses did not begin until 1801. A questionnaire is given to the head of every household in the UK and he or she is required to complete information on every occupant of the house. The type of information collected varies from census to census but basic demographic data are always included. A census is costly in money and the length of time it takes to plan and to execute. The analysis of the data also takes a long time. Studies using the survey approach nearly always use a proportion – a sample – of the population and seek to represent the characteristics of the population so that findings can be generalized.

There are broadly two types of surveys – descriptive and explanatory. Descriptive studies are designed to obtain detailed information on known variables so that current conditions and practices can be assessed and intelligent planning for health and social care provision can be made (LoBiondo-Wood and Haber 1994, Burns and Grove 1995). Researchers use this type of research design to obtain information on the characteristics of particular groups, subjects, institutions or the occurrences of particular phenomena. An excellent example of this type of research is the classic study of mothers' attitudes to childrearing practices (Newson and Newson 1974). Explanatory surveys seek to suggest cause and effect relationships. This can be achieved either by exploring associations across the whole range of variables, or preferably by focusing on associations suggested by the conceptual framework for the study. For example, McDonnell *et al* (1997) carried out a national survey of practice nurses to identify factors associated with their use of research-based knowledge in the prevention of cardiovascular disease and stroke. The analysis focused on individual, organizational and professional factors which the literature had suggested were associated with nurses' application of research-based knowledge. In this way, the researchers were able to add to existing knowledge by identifying factors which appear to have most influence.

There are three different types of survey design: one shot, time series and repeated contact. One shot is a term used by Campbell and Stanley (1963) to describe the survey which collects all the information needed during one approach to a sample of the population. Within one shot designs there are three further sub-divisions: cross-sectional, factorial and matched pairs. In a cross-sectional design the researchers examine groups of subjects simultaneously. This type of study relies on statistical control of variables (for example, Bond *et al* 1990). Factorial designs are modelled on experimental designs and use participants who have experienced a particular event or type of treatment (for example, Goldthorpe and Richman 1974). In matched pairs designs groups might be matched for particular characteristics. For example, a researcher trying to assess the effect of pregnancy on the mental health of women living in poverty might, having carefully defined poverty, select 50 women who are pregnant and living in poverty and compare their mental health with 50 pregnant women who are not living in poverty. This study could be extended to include non-pregnant women living in and out of poverty.

Time series (or trend) designs examine changes in the population, with regard to particular phenomena, over time. Information is collected from different samples of subjects at preset time intervals. The study of career patterns in midwives is an excellent example of this approach (Robinson and Owen 1994).

Repeated contact or longitudinal designs involve collecting data from the same sample on two or more occasions. These try to overcome the problem of retrospective data collection by collecting information at a relevant point in time. There are three styles of repeated contact designs; before and after studies, panel studies and longitudinal studies. Before and after studies are used to try and establish the effect of an event or stimulus and may involve the use of a control group as well. This type of study has some similarities with the experimental style and is referred to by some as quasi-experimental. Panel studies are particularly concerned with change over a period of time with respect to attitudes and behaviours. The same questions are asked of the same sample over a prescribed period of time. Longitudinal surveys seek to discover development or growth over a long period of time. Whilst the same sample is investigated, the information gathered will be different as data are collected at critical stages in development. An example of this type of study for nurses and midwives to consider is the Boyd Orr study which examined the relationship between the childhood energy intake of 1362 families between 1937 and 1939 and adult diseases in general and adult mortality from cancer specifically (Gunnell *et al* 1996; Frankell *et al* 1998).

Summary

Two broad types of quantitative design feature within research relevant to nursing and health care: experimental and survey. The main distinction is that experimental research aims to demonstrate a cause and effect relationship by manipulating an intervention and examining the effects on the variables of interest. Survey research aims to describe and quantify variables of interest and may seek to identify relationships between variables. However, it is not possible to impute a true cause and effect relationship on the basis of a survey.

Exercise 5.3

Obtain a copy of one of the research reports referred to in this section. Read the report carefully, and attempt to answer the following questions:

- Is the study at the level of exploration, description or prediction?
- What was the research strategy or design used in the study?
- Was it appropriate for the existing level of knowledge?
- Was it appropriate to answer the research questions?
- How could nurses and/or other health-care workers make use of the findings of the study?

Compare your answers with those to the reflective exercise on page 123. What does this tell you about the different ways in which qualitative and quantitative research approaches can contribute to knowledge for nursing and health care practice?

Bridging the gap

There are a number of approaches to research which, to answer the research question(s), use a combination of qualitative and quantitative research methods. Historical research, action research and case study are three approaches which often incorporate features of both types of design.

Historical research

Historical research attempts to explore events which have happened in the past in order to suggest solutions to current problems. For example, in her exploration of the work undertaken by domiciliary midwives in Nottingham in the period 1950 to 1972, Allison (1996) has shown that despite the fact that the midwives were providing care for a significant proportion of women who would now be classified as being at 'high obstetric risk' there was no excess of mortality or morbidity in the women for whom the midwives provided care. These findings add to the debate on the role of the midwife in the provision of maternity care in a developed country and fit in with the findings of some recent quantitative studies (Hundley *et al* 1994, Turnbull *et al* 1996).

Historical research is the 'systematic collection and critical evaluation of data relating to past occurrences' (Polit and Hungler 1991: 204). A knowledge of 'where we have come from' assists in knowing 'how we have got to where we are' and helps us to move forward so that we can capitalize on actions which have been positive in the past and helps prevent mistakes being replicated. However, to fully understand the history surrounding an event it is important to consider all the relevant factors. For example, Cowell and Wainwright (1981) wrote a narrative account of the history of the Royal College of Midwives (RCM). This did not put the development of the RCM into the context of other developments in health care provision at that time (Hannam and Maggs 1991) and therefore limits our understanding of the environs of the development of the RCM.

Polit and Hungler (1991) caution the research consumer not to confuse historical research with a literature review. Whilst reviewing the literature is an early step in this type of research it forms only part of the analysis and synthesis of data to explain the present or anticipate future events.

As most historical research is an examination of existing records, the records, or data, have to exist for the study to be undertaken. Historical research differs from other types of research in that the data have usually been created by someone other than the person undertaking the investigation (Glass 1989). The quality of the data is therefore subject to the vagaries of those who store records and the standard of storage methods.

Glass (1989) identifies seven steps in undertaking historical research. These are:

1. Think about and define a question
2. Identify the secondary sources
3. Locate and read the secondary sources
4. Frame and focus the research questions
5. Identify and locate the primary sources
6. Utilize the primary sources
7. Conduct analysis, synthesis, and exposition (Glass 1989: 184)

Secondary sources are items written about the subject and include books, journal articles and monographs. Primary sources are relevant documents and include birth, baptismal, marriage and death registers (Harley 1993, Hess 1993), sources containing accounts of witnesses (Ashford 1984, Harley 1993), letters (Hannam and Maggs 1991, Hannam 1996), diaries (Hannam and Maggs 1991, Hannam 1996), minutes of meetings (Hannam and Maggs 1991, Hess 1993, Hannam 1996), manuscripts (Evenden 1993), newspapers, legal documents (Harley 1993) and speeches (Hannam and Maggs 1991, Hannam 1996). Primary data sources particularly relevant to midwives (apart from birth registers) and nurses are records of statistics kept by county and borough councils and hospital management committees and the delivery registers which midwives are required to keep (Walmsley 1991, Allison 1996).

Data collection in historical research involves the gathering of the primary and secondary sources and can be very time consuming (Polit and Hungler 1991). Once the data have been collected they are subjected to external and internal criticism. External criticism relates to the authenticity of the sources and internal criticism is concerned with the relevance of the data to the research question.

A recent development in historical research has been the gathering of data from an older generation. In this an oral history is taken from those who have witnessed events. The advantage of this is that the researcher can record the events through the eyes of those who lived through a particular event or time. It also means that the researcher can ask questions which are particularly pertinent to the investigation. Oral history is increasingly popular in nursing and midwifery research (e.g. Leap and Hunter 1993, Allison 1996, Hemmings 1996).

Once the data have been gathered and assessed for authenticity and relevance the data are synthesized and organized, and conclusions and inter-relationships can be drawn. Generalizations can only be made with caution because events rarely replicate exactly (Polit and Hungler 1991).

Action research

Action research is a relatively new style of research in nursing and midwifery (Webb 1991) and there are comparatively few published examples. It is a different approach to investigation in that the study participants become equal participants in the study with the researcher (DePoy and Gitlin 1994). Based upon critical theory (see Chapter 4), the aim is to help practitioners, managers and researchers to make sense of problems in service delivery and to promote change and improvement (Hart and Bond 1994). Action research also attempts to avoid researchers 'using' practitioners as data gatherers without providing them with any further information or feedback from the study (Webb 1991). However, Greenwood (1994) cautions against seeing action research as just a method of change management and suggests it has a theory-generating function as well as a function in assisting with the management of change.

While action research is a relatively new approach in nursing and midwifery it has been used for some time in education (Hart and Bond 1995). Action research is different from other styles of research in that it aims to generate an equal partnership between the researcher and the researched. The aim is to improve service delivery through what Waterman (1995) describes as a spiral movement which is repeated on numerous occasions. This approach starts with the recognition of a problem and clarification of the questions to be addressed by undertaking baseline data collection. The issues which are amenable to change and the methods by which change can be achieved are agreed before the innovations are introduced and established. Monitoring and evaluation of the innovations feed cyclically into further assessment of the problem. During the data collection processes this approach uses the full gamut of research techniques and marries both qualitative and quantitative methods (Hart and Bond 1995). In this way the relationships and differences between theory and practice are subjected to systematic analysis (Waterman 1995). However, Waterman *et al* (1995) also suggest that action research is a method which can be adopted to ensure that research is incorporated into practice. Some of the action research projects which have been undertaken in nursing have assessed the feasibility of:

- The introduction of team nursing in an elderly care ward (Webb 1989)
- Improving the provision of care to those who have experienced a stroke (Gibbon and Little 1995)
- Improving ophthalmic nursing by understanding the meaning of visual impairment (Waterman 1994)
- A specialist nurse practitioner for children in accident and emergency departments (Jones 1996).

Case study   Case study is the intensive study of one person, group, institution or other social unit (Polit and Hungler 1991, 1993, DePoy and Gitlin 1994, LoBiondo-Wood and Haber 1994, Burns and Grove 1995). Burns and Grove (1995) report that the case study was used a lot in early nursing research, in particular to enhance understanding of nursing interventions. However, LoBiondo-Wood and Haber (1994) suggest that this method could be used more frequently in health services research to promote the understanding of a discipline.

The case study design involves an intensive exploration of a single unit of study or a very small number of subjects who are examined intensively (Burns and Grove 1993). Multiple case studies involve examination and comparison of a small number of such units. Case study research is particularly appropriate for evaluation purposes since it requires the analysis of contemporary phenomena within their 'real-life' context (Yin 1984) and thus provides a detailed and multiperspective account of experiences and processes resulting from an intervention.

Bergen (1992) used a multiple case study approach to evaluate the care of terminally ill people in the community of one health authority. Nine patients, and their visiting district nurses and Macmillan nurses, were interviewed to determine their different perspectives on needs identification and resolution. The health authority's *Standard on Care of the Dying* provided a framework for the interviews. Data were subjected to content analysis and categorized in relation to theory emerging from the literature. Needs were felt to be generally well met by the nurses, and patients indicated no serious areas of omission. However, a number of recurrent problems and issues were highlighted and recommendations put forward to redress them.

The advantage of a case study approach to answer Bergen's research questions was that it allowed a comparison of different perspectives in relation to the care of individual patients. Within-case analysis (in relation to the care of individual patients) and cross-case analysis (comparing the views of groups of participants across individual cases) were used to illuminate views and experiences of the care provided.

Maben *et al* (1997) used case study methods to evaluate the impact of Project 2000 (which led to the introduction of programmes for preregistration nursing preparation at Diploma level) on perceptions of the philosophy and practice of nursing. Data were collected in two case study centres, one in the north and one in the south of England. A combination of qualitative and quantitative data collection methods were used, including administration of self-completion questionnaires to students at intervals in their educational programme, focus group interviews with students, individual interviews with diplomates post qualification and review of course documentation. The longitudinal approach to data collection allowed the researchers to identify the students' changing perceptions of nursing as the course progressed.

Methodological triangulation (the combination of methods of data collection within a single study) is a common feature of case study research. Generalization of the findings of case study research in the statistical sense is rarely appropriate: however, the development of theoretical generalizations or propositions is important. It is important to distinguish between case study research and case study reports based on personal experience of a single incident or event. Such narrative accounts can be seen to contribute to experiential or personal knowledge (see Chapter 1) but lack the systematic approach and methodological rigour required to be classified as research.

Summary

Some types of research design may incorporate features of both qualitative and quantitative approaches. Examples include historical research, action research and case study. Triangulation, the process of combining methods of data collection within a single study, is becoming increasingly popular within research of relevance to nursing and midwifery practice.

Chapter conclusion

In this chapter the various research designs commonly used in research in nursing and midwifery have been considered. It is essential for the critical reader of research reports to identify the research design or strategy used at an early stage in their reading as this is of crucial importance to an appreciation of how the findings of the research might be used to inform practice.

The chapter includes references to methodological literature and reports of studies using the various approaches. By following up these references the reader will be able to gain a greater understanding of different research styles in order to appreciate the value of findings in a research report. The reader should not be dismayed at the suggestion that further reading might be needed since the study of research design is as exciting as the study of epidemiology, physiology, nursing theory or the practice of a discipline.

Exercise 5.4

Lathlean (1989) suggests that it is useful to think about research strategies according to where they fit on two polar dimensions. These are:

■ The extent to which the researcher attempts to manipulate reality within the research setting
■ The body of theory that is used to inform the research and interpret the findings – either social science theory or probability theory reflecting the qualitative/quantitative continuum.

These dimensions can be plotted as a matrix (Figure 5.3).

Where would you place each of the design types described in this chapter in relation to these polar dimensions?

Figure 5.3

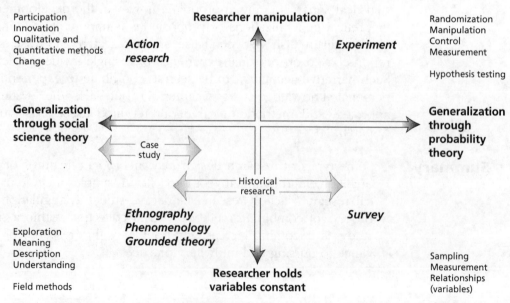

References

Alexander J (1996) The Southampton randomized controlled trial of breast shells and Hoffman's exercises for inverted and non-protractile nipples. In Robinson S, Thomson AM (eds) *Midwives, Research and Childbirth*, Vol 4. London: Chapman & Hall.

Allison J (1996) *Delivered at Home*. London: Chapman & Hall.

Ashford JI (ed) (1984) *Birth Stories, the Experience Remembered*. New York: The Crossing Press.

Berg M, Lundgern I, Hermansson E and Wahlberg V (1996) Women's experience of the encounter with the midwife during childbirth. *Midwifery* **12**(1): 11–15.

Bergen A (1992) Evaluating nursing care of the terminally ill in the community: a case study approach. *International Journal of Nursing Studies* **29**(1): 81–94.

Blumer H (1962) Society as symbolic interaction. In Rose AM (ed) *Human Behavior and Social Processes, an Interactionist Approach*. London: Routledge and Kegan Paul.

Booth C (ed) (1889–1902) *Labour and Life of the People of London*. London: Macmillan.

Bond S, Rhodes T, Phillips P and Tierney A (1990) HIV infection and community nursing staff in Scotland – 1. Experience, practice and education. *Nursing Times* **86**(44): 47–50.

Boyle JC (1994) Styles of ethnography. In Morse JM (ed) *Critical Research Issues in Qualitative Research Methods*. Thousand Oaks, CA: Sage Publications.

Brennan P and Croft P (1994) Interpreting the results of observational research: chance is not such a fine thing. *British Medical Journal* **309**: 727–730.

Brink P J and Wood M J (eds) (1989) *Advanced Design in Nursing Research*. London: Sage Publications.

Burns N and Grove SK (1995) *Understanding Nursing Research*. Philadelphia, PA: WB Saunders.

Callery P, Luker K (1996) The use of qualitative methods in the study of parents' experiences of care on a children's surgical ward. *Journal of Advanced Nursing* **23**: 338–340.

Campbell DT and Stanley JC (1963) *Experimental and Quasi-experimental Designs for Research*. Chicago: Rand McNally.

Chalmers I (1989) Evaluating the effects of care during pregnancy and childbirth. In Chalmers I, Enkin M and Keirse MJNC (eds) *Effective Care in Pregnancy and Childbirth*, Vol 1. Oxford: Oxford University Press.

Chamberlain M (1996) The clinical education of student midwives. In Robinson S and Thomson AM (eds) *Midwives, Research and Childbirth*, Vol 4. London: Chapman & Hall.

Chenitz WC and Swanson JM (1986) Qualitative research using grounded theory. In Chenitz WC and Swanson JM (eds) *From Practice to Grounded Theory*. Menlo Park, CA: Addison Wesley.

Cochrane A (1972) *Effectiveness and efficiency, random reflections on health services*. London: The Nuffield Provincial Hospitals Trust.

Cochrane A (1979) 1931–1971: a critical review with particular reference to the medical profession. In Teeling-Smith G and Wells N (eds) *Medicines for the Year 2000*. London: Office of Health Economics.

Cochrane WG and Cox GM (1957) *Experimental Designs*, 2nd edn. New York: John Wiley.

Cook TD and Campbell DT (1979) *Quasi-experimentation, Design & Analysis Issues for Field Settings*. Chicago: Rand McNally.

Cowell B and Wainwright D (1981) *Behind the Blue Door*. London: Baillière Tindall.

Davies R M (1996) Practitioners in their own right: an ethnographic study of the perceptions of student midwives. In Robinson S and Thomson AM (eds) *Midwives, Research and Childbirth*, Vol 4. London: Chapman & Hall.

Davies S, McDonnell A, Brown J and Shewan J (1997) *A detailed investigation of the implementation of research-based knowledge by practice nurses in relation to cardiovascular disease and stroke prevention*. Report to the NHS Executive, Northern and Yorkshire Region.

DePoy E, Gitlin NA (1994) *Introduction to Research: Multiple Strategies for Health and Human Services*. Mosley, St Louis.

Elliott B and Luker KA (1997) The experiences of mothers caring for a child with severe atopic eczema. *Journal of Clinical Nursing* **6**(3): 241–247.

Evans J (1979) Evaluation of research designs. In *Research Design*, Block 3B, Research Methods in Education and Social Sciences. Milton Keynes: Open University Press.

Evenden D (1993) Mothers and their midwives in seventeenth-century London. In Marland H (ed) *The Art of Midwifery: Early Modern Midwives in Europe*. London: Routledge.

Field PA and Morse JM (1985) *Nursing Research: the Application of Qualitative Approaches*. London: Croom Helm.

Frankel S, Gunnell DJ, Peters TJ *et al* (1998) Childhood energy intake and adult mortality from cancer: the Boyd Orr cohort study. *British Medical Journal* **316**: 499–504.

Gaskill D, Henderson A and Fraser M (1997) Exploring the everyday world of the patient in isolation. *Oncology Nursing Forum* **24**(4): 695–700.

Gibbon B and Little V (1995) Improving stroke care through action research. *Journal of Clinical Nursing* **4**: 93–100.

Glass LK (1989) Historical research. In Brink PJ and Wood MJ (eds) *Advanced Design in Nursing Research*. London: Sage Publications.

Gliksman M (1993) Methodological and political issues in occupational health research. In Colquhoun D and Kellehear A (eds) *Health Research in Practice*. London: Chapman & Hall.

Goldthorpe WO and Richman J (1974) Maternal attitudes to unintended home confinements: a case study of the effects of a hospital strike upon domiciliary confinements. *Practitioner* **212**: 845–853.

Grant A (1983) Evaluating midwifery practice: the role of the randomised controlled trial. In Thomson A and Robinson S (eds) *Proceedings of the 1982 Research and the Midwife Conference*. Manchester: School of Nursing Studies, University of Manchester.

Greene J (1979) Experimental design. In *Research Design*, Block 3A, Research Methods in Education and the Social Sciences. Milton Keynes: Open University Press.

Greenwood J (1994) Action research: a few details, a caution and something new. *Journal of Advanced Nursing* **20**: 13–18.

Gunnell DJ, Frankel S, Nauchahal K *et al* (1996) Life course and later disease: a follow-up study based on a survey of family diet and health in pre-war Britain (1937–9). *Public Health* **110**: 85–94.

Halldorsdottir S , and Karlsdottir SI (1996) Journeying through labour and delivery: perceptions of women who have given birth. *Midwifery* **12**(3): 48–61.

Hallett C (1995) Understanding the phenomenological approach to research. *Nurse Researcher* **3**(2): 55–65

Hammersley M and Atkinson P (1993) *Ethnography: Principles in Practice*. London: Routledge.

Hannam J (1996) Some aspects of the history of the Royal College of Midwives. In Robinson S and Thomson AM (eds) *Midwives, Research and Childbirth,* Vol 4. London: Chapman & Hall.

Hannam J and Maggs C (1991) A history of the Royal College of Midwives: research methods, networking and friendships. In Robinson S, Thomson AM and Tickner V (eds) *Proceedings of the 1990 Research and the Midwife Conference*. London: Nursing Research Unit, King's College, University of London.

Harley D (1993) Provincial midwives in England: Lancashire and Cheshire, 1660–1760. In Marland H (ed) *The Art of Midwifery, Early Modern Midwives in Europe*. London: Routledge.

Hart E and Bond M (1995) *Action Research in Health and Social Care: Guide to Practice*. Buckingham: Open University Press.

Heath C (1986) Speech and Body Movement in Medical Interaction. Cambridge: Cambridge University Press.

Hemmings L (1996) Vietnam memories: Australian army nurses, the Vietnam War and oral history. *Nursing Inquiry* **3**(3): 138–145.

Hess AG (1993) Midwifery practice among the Quakers in southern rural England in the late seventeenth century. In Marland H (ed) *The Art of Midwifery: Early Modern Midwives in Europe*. London: Routledge.

Hundley V, Cruikshank F, Lange G *et al* (1994) Midwife managed delivery unit: a randomised controlled comparison with consultant led care. *British Medical Journal* **309**: 1400–1404.

Hunt S (1990) The labour ward – a midwife's castle? Ethnography – more than just a snapshot. In Thomson AM, Robinson S and Tickner V (eds) *Proceedings of the 1989 Research and the Midwife Conference*. Manchester: School of Nursing Studies, University of Manchester.

Illingworth RS and Stone DGH (1952) Self demand feeding in a maternity unit. *Lancet* **i**: 682.

Jones S (1996) An action research investigation into the feasibilty of experienced registered sick children's nurses (RSCNs) becoming children's nurse practitioners. *Journal of Clinical Nursing* **5**: 13–21.

Lathlean J (1989) Action Research for Nursing. Unpublished paper. Oxford: Oxford University Department of Educational Studies.

Laryea M (1989) Midwives' and mothers' perceptions of motherhood. In Robinson S and Thomson AM (eds) *Midwives, Research and Childbirth*, Vol 1. London: Chapman & Hall.

Leap N and Hunter B (1993) *The Midwife's Tale*. London: Scarlet Press.

Leininger M (1985) Ethnography and ethnonursing: models and modes of qualitative data analysis. In Leininger M (Ed) *Qualitative Research Methods in Nursing*. Philadelphia, PA: WB Saunders.

LoBiondo-Wood G (1994) Introduction to design. In LoBiondo-Wood G and Haber J (eds) *Nursing Research, Methods, Critical Appraisal and Utilization*, 3rd edn. St Louis, MO: Mosby.

LoBiondo-Wood G and Haber J (1994) Non-experimental designs. In LoBiondo-Wood G and Haber J (eds) *Nursing Research, Methods, Critical Appraisal and Utilization*, 3rd edn. St Louis, MO: Mosby.

Luker KA (1980) *Health visiting and the elderly: an experimental study to evaluate the effects of focused health visitor intervention on elderly women living alone at home*. Unpublished PhD thesis. Edinburgh: University of Edinburgh.

Maben J and Macleod Clark J (1997) The impact of Project 2000. *Nursing Times* **93**(35): 55–58.

Mackenzie A (1992) Learning from experience in the community: an ethographic study of district nurse students. *Journal of Advanced Nursing* **17**: 682–691.

MAIN Trial Collaborative Group (1994) Preparing for breast feeding: treatment of inverted and non-protractile nipples. *Midwifery* **10**(4): 200–214.

Mallett J (1990) Communication between nurses and post-anaesthetic patients. *Intensive Care Nursing* **6**(1): 45–53.

McDonnell A, Davies S, Brown J, Shewan J, Crookes P (1997) *A detailed investigation of factors associated with the implementation of research-based knowledge by practice nurses in the prevention of cardiovascular disease and stroke*. Report to NHS Executive R&D Programme (Cardiovascular Disease and Stroke), University of Sheffield.

McGurk H (1979) Visual perception in young infants. In Oates J (ed) *Early Cognitive Development*. London: Croom Helm.

Morse J (1994a) Qualitative research: fact or fantasy? In Morse J (ed) *Critical Research Issues in Qualitative Research Methods*. Thousand Oaks, CA: Sage.

Morse J (1994b) 'Emerging from the data': the cognitive processes of analysis in qualitative inquiry. In Morse J (ed) *Critical Research Issues in Qualitative Research Methods*. Thousand Oaks, CA: Sage.

Morse JM and Field PA (1996) *Nursing Research: The Application of Qualitative Approaches*. London: Chapman & Hall.

Moser C and Kalton G (1979) *Survey Methods in Social Investigation*, 2nd edn. London: Heinemann Educational.

Mugford M, Somchiwong M and Waterhouse IL (1986) Treatment of umbilical cords: a randomised trial to assess the effect of treatment methods on the work of midwives. *Midwifery* **2**(4): 177–186.

Nay R (1995) Nursing home residents' perceptions of relocation. *Journal of Clinical Nursing* **4**(5): 319–325.

Newson J and Newson E (1970) *Four Years Old in an Urban Community*. Harmondsworth: Penguin.

Olsson P, Sandman P and Jansson L (1996) Antenatal 'booking' interviews at midwifery clinics in Sweden: a qualitative analysis of five video-recorded interviews. *Midwifery* **12**(2): 62–73.

Parahoo K (1997) *Nursing Research: Principles, Process and Issues*. London: Macmillan.

Patterson B (1995) The process of social support: adjusting to life in a nursing home. *Journal of Advanced Nursing* **21**: 682–689.

Phillips R (1996) Choice or chance? The selection of student midwives. In Robinson S and Thomson AM (eds) *Midwives, Research and Childbirth*, Vol 4. London: Chapman & Hall.

Polit DE and Hungler BP (1991) *Nursing Research, Principles and Methods*. Philadelphia, PA: Lippincott.

Polit DF and Hungler BP (1993) *Essentials of Nursing Research*. Philadelphia, PA: Lippincott.

Robinson S (1985) Responsibilities of midwives and medical staff: findings from a national survey. *Midwives Chronicle* **98**(1116): 64–71.

Robinson S (1989) Caring for childbearing women: the inter-relationship between midwifery and medical responsibilities. In Robinson S and Thomson AM (eds) *Midwives, Research and Childbirth*, Vol 1. London: Chapman & Hall.

Robinson S, Golden J and Bradley S (1983) *A study of the role and responsibility of the midwife*. London: NERU Report No 1, Nursing Research Unit, King's College, University of London.

Robinson S and Owen H (1994) Retention in midwifery: findings from a longitudinal study of midwives' careers. In Robinson S and Thomson AM (eds) *Midwives, Research and Childbirth*, Vol 3. London: Chapman & Hall.

Roethlisberger FJ and Dickson WJ (1939) *Management and the Worker*. Harvard, MA: Harvard University Press.

Rosenthal T (1989) Using ethnography to study nursing education. *Western Journal of Nursing Research* **11**: 115–127.

Rowntree SB (1971) *Poverty: A Study of Town Life*. Howard Fertig.

Rowntree SB (1941) *Poverty and Progress*. London: Longmans, Green & Co.

Siegel S and Castellan NJ (1988) *Nonparametric Statistics for the Behavioral Sciences*. New York: McGraw-Hill.

Sleep J, Grant A, Garcia J, Elbourne D, Spencer J and Chalmers I (1984) West Berkshire perineal management trial. *British Medical Journal* **289**(8): 587–590.

Thomson AM (1990) *A comparison of pushing techniques in the second stage of labour: a pilot study*. Unpublished MSc thesis. Manchester: University of Manchester.

Thomson AM (1993) Pushing techniques in the second stage of labour. *Journal of Advanced Nursing* **18**: 171–177.

Treece EW and Treece JW (1986) *Elements of research in nursing*, 4th edn. St Louis: CV Mosley.

Turnbull D, Holmes A, Shields N *et al* (1996) Randomised controlled trial of efficacy of midwife-managed care. *Lancet* **348**: 213–218.

United Kingdom Central Council for Nurses, Midwives and Health Visitors (1992) *Code of Professional Conduct*. London: UKCC.

Walker JM, Hall S and Thomas M (1995) The experience of labour: a perspective from those receiving care in a midwife-led unit. *Midwifery* **11**(3): 120–129.

Waller H (1946) The early failure of breast feeding: a clinical study of its causes and their prevention. *Archives of Diseases in Childhood* **21**: 1–12.

Walmsley W (1991) The changes in work load of Manchester domiciliary midwives 1960–1972. In Robinson S, Thomson AM and Tickner V (eds) *Proceedings of the 1990 Research and the Midwife Conference*. London: Nursing Research Unit, King's College, University of London.

Waterman H (1994) *Meaning of visual impairment: developing ophthalmic nursing practice*. Unpublished PhD thesis. Manchester: University of Manchester.

Waterman H (1995) Distinguishing between 'traditional' and action research. *Nurse Researcher Compendium* **2**: 197–205.

Waterman H, Webb C and Williams A (1995) Parallels and contradictions in the theory and practice of action research and nursing. *Journal of Advanced Nursing* **22**: 779–784.

Webb C (1989) Action research: philosophy, methods and personal experience. *Journal of Advanced Nursing* **14**: 403–410.

Webb C (1990) Partners in research. *Nursing Times* **86**(32): 40–44.

Webb C (1991) Action research. In Cormack DFS (ed) *The Research Process in Nursing*, 2nd edn. London: Blackwell Scientific Publications.

Yin R. (1984) *Case Study Research: Designs and Methods*. London: Sage.

6 Evaluating methods for collecting data in published research

Nigel Mathers, Yu Chu Huang

Introduction

In reading any piece of research, it is important to consider how the data have been collected. Without appropriate and rigorous methods any conclusions drawn from the data will not stand up to critical appraisal.

Data collection in its broadest sense is gathering information about something which the researcher has chosen to explore or investigate. However, depending on the research question which has been asked, different ways of gathering information are appropriate. There is an important distinction to be made between research design and data collection methods. Research design is an overall structure within which data are collected – a randomized controlled trial, for example, is *not* a data collection method but a structure within which different methods can be used to gather information. These methods could be, for example, self-reporting by subjects, researcher observations or laboratory measurements of blood chemistry. Research design and data collection methods are often subsumed under the overall heading of methodology.

Broadly speaking, quantitative data collection methods express the information collected about a particular topic using numbers. Qualitative data collection methods use words to express the information gathered to answer a particular research question.

There are four main characteristics of data collection methods which the critical reader needs to consider:

- Degree of structure
- Approach to measurement
- Effects of observation
- Objectivity.

Degree of structure

It is usually necessary to be able to make observations about subjects in such a way that some sort of comparison between subjects may be made. Even if a qualitative method is used some minimum structure is needed to make sense of the observations.

Approach to measurement

The way in which data have been collected will, to a large extent, affect the way it is analyzed at the end of the study. It may be clear from some published studies that attempts have been made to quantify data *after* it has been collected. Such studies can be used by the critical reader to reflect on the importance of a prespecified data collection method before starting to collect data for a study. It is also important that appropriate matching methods of data collection and analysis have been chosen (see Chapter 7). Even if qualitative data have been collected, some form of categorization is essential at the analysis stage of most studies.

Effects of observation

The method of data collection chosen for a study may affect the subjects' responses. Using a questionnaire with leading questions, for example, may confirm the researcher's prejudices but actually won't advance knowledge very much! Whether the researcher has been a 'fly on the wall' or conducted a structured interview is an important consideration for the critical reader.

Objectivity

It is important to be able to assess how 'objective' a researcher has tried to be in their data collection method(s). By this, we mean the extent to which the researcher has tried to distance him or herself from the data and minimize their influence on the observations. Of course, some qualitative data collection methods rely on an observer's 'subjectivity' and indeed make it a virtue! Webb (1989) offers a good explanation of this.

By the time you have finished reading this chapter and working through each of the reflective exercises, we hope that you will understand the principles of the different methods of quantitative and qualitative data collection, be able to match appropriate data collection methods to particular research questions and apply your knowledge of data collection methodology to the critical appraisal of published literature.

Key issues

- Quantitative data collection methods
- Validity and reliability in quantitative data collection
- Sample size and quantitative methods
- Sampling in qualitative research
- Validity and reliability in qualitative data collection
- Qualitative data collection methods
- Critical appraisal of methods of data collection

Quantitative data collection methods

The Questionnnaire

All too often when reading a published paper you will find that only a single sentence refers to the design or piloting of a questionnaire – giving the impression that all one needs to construct a questionnaire is common sense and enthusiasm. However, constructing a reliable and valid questionnaire to collect high quality data is a subtle and sophisticated art. Poorly designed questionnaires collect poor quality data. Lydeard (1991) describes a number of steps necessary for developing a questionnaire to use as a research tool which are as follows:

- Define the area of investigation
- Formulate the questions
- Choose the sample and maximize the response rate
- Pilot and test for validity and reliability
- Recognize sources of error.

However, there is little to be gained in trying to reinvent the wheel! There are many 'off the peg' questionnaires which can be used for particular purposes whose authors have established both the reliability and validity of specific instruments. When reading a published study which has used a well-established questionnaire to collect data it is probably more important to make a judgment as to whether it has been used appropriately rather than assess how it has been developed. This information is readily available from the texts referenced at the end of this chapter (for example, McDowell and Newell 1987).

For example, there are a number of versions of the General Health Questionnaire (GHQ) which is one of the most widely used mental health questionnaires and has high validity and reliability. A manual for its use is available. However, it is designed to collect data with reference to the past two weeks only, rather than for any longer period. It should be clear from a published study that this is, in fact, how it has been used. Stoate (1989), for example, used the GHQ to assess the psychological impact of well person screening in primary care. He reported that significantly fewer of those attending for screening had psychological distress than a control group. Three months after screening, however, significantly more of the screened groups had a high GHQ score. Stoate concluded that screening *per se* may result in psychological harm to the participants. However, the assumption is made by the author that a GHQ score three months after the intervention (i.e. screening) accurately reflects the psychological state of the subjects during the whole of the intervening period rather than the preceding two weeks. Questionnaires should only be used for the purposes for which they were designed!

Some studies are concerned primarily with the development and psychometric testing of a questionnaire rather than its implementation. Hagerty and Patusky (1995) for example, in a careful and well written paper describe the process of developing a questionnaire to measure a 'sense of belonging' (SOB).

- Initially, the area of investigation was defined by reviewing the relevant literature
- The questions were formulated from a number of sources, including the literature review, clinical experiences and statements by people who had participated in earlier focus group interviews
- The process of sampling and piloting took place initially amongst community college students and clients in hospital diagnozed with major depression. A third group of Roman Catholic nuns was subsequently sampled. Details of how response rates were maximized – such as paying respondents $5.00 for completed questionnaires, are also given
- A good description of how the validity and reliability testing of the questionnaire was established is included. For example, content validity (see page 145) was assessed by a panel of experts and retest reliability (page 144) was examined through the studies with the three subject groups
- Finally, some consideration is also given to reflection on the possible sources of error in the whole process of developing the instrument.

See *Reliability*, page 144.

When reviewing a study which has used a self-developed instrument for data collection, there should be sufficient detail given for an appraisal of how it was developed before application. Timms and Ford's paper on nurses' perceptions of the need for continuing education in gerontology (Timms and Ford 1995) is a further example of a research report which gives sufficient detail about the development of a questionnaire to allow an assessment by the critical reader. For example, the questionnaire was pilot tested by a convenience sample of 30 nurses for clarity, completeness, readability and for test/retest reliability (see page 144). The use of a convenience sample may be criticized on the grounds of representativeness but the important point is that the reader can find out from the paper how the instrument was piloted and make an assessment of this process.

For those readers old enough to remember the 1950s American TV series *Dragnet*, the policeman Joe Friday's catchphrase was always 'Give me the facts, Ma'am, just stick to the facts'. It may be just so with questionnaires. Respondents can be forced into categories by questionnaires although this may often be entirely appropriate. The alert reader will, at this point, recognize that whether or not a questionnaire is an appropriate data collection method depends on the research question which has been asked. For example, Younger *et al* (1995) considered the relationship of health locus of control and cardiac rehabilitation to mastery of illness-related stress. This was a highly focused study in which a sample of 111 subjects completed two questionnaires – the Master of Stress Instrument and the Multidimensional

Health Locus of Control Scale. In this study, because of the specific nature of the research question being asked and the fact that a well-defined hypothesis was being tested, it is entirely appropriate that specific questionnaires were used to collect the data.

However, Seidemann and Kleine (1995), in developing a theory of parenting for children with developmental delay, used semistructured interviews as their method of data collection. Using the data so collected they were able to present a particular model grounded in the data. In this case, because of the nature of the research problem and the existing level of knowledge about the topic in which they were interested, it would have been entirely inappropriate to have used highly structured questionnaires to collect the data.

The pilot study

Hanson *et al* (1995) conducted a pilot study of the psychological support role of night nursing staff on an acute care oncology unit. This impressive paper used observation field techniques (see page 153) to explore the nature of the nurse–patient relationship. The study revealed 11 main categories leading to indicators distinctive to night nursing which needed to be explored through further research. Such a pilot study is usually the preliminary to a main study and as such should follow the design of the main study closely. The sample used should also consist of subjects who resemble as closely as possible those who will be used in the main study. Another criterion a pilot study should meet is the extent to which the areas covered or the questions asked by interview or questionnaire measure what they are supposed to measure. In Hanson *et al's* excellent paper, considerable attention is paid to this criterion and it could be considered a 'benchmark' by which you can appraise any published pilot study.

Summary

- There is an important distinction between research design – the overall structure of the research – and methods for data collection (the methods used to gather information within the project)
- The main characteristics of data collection methods which the critical reader of research needs to consider are the degree of structure, the approach to measurement, the effect which data collection might have on those being studied and the objectivity of data collection
- In quantitative research, careful questionnaire design is essential for the collection of good quality data
- Critical readers should look for evidence that research methods were piloted and modified accordingly.

Validity and reliability in quantitative data collection

The concepts of reliability and validity have become increasingly well defined and more complex to assess over the past 30 years. For example, Blalock and Morse (1960) briefly introduce the concept of validity and discuss how to use it, whilst Steiner *et al* (1989) sets out in some detail clear operational definitions of the concepts. Unfortunately much of the published literature glosses over these important issues although they are crucial in appraising a piece of work.

Reliability

Test/retest reliability

Within quantitative research studies, reliability is the extent to which a test or an instrument such as a questionnaire gives consistent results. For example, a questionnaire can be given to the same person on two separate occasions and the consistency of their responses examined. A good correlation between the results would suggest that the test/retest reliability of the questionnaire was good. However, if the correlation coefficient (a measure of the degree of association between two sets of responses) is low (e.g. < 0.5), one should question any conclusions the author has drawn from data collected using such a questionnaire. It is important to remember that the time between administrations of the questionnaire is key. If it is too long, what is being measured may have changed. If it is too short, then the second set of results will be affected by the individual's memory of the previous administration of the questionnaire.

Interobserver (between) reliability

If two different people administer the same questionnaire or interview to the same person, to what extent is there agreement between the results obtained? This agreement or otherwise is usually reported in the literature as a **Cohen's Kappa** (or **K coefficient**). This expresses the level of agreement that is greater than that expected by chance alone. In reviewing the literature a K coefficient of 1 is perfect agreement. Such a statistical analysis can also be used to assess the intraobserver (within) reliability of an instrument such as a questionnaire. The **Pearson correlation coefficient** may also be used for this purpose. This statistical test is based on a regression analysis and measures the extent to which the relationship between two variables can be described by a straight (regression) line.

'Internal' or 'split-half' reliability

This is a measure of how much a subject gives similar answers to similar questions. For example, a subject may be asked in a questionnaire whether he or she agrees with the statement that the Government should regulate chemical additives in food. Towards the end of the questionnaire, the subject is asked if he or she agrees with the statement that the Government should not regulate chemical additives in food. Agreement by the subject with the first statement but disagreement with the second gives an indication of the internal reliability or consistency of the questionnaire. This would typically be expressed as **Cronbach's alpha**, with a result greater than 0.5 indicating an acceptable level of consistency between responses. The same process can be used to look at a series of questions or a subscale to assess the extent to which a questionnaire reliably reflects an attitude, for example.

Phillips and Wilbur (1995) evaluated adherence to breast cancer screening guidelines among African-American women of differing employment status. Data were collected using the Breast Cancer Screening Questionnaire (BCSQ). This was developed using published instruments and a review of the literature. The reliability of the published instruments was quoted as previously established, and although the individual components of test/retest or intra/inter observer reliability were not specified, they were expressed as a Cronbach's alpha coefficient. For example, the alpha coefficients for Champion's Health Belief Model Scale (1991) ranged from 0.72 to 0.88 in the study and this was judged acceptable. However, the Knowledge Scales of Dickson's Breast Cancer Screening Inventory (1990) produced alpha coefficients of 0.22, 0.30 and 0.29 and as a result these measures were dropped from further analysis. The paper is a good example of the care which is necessary in choosing and applying a questionnaire. When appraising a piece of literature, such efforts give added credibility to the conclusions drawn from a particular piece of research. It is unfortunate that much of the published literature only pays 'lip service' to the concept of reliability. However, Phillips and Wilbur's paper is again a standard against which others can be measured.

Validity

In its broadest sense, validity is the extent to which a study using a particular instrument measures what it sets out to measure. Reliability is an important precondition for validity – if an instrument is unreliable, it lacks adequate validity. However, a reliable instrument is not necessarily valid since it may be measuring something other than what it is supposed to measure.

Unlike reliability there are no simple statistical tests to assess validity. The relationship between validity and reliability is best shown by Figure 6.1.

Three main aspects of validity are recognized:

Face or content validity

This relates to whether 'on the face of it' the instrument or study measures what it is supposed to measure. For example, Yamashita (1995) used an instrument for measuring the occupational satisfaction of hospital nurses developed by Stamps *et al* (1978). The face or content validity of this instrument used in her

Figure 6.1
*The relationship
between reliability
and validity*

	RELIABILITY	
	HIGH	LOW

Key

✪ is the 'true' result
× represents attempts to measure the 'true' result

❶ High reliability/high validity
This is the 'ideal' situation where measurements
are clustered around the true result.

❷ High reliability/low validity
In this situation the measure produces a
consistent result but this is not close to the
true result.

❸ Low reliability/high validity
The measure hits the target (true result)

occasionally but not consistently. The validity of
such a measure is likely to be inadequate even
if it is the instrument available which hits
the target.

❹ Low reliability/low validity
This is the worst of all worlds where the measure
not only fails to give a consistent result
but also there may be evidence of systematic
bias in that the target or 'true' result is missed.

particular setting was established by submitting an appropriately
modified version of the questionnaire to a panel of experts for
content analysis. Since the assessment of face validity is essentially subjective, a panel of experts should be used for this
process rather than the individual researcher.

*Criterion or
convergent validity*

This assesses a measure against another measure of the same phenomenon. This is usually an already existing and well accepted measure. For example, the General Health Questionnaire (GHQ), a
mental health screening instrument, was developed by independent
comparison of the score on the questionnaire with the *mental state
examination* by an experienced psychiatrist (Manual of the GHQ
1991). This process established the **concurrent convergent** or **criterion validity** of the instrument. **Predictive convergent validity**
assesses the degree to which a measure can predict future events.
For example, risk scales are often used to predict the probability of
ischaemic heart disease and the agreement of the scales with subsequent cardiac events gives a measure of their predictive convergent
validity.

Construct (or hypothesis) validity

This is the most important and highest level of validity in quantitative research. It expresses the confidence we can have in a particular construct or hypothesis. It can be used to find out how closely an instrument correlates with another variable to support an hypothesis. For example, if an hypothesis that wheezy children had unhappy parents was correct, then a questionnaire to measure degrees of unhappiness in parents which was able to distinguish between the parents of wheezy and non-wheezy children would give the hypothesis construct validity. The more ways the construct validity of an hypothesis has been tested the more confidence we can have in the conclusions drawn by particular authors in relation to their hypothesis.

Note

Some authors use the term convergent validity to express a component of construct validity rather than criterion validity. Convergent validity is defined in this case as the agreement (high correlation) of the scores on an instrument with other instruments which are assumed theoretically to measure the same thing. It is contrasted with discriminant validity which expresses the disagreement (low correlation) of the scores on an instrument with other instruments which are believed to measure different constructs.

Summary

The validity and reliability of data collection methods are important aspects of the rigour of a quantitative research study. The validity of such a research method is the extent to which it measures what it sets out to measure. The reliability of a method refers to the consistency of measurement. Critical readers of research should look for evidence of the extent to which different aspects of the validity and reliability of data collection methods have been established with the population under study.

Sample size and quantitative methods

The question of sample size is inextricably linked to the subject of statistical power which is discussed in some detail in the next chapter on data analysis. Moody *et al* (1988) reported that many quantitative studies in nursing use sample sizes of lower than 100 subjects. Axton and Smith (1995) for example, in their comparison of brachial and calf blood pressures in infants, used a convenience sample of 79 infants. They reported no statistically significant differences in their measurements when assessed by a paired t-test (see page 166). Although less than 100 subjects, this sample size allowed for more than adequate power for this particular statistical test when both effect size and level of significance were taken into account (see Chapter 7).

However, in many studies, not only are inappropriate sampling methods used but also the size of the sample is also inadequate to demonstrate the effect of one variable on another (Sherman and Polit 1990). In other words the confidence one can have that there is a link between a cause (the independent variable) and an effect (the dependent variable) must be tempered by the knowledge that the sampling method used – as well as the size of the sample – are crucial in establishing this relationship and its generalizability.

Types of sampling

Convenience (opportunistic) sampling

Snowdon and Kane (1995) obtained a convenience sample from the paediatric ward of a large, acute care hospital in Canada to identify the needs of parents following the discharge of a child from hospital. This was a descriptive study of 16 families. The authors, quite rightly in our view, are cautious about the conclusions which can be drawn from such a small convenience sample and describe the study as preliminary. A convenience, or opportunistic sample is just that – resources may only allow for a sample drawn from a convenient population and any conclusions drawn need to be cautious. Even when considering a study with a much larger non-probability convenience sample such as that by Stein (1995) who had a sample of 149 children in an investigation of the pain intensity experienced, the critical reader needs to have considerable reservations about the generalizability of the results, since whatever makes the sample 'convenient' may be related to the variables of interest. This could introduce bias into a study.

Random sampling

If a study reports an association between an independent variable (cause) and a dependent variable (effect), we can be more confident that this association is real if the sample was drawn randomly. This is because a relationship between two variables will never be perfect in the real world – confounding variables (variables you haven't thought of or controlled for) will always be present to influence the results. A random sample allows for this in that anything you haven't thought of should be influencing both groups equally (for example, an intervention and a control group) and one can have more confidence that there actually is an association between the two variables (see Chapter 7).

For some research questions, such a sampling method may be inappropriate, particularly if the study is primarily qualitative. Vehuilainen-Julkunen (1994), for example, examined the function of home visits in maternal and child welfare as evaluated by service providers and users. Clearly, random sampling would have been inappropriate in this qualitative study without an intervention.

However, even though the sample was relatively large (263 public health nurses and 323 clients), the results are not generalizable although they do describe, to a certain extent, Finnish home visiting nursing practice. In general, if a study has used random sampling, the sample size necessary to establish an association between independent and dependent variables (cause and effect relationship) is smaller.

Berg *et al* (1994) compared two groups of nurses following an intervention designed to increase creativity and reduce tedium and burnout. The sample size was small (experimental group 19, control group 20) and no attempt was made at randomization. The results showed a lower degree of conflict amongst the experimental group; a difference which persisted and increased at 12-month follow up. The authors report that this difference could mean that their samples were different from one another, that is, conflict could be a confounding variable influencing the association they found between the intervention (independent variable) and the change in the experimental group of nurses (dependent variable). A larger, random sample would have enabled the reader to have more confidence in the claimed association between the intervention and the nurses' well being.

Representative and stratified sampling

Sometimes, to make the results of a study generalizable to a particular population with a specified condition, researchers may choose a representative sample. In a random sample, all members of a population have an equal chance of being included in the study. In a representative sample, participants are selected to ensure that all possible subcategories of the population have an equal chance of being included since randomization may result (by chance!) in the over- (or under-)representation of one particular group within the population. If a representative (stratified) sample is big enough, then randomization can occur within those samples or subcategories of the population. Such a sampling strategy gives the critical reader more confidence in a claimed association between two variables.

How big should a sample be?

This is a bit like asking 'how long is a piece of string?' Most nursing studies continue to rely on relatively small convenience or opportunistic samples. Brown *et al* (1984) looked at four journals between 1952 and 1980 and reported a median sample size of 84 in 1952 and 80 in 1980. Clearly, it is the nature of nursing research to ask research questions whose answers are both complex and difficult to measure. However, for a quantitative study to have enough statistical power to give the critical reader confidence that a relationship exists between two variables requires larger sample sizes than are currently used in much nursing research. Sherman and Polit (1990) looked at 62 articles in nursing research published in 1989 and concluded that 'a substantial number of nurse studies ... have insufficient power to detect real effects primarily because the samples used are too small'. They calculated that for two-thirds of the articles reviewed which had sample sizes less than 100 to demonstrate sufficient power, an average sample size of 218 subjects per group was required rather than the actual average of 83. Does this mean 'the larger the better?' For some quantitative research questions this is the case up to a point since a study can be 'over-powered'! However, the confidence one can have in a claimed association between two variables in a quantitative study also depends on the data collection methodology, the design of the study and the use of valid and reliable measuring instruments. For a further discussion on power, statistical analysis and sample size, the critical reader is referred to Chapter 7.

Sampling in qualitative research

When collecting qualitative data it is often impractical and inappropriate to use a probability (random or representative) sample because such data collection methods require a list of the total population, take longer, and hence are more expensive on resources. It is also true that when the objective of research is to understand and give meaning to a social process it is inappropriate to use a random sample since the intention is not to apply statistical tests and generalize the findings to the wider population. For this reason qualitative data are often collected using a **purposive**, **non-probability** sample.

This is different from a convenience sample since its purpose is to identify specific groups of people who exhibit the characteristics of the social process or phenomenon which is being investigated. The researcher can then include all sorts of people who have particular knowledge of the topic under investigation.

If a nursing researcher wishes to develop a social theory, a 'theoretical' sampling technique may be used. The idea here is that the researcher selects the subjects and collects and analyzes data to produce an initial theory, which is then used to guide further sampling and data collection from which further theory is developed. Lucas *et al* (1993) in a paper entitled *Replication and Validation of an Anticipated Turnover Model for Urban Registered Nurses* were able to validate with younger, more educated staff, the major findings from an original study. Substantial support for the stability and generalizability of the theoretical model was found.

Sometimes, however, in a desire to increase their 'street credibility' researchers will allow a particular methodology to 'drive' a particular research question. For example, a research group might be interested in diabetes and choose a randomized, controlled design to try and answer a particular question. Although such quantitative designs have yielded much useful data about, for example, outcomes of diabetic interventions, the difficulty arises when a qualitative research question is being asked but a quantitative data collection method is used to answer it. It would be very difficult, for instance, to evaluate the impact of professional health care education on the quality of life experienced by diabetic patients using a randomized, controlled design. However, a mixed qualitative and quantitative data collection method could be used as part of a validation process such as **triangulation** (e.g. Denzin and Lincoln 1994). Here, more than one method is used to collect the data and the results are analyzed for agreement (see *confirmability* later in this chapter). The sample of diabetics could be interviewed for their experience of, and their attitudes towards, 'empowerment' by health care professionals. At the same time, quantitative data would be collected such as the number of admissions to hospital and details of adjustments to insulin regimens. These data could be used in conjunction with the data from the interviews to illustrate the quality of life experienced by diabetic patients.

See *Confirmability*, page 152

Summary

Different approaches to sampling are appropriate for different research designs. In general, quantitative research relies on large samples which are randomly selected in order to produce findings which can be generalized with a known degree of accuracy to the population from which the sample is drawn. However, many quantitative studies in nursing use sample sizes which are too small to either enable accurate generalization or to detect the effects of a specific intervention. It is crucial therefore that the critical reader should consider how the sample size and approach to selection are justified. Qualitative research designs are more likely to use convenience or purposive samples, since the main intention is to identify participants who can provide a range of experiences of the phenomena under investigation. Again, it is important for the critical reader to consider how the sample was selected in order to identify any potential sources of bias.

Validity and reliability in qualitative data collection

Britten and Fisher (1993) summarize the relationship between quantitative and qualitative data collection methodology rather well when they write:

'There is some truth in the quip that quantitative methods are reliable but not valid and qualitative methods are valid but not reliable'

(Britten and Fisher 1993: 270)

In their standard text on naturalistic enquiry, Lincoln and Guba (1985) draw parallels between the concepts of validity and reliability as used in quantitative research and their qualitative equivalents (Table 6.1) It is probably easier to publish 'bad' qualitative research than 'bad' quantitative research. The basic strategy needed to ensure rigour in qualitative research is the application of a systematic and self-conscious methodology (Mays and Pope 1995a). In the evaluation of published literature, it is important for the critical reader to review the data collection methodology of a particular study with particular reference to the parallel concepts of validity and reliability used in qualitative research (Table 6.1).

Table 6.1
A comparison of concepts of rigour between quantitative and qualitative research

Quantitative concept	Equivalent in qualitative research
Validity	Credibility
Reliability	Dependability
Generalizability	Transferability
Objectivity	Confirmability

Credibility (validity)

This concerns the accuracy of description. By stating the precise parameters of the study (who, where, when) accurately, the data can only be claimed to be valid for that particular setting. Credibility is enhanced by detailed and accurate description of the setting and research participants.

Dependability (reliability)

Quantitative researchers often assume an objective reality or unchanging world which can be consistently described by more than one observer. In qualitative research, however, the continually changing social world is acknowledged and the researcher should try to account for changes rather than to demonstrate the reliability of their findings.

Transferability (generalizability)

Qualitative researchers should be cautious about making claims for other settings. If other researchers investigate the same phenomenon to generalize a study's findings, they must themselves demonstrate its applicability to the new setting.

Confirmability (objectivity)

Despite the best attempts of researchers not to influence the data they collect by the way they collect it, some 'Hawthorne effect' is a fact of life. Whenever possible, researchers should try to fault their own methodologies and attempt to find alternative methods of collecting the data. **Triangulation** describes how qualitative data collection methodologies may be applied to increase but not capture 'objectivity'. Between-method triangulation uses differing but complementary methods to get 'a better fix on the subject matter' (Nolan and Behi 1995). Carson *et al* (1995) looked at stress in mental health nurses by comparing data obtained from ward and community staff using semistructured interviews and focus groups. Within-method triangulation uses two or more variants of the same method: for example, two different rating scales may be used to measure the same concept (such as stress or anxiety) or a combination of open and closed questions are used in the same questionnaire.

Knafl and Breitmayer (1991) contrast confirmability with completeness – the latter concept does not assume that varying approaches will confirm each other, rather that they will identify different aspects of the same subject. The concepts of confirmability and completeness are the subject of much debate at the time of writing, and no clear consensus has yet emerged. For an alternative view, see Denzin and Lincoln (1994).

Summary

As with quantitative research, it is just as important to assess the rigour of qualitative research designs to make a decision about the most appropriate way to make use of the findings. However, a number of authors have questioned the relevance of the notions of 'validity' and 'reliability' in the context of qualitative research which is based upon different assumptions about the world. Alternative criteria for assessing the rigour of qualitative research methods have been identified: these include credibility, confirmability, dependability and transferability. Researchers often combine a number of techniques to enhance the rigour of their methods, including triangulation and detailed and accurate description of the setting and research participants.

Qualitative data collection methods

The methods of data collection used in qualitative research include:

- Observational methods
- Interviews
- Focus groups
- Consensus methods.

Observational methods

Observational methods generally use the researcher as the research instrument to collect the data. Although observational methods of collecting data may involve questioning or analysis of documentary evidence, they are primarily based on observation *per se*, either as complete participant (covert observation), participant as observer (overt observation) or observer as participant (Mays and Pope 1995b). Patterson (1995), for example, collected qualitative data during participant observation in a nursing home over a period of 12 months, with the objective of examining the process of social support, in particular how residents adjusted to life in a nursing home. All observations were recorded daily in computerized field notes using a strategy developed by Schatzman and Strauss (1973) which included observational, theoretical and methodological notes.

In reviewing the findings, Patterson quotes examples from the observational data for illustrative purposes. She was able to conclude that emotional support and practical assistance are primary supportive behaviours from others. Although she does not use the terms credibility, dependability, transferability and confirmability, some of these concepts are embodied within the research. For example, in addition to observation, she also conducts informal and semistructured interviews to increase the confirmability of her study. She also states the precise parameters of her research (including details of the interview guide, for example) to improve the study's credibility. She suggests some supportive interventions for others and her confidence that her findings are transferable is based on the rigour of her data collection methodology. Good qualitative researchers are cautious about the generalizability of their findings and often can only *suggest* that interventions *may* be appropriate in other settings.

The details of how field notes are recorded can be very helpful when appraising published qualitative research. In an excellent paper on the field experience of a white researcher 'getting in' a poor black community, Kauffman (1994) gives a good example of how a field note can be used to illustrate one of the central themes of a piece of research when she describes how an 'outsider' can appear non-judgmental:

'. . . Yep, ev'rybody like' you in there 'cause you like ev'rybody!'
(Kauffman 1994)

This is a highly appropriate use of field notes within a publication which enables the critical reader to appraise the quality of the data collection.

Participant observation is also commonly used as a data collection method within action research (see Chapter 5, page 131).

Interviews   A great deal of the qualitative data in published literature is collected by interviews. White (1995) undertook an in-depth series of interviews amongst a small group of older, Caucasian women in Auckland, New Zealand to determine how perceptions of cervical cancer and cervical screening services might be affecting health-seeking behaviour. She gives a good description of her interview schedule in sufficient detail to enable the critical reader to assess this part of her methodology. However, this is not the case with many published studies. For example, Kyngas and Hentinen (1995) in their study of self-care in young diabetics, merely describe the circumstances of the interviews rather than giving details of their process. It may be, of course, that interview details are omitted from a published paper because of editorial policy! Nonetheless, it is often useful to see at least some detail of how an interview has been conducted when appraising the quality of a piece of published research.

Interviews may be classified as shown in Box 6.1.

To conduct a good in-depth or indeed any interview, interviewers

Box 6.1
Types of interview

- Structured – questionnaire-based
- Semistructured – open-ended questions
- Depth – reflective questioning, covering few issues in great detail

need to be trained. This training includes familiarizing a researcher with the skills of, for example, reflective questioning, summarizing and 'controlling' an interview. Whyte (1982), for example, gives a 'directiveness scale' for analyzing interview technique. Authors who report data from interviews should normally also give details of the training which interviewers received.

Details of how the data were recorded are also important in evaluating the research. For example, field notes written at the time may interfere with the data collection but field notes written afterwards may miss out on some details! For most situations, audiotaping is an appropriate method for recording the data, although transcription is an immensely time-consuming activity.

Focus groups   The idea of focus groups is to collect qualitative data by encouraging group interaction and recording that interaction rather than a researcher asking individuals questions in turn (Kitzinger 1995). Such groups can encourage participation from reluctant interviewees or those who feel they have nothing to say as well as monitoring changes in the group's opinions or attitudes. As with individual interviews, this method does not discriminate against those who cannot read or write. In her study of family caregivers of people with AIDS, Powell-Cope (1994) used a focus group to assess the content validity of her method. The focus group consisted of three family caregivers who were in an original study but not part of the 12 subjects whose transcripts were used for the analysis. The focus group participants were asked to determine how closely descriptions of categories reflected their own experiences with professional caregiving, how well the categories described their own experiences and whether or not they agreed with the conclusions. This is an excellent example of how a focus group can be part of a qualitative data collection methodology. To ensure the credibility of the findings, and the dependability (reliability) of the coding, a 'nurse expert in caring' was consulted regularly. Such details are important in the appraisal of published nursing research.

Consensus methods

These methods of data collection include:

- The Delphi technique
- Nominal group technique
- Consensus development conferences.

The Delphi technique is not new and has developed into an accepted method of achieving consensus between experts. However, concern has been expressed about the subjectivity associated with its use and perhaps the major deficiency in studies using the Delphi technique is the question of what is meant by 'consensus' (Duffield 1993). Mobily *et al* (1993) report a validation study of cognitive–behavioural techniques to reduce pain. Using a Delphi survey, nurses selected for their expertise in pain management were asked to validate definitions and activities considered important in the implementation of three non-pharmacological pain management interventions. Considerable care was taken in the selection of subjects to provide expert opinion and 42 out of 97 completed a first round of the Delphi survey. As the authors correctly pointed out, the actual response rate is not critical in this type of study where the most important factor is expertise rather than representation.

Space does not permit detailed examination of nominal group techniques, and consensus development conferences which are similar in principle to the Delphi technique. The interested reader is referred to Mays and Pope (1995c).

Case studies

See *Case study*, page 132

See *Grounded theory*, page 122

Case study could be considered to be a type of research design as well as a method for data collection and is also discussed in Chapter 5. Case studies usually focus on one or a limited number of settings and are used to explore specific social processes, especially where complex, inter-related issues are involved. Kearney *et al* (1995) developed a grounded theory methodology (see Chapter 5) to describe how pregnant crack cocaine users perceived and responded to their problems. They collected their data using in-depth interviews with 60 pregnant or postpartum women (cases) who used crack cocaine, on average, at least once per week in pregnancy. Their sample was derived from a larger study of pregnant drug users and all participants were screened for eligibility including confirmation of pregnancy or postpartum status. This was particularly important, not only for reasons of credibility, but also because the sources of referrals which resulted in interviews were paid. This paper is an excellent example of the detail which is necessary for a critical reader to appraise the rigour with which a data collection methodology has been used.

A further example of a case study involving the collection of qualitative data is the paper by Thomas and DeSantis (1995) on the feeding and weaning practices of Cuban and Haitian immigrant mothers in South Florida. Once again, inclusion criteria are detailed to enable evaluation of the credibility of the data collection. Conclusions drawn from publications which omit such criteria should be treated with great caution by the critical reader.

Summary

A range of methods is used to collect data within qualitative research studies including interviews, observation and focus groups. Since these methods invariably involve the researcher directly, there is a greater potential for the researcher to influence the data which is collected. It is important, therefore, that qualitative researchers reflect upon – and acknowledge within reports – the effect which their presence or their own views and experiences may have had on the data.

Chapter conclusion

Which questions should the critical reader ask about a data collection method in the nursing literature?

Quantitative or qualitative?

Neither method of data collection is superior to the other – authors should have chosen an appropriate method for a particular research question. Quantitative methods only help in the discovery of quantifiable information. Qualitative methods should be used for exploring complex social processes. Using mixed methodologies, as in **triangulation**, can be powerful in establishing the credibility or validity of a piece of published research. The interested reader is referred to Carr (1994) for a fuller discussion of this issue.

Quantitative data collection

- Has an 'off the peg' questionnaire been used appropriately by the researchers?
- If a questionnaire has been developed by the authors, has the process been described in sufficient detail for an assessment of its reliability and validity?
- Has it been piloted?

■ If an interview has been used to collect the data, has enough information been given, for you the critical reader, to conduct a similar interview?

Sampling

■ Has an appropriate method of sampling for the research question been used to collect the data?
■ Was the sample size big enough to demonstrate an association between variables? (See Chapter 7, page 170, and Chapter 8)

Qualitative data collection

■ Has an appropriate method of data collection been used for the research question which has been asked?
■ Have the authors incorporated the concepts of credibility/dependability/transferability and confirmability into their study?
■ Finally, for both quantitative and qualitative data collection methodologies, have the limitations of the methodology used been considered and discussed?

Exercise 6.1

Task: Obtain this article from your library and answer the following questions:

Gullicks JN and Crase SJ (1993) Sibling behaviour with a newborn: parents' expectations and observations. *Journal of Obstetric, Gynecologic and Neonatal Nursing* **22**: 438–444.

■ How was the data collection method chosen and developed?
■ How was the 'internal' or 'split-half' reliability of the questionnaire determined?
■ Was the assessment of this satisfactory?
■ If not, why not?
■ What level of validity do the authors claim for their study and how has it been established?

Exercise 6.2

Task: Read the following article and answer the questions below:

Oleson M, Heading C, McGlynn Shadick K and Bistodeau J (1994) Quality of life in long-stay institutions in England: nurse and resident perceptions. *Journal of Advanced Nursing* **20**: 23–32.

■ Which sort of sampling have the authors used?
■ Is this an appropriate sampling method for the research question asked?
■ If not, why not?
■ Is the sample large enough?
■ If not, why not?
■ Which details of the interviews do the authors report to help a critical reader have confidence in the instruments used?
■ What else might you want to know about these instruments?

Further reading

The main topics outlined in this chapter are covered in greater depth in these texts. Denzin and Lincoln (1994) is a comprehensive review of qualitative research methodology. McDowell and Newell (1987) contains a large number of questionnaires particularly suitable for the collection of data in nursing research.

Baker C, Wuest C and Stern PN (1992) Method slurring: the grounded theory/phenomenology example. *Journal of Advanced Nursing* **11**: 1355–1360.

Behi R and Nolan M (1995) Reliability: consistency and accuracy in measurement. *British Journal of Nursing* **4**(8): 472–475.

Carr LT (1994) The strengths and weaknesses of quantitative and qualitative research: what method for nursing? *Journal of Advanced Nursing* **20**: 716–721.

Denzin NK, Lincoln YS (eds) (1994) *A Handbook of Qualitative Research*. Thousand Oaks, CA: Sage.

Gibbon B (1995) Validity and reliability of assessment tools. *Nurse Researcher* **2**(4): 48–55.

Howe T (1995) Measurement scales in health care settings. *Nurse Researcher* **2**(4): 30–37.

Lynn MR (1988) Should you believe what you read? Reliability and validity in published paediatric nursing research. *Journal of Paediatric Nursing* **3**(3): 197–199.

McDowell I and Newell C (1987) *Measuring Health: A Guide to Rating Scales and Questionnaires*. Oxford: Oxford University Press.

Morse JM (ed) (1991) *Qualitative Nursing Research: A Contemporary Dialogue*. Newbury Park, CA: Sage.

Oldham J (1995) Biophysiologic measures in nursing practice and research. *Nurse Researcher* **2**(4): 38–47.

Pretzlik U (1994) Observational methods and strategies. *Nurse Researcher* **2**(2): 13–29.

Wilkin D, Hallam L and Doggett M (1992) *Measures of Need and Outcome for Primary Health Care*. Oxford: Oxford University Press.

Webb C (1989) Action research: philosophy, methods and personal experiences. *Journal of Advanced Nursing* **14**: 403–410.

References

Axton SE and Smith LF (1995) Comparison of brachial and calf blood pressures in infants. *Paediatric Nursing* **21**(4): 323–326.

Berg A, Hansson UW and Hallberg IR (1994) Nurses' creativity, tedium and burnout during 1 year of clinical supervision and implementation of individually planned nursing care: Comparisons between a ward for severely demented patients and a similar control ward. *Journal of Advanced Nursing* **20**: 742–749.

Blalock HM and Morse H (1960) *Social Statistics*. London, New York: McGraw-Hill.

Blalock HM (1960) *Social Statistics* (2nd edn). London: McGraw-Hill Kogakusha.

Britten N, Fisher B (1993) Qualitative research and general practice (editorial). *British Journal of General Practice* **43**: 270–271.

Brown JS, Tanner CA and Padrick KP (1984) Nursing's search for scientific knowledge. *Nursing Research* **33**(1): 26–34.

Carr LT (1994) The strengths and weaknesses of quantitative and qualitative research: what method for nursing? *Journal of Advanced Nursing* **20**: 716–721.

Carson J, Leary J, De Villiers N, Fagin L, Randmall J (1995) Stress in mental health nurses: a comparison of ward and community staff. *British Journal of Nursing* **4**(10): 579–582.

Denzin NK and Lincoln YS (eds) (1994) *A Handbook of Qualitative Research*. Thousand Oaks, CA: Sage.

Duffield C (1993) The Delphi technique: A comparison of results obtained using two expert panels. *International Journal of Nursing Studies* **30**(3): 227–237.

Goldberg D and Williams P (1991). *A Users Guide to the General Health Questionnaire*. Windsor: Nfer-Nelson.

Hanson EJ, McClement S and Kristjanson LJ (1995) Psychological support role of night nursing staff on an acute care oncology unit. *Cancer Nursing* **18**(3): 237–246.

Hagerty BMK and Patusky K (1995) Developing a measure of sense of belonging. *Nursing Research* **44**(1): 9–13.

Kauffman KS (1994) The insider outsider dilemma: Field experience of a white researcher 'Getting in' a poor black community. *Nursing Research* **43**(3): 179–183.

Kearney MH, Murphy S, Irwin K and Rosenbaum M (1995) Salvaging self: a grounded theory of pregnancy on crack cocaine. *Nursing Research* **44**(4): 208–213.

Kitzinger J (1995) Introducing focus groups. *British Medical Journal* **311**: 299–302.

Knafl KA, Breitmayer BJ (1991) Triangulation in qualitative research: issues of conceptual clarity and purpose. In Morse J (ed) *Qualitative Nursing Research: A Contemporary Dialogue*. Revised edn. Newbury Park, DC: Sage, 266–239.

Kyngäs H and Hentinen M (1995) Meaning attached to compliance with self-care, and conditions for compliance among young diabetics. *Journal of Advanced Nursing* **21**: 729–736.

Lincoln YS and Guba EG (1985) *Naturalistic Enquiry*. Thousand Oaks, CA: Sage.

Lucas MD, Atwood JR and Hagaman R (1993) Replication and validation of anticipated turnover model for urban registered nurses. *Nursing Research* **42**(1): 29–35.

Lydeard S (1991) The questionnaire as a research tool. *Family Practice* **8**(1): 26–33.

McDowell I and Newell C (1987) *Measuring Health: a Guide to Rating Scales and Questionnaires*. Oxford: Oxford University Press.

Mays N and Pope C (1995a) Rigour and qualitative research. *British Medical Journal* **311**: 109–112.

Mays N and Pope C (1995b) Observational methods in health care settings. *British Medical Journal*. **311**: 182–184.

Mays N and Pope C (1995c) Qualitative interviews in medical research. *British Medical Journal* **311**: 251–253.

Mobily PR, Herr KA and Kelley LS (1993) Cognitive–behavioural techniques to reduce pain: a validation study. *International Journal of Nursing Studies* **30**(6): 537–548.

Moody LE *et al* (1988) Analysis of a decade of nursing practice research: 1977–1986. *Nursing Research* **37**(6): 374–379.

Nolan M and Behi R (1995) Triangulation: the best of all worlds? *British Journal of Nursing* **4**(14): 829–832.

Patterson BJ (1995) The process of social support: adjusting to life in a nursing home. *Journal of Advanced Nursing* **21**: 682–689.

Phillips JM and Wilbur J (1995) Adherence to breast cancer screening guidelines among African-American women of differing employment status. *Cancer Nursing* **18**(4): 258–269.

Powell-Cope GM (1994) Family caregivers of people with AIDS: negotiating partnerships with professional health care providers. *Nursing Research* **43**(6): 324–330.

Schatzman L and Strauss AL (1973) *Field Research: Strategies for a Natural Sociology*. Englewood Cliffs and NJ: Prentice-Hall.

Seideman RY and Kleine P (1995) A theory of transformed parenting: parenting a child with developmental delay/mental retardation. *Nursing Research* **44**(1): 38–44.

Sherman RE and Polit DF (1990) Statistical power in nursing research. *Nursing Research* **39**(6): 365–369.

Snowdon AW and Kane DJ (1995) Parental needs following the discharge of a hospitalised child. *Paediatric Nursing* **21**(5): 425–428.

Stamps PL, Piedmont EB and Haase AM (1978) Measurement of work satisfaction among health professionals. *Medical Care* **XV**(4): 337–352.

Stein PR (1995) Indices of pain intensity: construct validity among pre-schoolers. *Paediatric Nursing* **21**(2): 119–123.

Stoate HG (1989) Can health screening damage your health? *Journal of Royal College of General Practitioners.* **39**(322): 193–195.

Steiner DL, Norman GR and Blum HM (1989) *Epidemiology.* Philadelphia, PA: BC Decker.

Thomas JT and DeSantis L (1995) Feeding weaning practices of Cuban and Haitian immigrant mothers. *Journal of Transcultural Nursing* **6**(2): 34–41.

Timms J and Ford P (1995) Registered nurses' perceptions of gerontological continuing education needs in the United Kingdom and in the USA. *Journal of Advanced Nursing* **22**: 300–307.

Vehvilaineu-Julkunen K (1994) The function of home visits in maternal and child welfare as evaluated by services providers and users. *Journal of Advanced Nursing* **20**: 672–678.

Webb C (1989) Action research: philosophy, methods and personal experiences. *Journal of Advanced Nursing* **14**: 403–410.

White GE (1995) Older women's attitudes to cervical screening and cervical cancer: a New Zealand experience. *Journal of Advanced Nursing.* **21**: 659–666.

Whyte WF (1982) Interviewing in field research. In Burgess RG (ed) *Field Research: a Sourcebook and Field Manual.* London: George Allen and Unwin: 111–122.

Yamashita M (1995) Job satisfaction in Japanese nurses. *Journal of Advanced Nursing* **22**: 158–164.

Younger J, Marsh KJ and Grap MJ (1995) The relationship of health locus of control and cardiac rehabilitation to mastery of illness-related stress. *Journal of Advanced Nursing* **22**: 294–299.

7 Evaluating methods for analyzing data in published research

Nigel Mathers, Yu Chu Huang

Introduction

When reading a piece of research the critical reader should consider the methods used by the authors to analyze their data. Without appropriate and rigorous analysis of data, the conclusions which have been drawn may not be supported. In the broadest sense of the term, methods of analysis are the way researchers interpret the data they have collected to support their claims. If, for example, in a piece of quantitative research it is claimed that Y is caused by (or associated with) X, the critical reader must ask:

- Has an appropriate method been used to analyze the data?
- How valid is the link claimed between X and Y?
- In statistical terms, how robust is the statistical test which has been used to establish such a link?

By the time you have finished reading through this chapter, and working through each of the reflective exercises, we hope that you will be able to describe the principles underlying the analysis of quantitative and qualitative data, match appropriate methods of analysis to particular types of data and apply your knowledge of different data analysis methodologies to the critical appraisal of published literature.

Key issues

- Approaches to the analysis of quantitative data
- Types of variables and their measurement
- The null hypothesis, statistical significance and statistical power
- Approaches to the analysis of qualitative data
- The contribution of quantitative and qualitative research to nursing

Quantitative data analysis

When reading a published study which has collected quantitative data, the critical reader should ask themselves which sort of data has been collected. Different methods of statistical analysis are used for different types of data and so, in deciding if an appropriate test has been used, it is necessary to be clear about the type of data which has been collected. The different methods of statistical analysis for quantitative data may be broadly classified into **parametric statistics** which assume the data have a normal distribution and which are used to manipulate **interval** or **ratio** data and nonparametric statistics which make no assumptions about distribution, and are used to analyze **ordinal** or **nominal** data.

Interval and ratio data

An interval or ratio scale is one in which data are recorded on a measurement scale where the gaps between the numbers are the same wherever you are on the scale. For example, in measuring the level of iron in the blood, data are recorded in milligrams. Wherever you are on the scale 'a milligram (mg) is a milligram', i.e. the difference between 3mg and 4mg is the same as between 11mg and 12mg. This is an interval or ratio scale. A ratio scale specifically is one which has an absolute zero (i.e. there is a meaningful zero point on the scale such as nil volume) which allows you to make meaningful ratio comparisons such as 100ml is twice as much as 50ml. The distinction between interval and ratio data is not important as far as critical appraisal is concerned, since interval and ratio data may be analyzed statistically in the same way.

Ordinal data

Here, data are collected on a scale which has an order but there is no mathematical relationship between different points on the scale. For example, the classification of Social Class stretches from Social Class V to I. However, although the measurement has an order, in no sense can Social Class II be regarded as twice Social Class I.

Nominal data

When nominal data are collected, there is no mathematical relationship at all between the different categories. For example, in the Registrar General's classification of occupation, although one may wish to categorize and number the different occupations for analysis, there is no sense of a mathematical relationship between the categories – a refuse collector is not twice a teacher!

Which statistical test for which type of data?

When comparing two samples to see if there is any statistically significant difference between them (i.e. differences which are highly unlikely to have occurred by chance), appropriate statistical tests for interval or ratio data are the t-tests for matched or unmatched pairs. Matched pairs of samples are used, for example, for assessing the effect of an intervention before and after in the same subjects. If more than two samples are being compared, then an ANOVA test (*Analysis of Variance*) should be used to analyze the data.

Janke (1994) in her development of a breastfeeding attrition prediction tool reports a one-tail t-test of mean instrument scores of women with and without prior breastfeeding experience. Statistically significant ($p = 0.001$) group differences were found in two components of the instrument (the negative breastfeeding sentiment and the breastfeeding control contrast). Although the scales of her instrument are chosen to measure the attitudes of women (nominal data), she has treated these data as interval in her analysis. This is because it is possible – although controversial – to sum the items of a subscale in a questionnaire to create an index which, although it is derived from nominal data, may be treated as interval data for analysis.

In her study of job satisfaction in Japanese nurses Yamashita (1995) used a one-way ANOVA to look for differences among medical ($n = 175$), surgical ($n = 199$) and ICU ($n = 240$) nurses. She was able to demonstrate statistically significant differences among the three practice areas of nurses in terms of their job satisfaction.

A **one-way** ANOVA is used when there are sets of data from three separate groups of subjects and we want to know whether there is a difference between the three groups. A **two-way** ANOVA is used when there are two or more independent (cause) variables and we wish to test an hypothesis that they affect a dependent (effect) variable. The interested reader is referred to Campbell and Machin (1990) for a more detailed discussion of these issues.

Berg *et al* (1994) performed a two-way ANOVA to analyze the differences in nurses' creativity, tedium and burnout between a ward for severely demented patients and a similar control ward. The comparisons over time within each sample showed that the creativity and innovative climate of an intervention group which consisted of systematic clinical supervision and individualized planned care increased during the year of the study. In this example, two independent variables (the intervention and time) are examined for their effect on the dependent variables of creativity, tedium and burnout. Their results are tabulated very clearly in the original paper and this is a good example of the necessary transparency for the critical reader to assess a data analysis methodology.

One- and two-tailed hypotheses

If the aim of a particular study is to test an hypothesis (H_1) that there is a difference between the scores of two groups of subjects, then the corresponding null hypothesis (H_0) is that there is no such difference. The original hypothesis (H_1) therefore merely states that there is a difference. It does *not* say, for example, that group 2 will score higher or lower than group 1, only that group 1 and 2 will differ. This is called a two-tailed hypothesis: group 2 could score less than or more than group 1. If, however, the original hypothesis was that group 1 would score less than group 2 (i.e. if the direction of the difference between the two groups is predicted) then this would be a one-tailed hypothesis. Similarly, if H_1 was that group 1 would score more than group 2, this would also be a one-tailed hypothesis since the direction of the difference would still be predicted. This distinction may seem arcane to the uninitiated but it is important when applying significance tests. Statistical printouts usually show the two-tailed probability of a calculated statistic. One-tailed probabilities are the two-tailed probabilities divided by two.

The appropriate statistical tests for comparison of ordinal data sets are the Wilcoxon test for paired or related samples and the Mann–Whitney test for unpaired or independent samples. For example, a researcher wishes to find out if there is an improvement in the quality of life for hypertensive patients following the introduction of new clinical guidelines. Ordinal data are collected to assess the impact of the intervention and the scores of the patients are compared before and after the intervention. In this situation the Wilcoxon test for paired or related samples should be used. The point here is that the Wilcoxon is used when the subjects are the same.

However, if a researcher wished to compare the performance of two groups of nurses, one of whom used the new clinical guidelines and the other who did not, then, assuming once again that ordinal data have been collected, the Mann–Whitney test should be used to make comparisons between the groups since they contain *different* subjects. The Claybury community psychiatric nurse stress study (Fagin *et al* 1995) asked the question: is it more stressful to work in hospital or the community? The authors collected data on the stress levels of 250 community-based and 323 ward-based psychiatric nurses. The Mann–Whitney test was used to compare the mean scores for each group for job satisfaction and occupational burnout. By means of this analysis, the authors were able to conclude that the ward-based psychiatric nurses were achieving less personal fulfilment from their work and that 'stress was reaping its toll on mental health nurses'. This is a well-written paper which gives the critical reader plenty of information to evaluate the methods of data analysis which the authors have used.

The statistical test used for comparing groups when nominal data have been collected is generally χ^2 (chi-squared). A good example of the use of χ^2 may be found in Dealey's paper (1994) on monitoring pressure sore problems in a teaching hospital. Using the χ^2 test, each grade of pressure sores was assessed for any differences between two surveys done in 1989 and 1993. There was no statistically significant difference in pressure sores although the survey did show an improvement in the management of established pressure sores. The paper itself is well written and sufficient detail is given for the critical reader to evaluate the appropriateness of the statistical tests used.

Analyzing different types of data

The critical reader will find that some authors use nonparametric tests (e.g. Mann-Whitney U test) for interval data and this is accepted by the editors of journals. The difficulty is, however, that if a nonpara-

Figure 7.1 *The statistical flow chart*

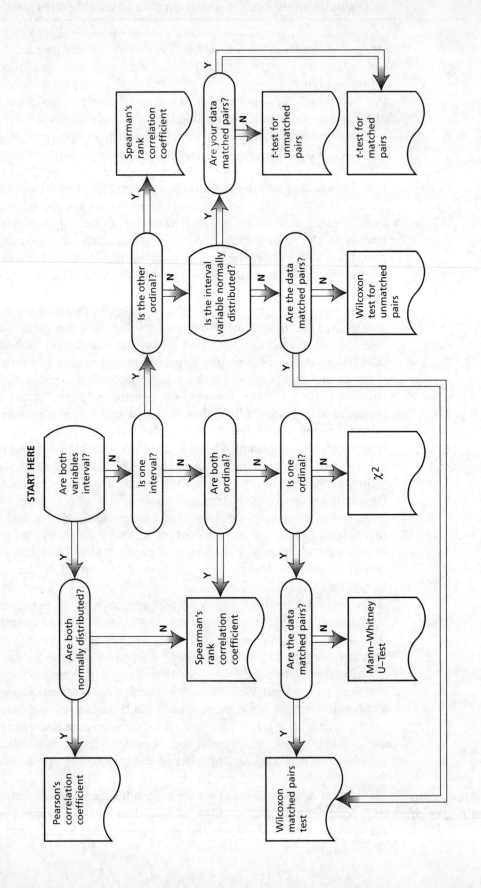

(From Armstrong et al 1990: 158, by permission of Oxford University Press)

metric test is used for interval data, then the calculated P-value (significance level) will always be greater than that obtained using, for example, the t-test. This means that one is less likely to find a significant result with a non-parametric test using the same data, so such tests are less powerful. Non-parametric tests are also much less flexible when used to analyze interval data. For example, multiple regression and analysis of covariance are not possible with such tests.

Sometimes it is necessary for a researcher to compare interval with ordinal data rather than the same type of data (i.e. interval). More detailed discussion of the statistical manipulations which then become necessary is unfortunately beyond the scope of this text. However, a statistical flow chart is shown on page 166 (Armstrong *et al* 1990) which is an easy guide for the novice through the bewildering world of statistics.

A note on confidence intervals

The published literature often reports confidence intervals for populations. These are the range of values within which a researcher can be confident that the population value falls. Confidence intervals can be set at different levels. A 95% confidence interval (CI 95) means that one can be 95% confident that the population value falls within a certain range. These values should not be too wide for the critical reader to be confident that the sample represents the attributes of the rest of the population. A study might report, for example, that 40% of a sample of 1000 people were smokers and that the calculated 95% confidence interval was plus or minus 3% of this value. The critical reader could then be 95% confident that the frequency of smoking in the population was between 37% and 43%. However, sample sizes have a crucial influence on confidence intervals. If the sample size was only 100 and the percentage of smokers was still 40%, the corresponding 95% confidence interval might be 12% either side: a range of between 28% to 52% for the population. Unfortunately, much of the published literature does not include confidence intervals and it is often difficult to evaluate this aspect of data analysis in a study. The interested reader is referred to Gardner and Altman (1989).

Summary

A number of factors determine the appropriate statistical test for the analysis of quantitative data in a given set of circumstances. These include the level of measurement of the data (ratio, interval, ordinal or nominal), the question to be answered (i.e. is a description of the data required or an indication of the relationship between variables?) and the number of groups in the study. Although decisions about the use of different methods of analysis often require advanced statistical knowledge, it is possible for the novice critical reader to assess whether a researcher has provided sufficient justification for the approach they have used.

Independent and dependent variables

In addition to suggesting population parameters the aim of quantitative data analysis is often to establish an association between two variables: the independent variable (cause) and the dependent variable (effect). The strength of the association is determined partly by the 'robustness' of the statistical test used. In a perfect world variable X causes effect Y as shown in Figure 7.2.

However, when data are analyzed in the real world, such 'perfect' relationships are rarely found! This is illustrated in Figure 7.3 where variable X is sometimes present when Y is absent and Y is sometimes present when X is absent.

These sorts of data imply that 'something else' is disturbing the relationship between X and Y. This 'something else' may be another variable often referred to as the 'confounding variable'. The influence of a confounding variable on a relationship between an independent and dependent variable is known as 'Simpson's paradox' and the process of taking it into account when inferring a cause and effect relationship is known as **specification** or **elaboration**. The interested reader is referred to Campbell and Machin (1993) for a far more detailed discussion of this topic. Such an analysis of three variables (dependent, independent and confounding) is also admirably presented in Lauver and Tak's paper (1995) on optimism and coping with a breast cancer symptom.

Figure 7.2
'Perfect' relationship between X and Y

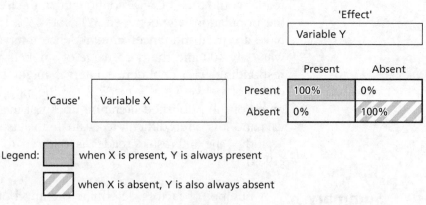

Legend:
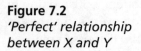 when X is present, Y is always present
when X is absent, Y is also always absent

Figure 7.3
Relationship between variables in the 'real' world

'Effect' Variable Y		
	Present	Absent
Present	80%	20%
Absent	20%	80%

'Cause' Variable X

However, for the critical reader the key issues are:

- Has an appropriate statistical test been used by the authors for the particular type of data which have been collected?
- Have justifiable statistical inferences been made about a relationship between different variables?
- In other words, are the authors justified in their claim that an intervention (variable X) has resulted in a particular effect (variable Y)?

The distinction between the independent and the dependent variables is crucial. A hypothetical example may make this clearer: a research question might be: *do female babies have higher concentrations of C-reactive protein (an indicator of infection) in their blood when they are born than male babies?* Data are collected and tabulated as shown in Figure 7.4.

In Figure 7.4 the gender of the baby was totalled to 100% of the observations. In Figure 7.5 it is the CRP concentrations.

Figure 7.4
Concentrations of C-reactive protein (CRP) in the blood of newborn babies: (1)

		CRP Concentration		
		Low	High	Total
Gender	Male	85%	15%	100%
	Female	67%*	33%	100%

*Note: This means 67% of the female babies had low CRP concentrations.

Figure 7.5
Concentrations of C-reactive protein (CRP) in the blood of newborn babies: (2)

		CRP Concentration	
		Low	High
Gender	Male	85%	67%
	Female	15%*	33%
	Totals	100%	100%

*Note: This means 15% of the low CRP concentrations were found in female babies.

Exercise 7.1   Which hypothesis is being tested by each table? (Clue: the independent variable must total 100%.)

Summary   When reading reports of research investigating the relationship between one or more variables, it is important to identify which is the independent variable (or presumed cause) and which the dependent variable(s) (or presumed effect). It is also important to be aware of the effects of confounding influences which mean that, in the real world, 'perfect' relationships between variables are rarely observed. An important function of quantitative analysis is to determine the probability or 'likelihood' that a relationship between variables observed in the context of a research study could have occurred simply by chance.

The null hypothesis, statistical significance and statistical power

When quantitative data are analyzed for relationships between variables a **null hypothesis** is tested. The null hypothesis (H_o) states that there is no difference between the two groups which are being compared. If the null hypothesis can be rejected on the basis of analysis using appropriate statistical tests (see above) then one can infer that there *is* an association between two variables which *may* be cause and effect. The strength of such an association depends on the statistical test used and the statistical power of the study. Sherman and Polit (1990) reviewed a large number of published studies in nursing research and concluded that 'a substantial number of nurse studies ... have insufficient *power* to detect real effects primarily because the samples used are too small'.

The concept of statistical power is at the heart of quantitative research and may best be understood in conjunction with the null hypothesis. There are four situations which can arise when the data from a particular study have been analyzed. These are illustrated in Figure 7.6. Each cell of Figure 7.6 is discussed below.

Cell 4. The null hypothesis is not supported by the results of the study (i.e. found to be false) and this is also the situation in the 'real' world. There are no problems with this and there *is* an association between the variables.

Cell 2. If, however, the null hypothesis is supported by the results of the study (i.e. found to be true), but in the 'real' world, the null hypothesis is in fact incorrect this is known as a Type II error (beta).

Figure 7.6
The null hypothesis (H_o) statistical significance and statistical power

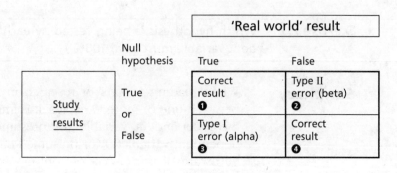

The concept of statistical power is used to try and minimize the likelihood of this Type II error. The lower the power of the study, the more likely it is that any lack of association which has been found between two variables is due to chance. Clearly, sample size is crucial here in determining the power of a study and the smaller the sample the greater the likelihood of the negative results being due to chance. Conventionally, a value of 0.80 is acceptable as a measure of sufficient statistical power to minimize the chances of such a Type II error.

Cell 1. A third possibility is that the results from a study support the null hypothesis and this is, in fact, the situation in the 'real' world. Again there are no problems with this since the results reflect 'reality' and there is *no* association between the variables demonstrated either by the study or in the 'real' world.

Cell 3. However, the situation may also arise that the study results show the null hypothesis to be false (i.e. it shows that there is an association between two variables) but in 'reality' the null hypothesis is true (i.e. there is *no* association between the variables). This is known as a Type I error (alpha). Again, sample size is crucial here, in determining the likelihood of a statistically significant result and whether such results might have arisen by chance. This is usually expressed in the published literature as a p value. The higher the p value, the more likely it is that such results have occurred by chance and there is no 'real' association between the variables. Conventionally, a value of < 0.05 is acceptable as a measure of sufficient statistical significance to demonstrate a 'real' association between two variables (i.e. a statistically significant difference between two groups).

Apart from sample size, two other factors affect the statistical power of a study. The first is the significance level or alpha. Power increases with higher Type I errors. However, if the significance level which is required is less than the conventional 0.05 (i.e. the risk of a Type I error is required to be lower than is conventionally acceptable, e.g. 0.01) then the statistical power would also decrease.

The second factor affecting statistical power is effect size. The effect size is merely a measure of how 'wrong' the null hypothesis is, i.e. it measures the strength of the association between the independent and the dependent variable. There is a reciprocal relationship between effect size and sample size: the larger the effect size, the smaller the sample size needs to be and the greater the power. Of course, in non-experimental (or non-intervention) research, the researcher does not manipulate or control the independent variable but nevertheless its value can be estimated.

Much of the published literature is based on relatively small sample sizes. This means that unless effect sizes are large, many of these studies are underpowered and have a high probability of committing a Type II error (showing no association between two variables, when 'in reality' there is an association). Some assessment of statistical power by the critical reader is particularly important when non-significant results are reported and the study inconclusive. In addition, many research studies in nursing are concerned with small effect sizes and consequently are likely to be underpowered. When a study is designed, a statistical power of about 0.80 should be aimed for which means that only one in five times would a false null hypothesis be accepted. Lower values, for example 0.66, would mean that the chance of accepting a false null hypothesis would be one in three.

The calculations of statistical power are complex but tables are available (e.g. Cohen 1977) to identify the necessary sample size to achieve a statistical power of 0.80 for each of the different statistical tests. Some estimate of effect size is also necessary and as a 'rule of thumb' a medium effect size is visible to the naked eye: anything less clear should be counted as a small effect. In other words a medium effect can be discerned from everyday experience without recourse to formal measurement. For example, the difference between male and female adult heights in the UK would be counted as medium effect size. Most effects encountered in biomedical and social research should be assumed to be small unless there is a good reason to claim a medium effect, while a 'large' effect size would probably need to be defined as one which is so large that it hardly seems necessary to undertake research into something so well established. Cohen (1977) offers the example of the difference between the heights of 13 and 18 year old girls as a large effect. For a fuller discussion of these issues the reader is referred to Sherman and Polit (1990).

Summary

Further questions which a critical reader needs to ask about the data analysis methodology in a published paper are as follows:

- What is the level of statistical significance which has been chosen by the authors?
- Is there sufficient statistical power in the study to support any claimed association between an intervention and a result?
- Has 'real world' (or clinical) significance been considered as well as statistical significance?

The last question is particularly relevant for the weary critical reader of the academic literature. If the results of a study have statistical significance but not 'real world' (or clinical) significance, so what?! (See Figure 7.7.)

Figure 7.7
*Statistical significance
and the 'real' world*

'Real world' importance

		High	Low
Statistical Significance (p < 0.05)	Yes	Great!	So what?!
	No	Chance! (Larger sample?)	Reject! (Power?)

Qualitative data analysis

In Chapter 6 we defined qualitative data collection methods as using words to express the information gathered to answer a particular research question. This is a loose definition of 'qualitative' and it is important to be clear about what a 'qualitative' study is not. A paper reporting a small number of subjects is not a qualitative study simply because the sample size is too small for statistical analysis, nor is it qualitative because it is based on questionnaire responses to subjective material or collected by interview. Qualitative data analysis depends on conceptual analysis and is used where the purpose is to understand the meaning and interpretation of complex social phenomena. There are a considerable number of qualitative data analysis methodologies. Those which the critical reader is most likely to encounter in the published literature are outlined below.

Grounded theory

If 'grounded theory' (Strauss and Corbin 1990) has been used as a method of data analysis, the data have been collected without a pre-existing theoretical framework (see Chapter 4). In other words, there have been no preconceptions about the data. This means that, during the analysis of interview transcripts, for example, theoretical propositions will have been generated. A theory grounded in this way should be able to fully explain the data.

Donovan (1995) used such a grounded theory approach to study men during their partners' pregnancies. One antenatal group consisting of six men, whose partners were in the second trimester of pregnancy, attended a series of five meetings and subsequent individual interviews. Additional data and insights were gained by the researcher and the research assistant attending other antenatal classes with men and women present. The data which they collected consisted of transcripts of tape-recorded interviews, group discussions, and observations and field notes made by the researcher and co-leader following each of the group sessions. The aim was to develop a substantive grounded theory which was drawn from the experiences of the men during this transitional period in their lives.

This excellent paper discusses the process of analysis which led to identification of the central phenomenon – *disequilibrium in the relationship with their female partner* – the core category of the research, around which the grounded theory is built. The process of analysis is transparent and allows the critical reader to evaluate the methodology in detail. It is of a standard by which other published research may be judged and as such is highly recommended.

Despite the fact that Donovan did not use a pre-existing theoretical framework, some structure with which to approach her data was essential. Data were entered into the NUDIST (Non-numerical Unstructured Data Indexing, Searching and Theorising) computer programme which is a system for managing, organizing and supporting research in qualitative data analysis. When printed, all the lines of data were numbered which helped in the processes of re-ordering and re-entering the data into the computer in a form which could be retrieved in any order or combination. The process she used subsequently for coding and categorizing and then analyzing the data followed the standard procedure recommended by Strauss and Corbin (1990).

The advantages of grounded theory as a method of data analysis are that it tries to minimize researcher bias, is probably the best method to identify 'meanings' from participants' perspective and is particularly useful when there are multiple cycles of data collection and analysis. In reviewing a published paper, the critical reader should look for such justifications in the rationale for the choice of the method and decide whether such a method is appropriate for the research question which is being asked.

One of the main disadvantages of such a methodology is the impossibility for researchers to be free of 'conceptual baggage' and pre-existing assumptions about the data. Also, the analysis, if done well, is complex. The perceptive reader should also be able to appreciate that grounded theory makes the assumption that life is holistic in the sense that all observations about the world can be explained theoretically: in the 'real' world of data analysis, however, some data will never 'fit' the theory. It is probably much easier to have poor qualitative research published than poor quantitative research since, unless the processes of data collection and analysis are transparent to the critical reader, can he or she conclude that a piece of work is any more than a 'believable fiction'?!

Constant comparative methods

Theoretical sampling

Such methods of data analysis use two linked strategies – *theoretical sampling* and *analytic induction*. The idea here is to minimize and maximize differences between the two groups which are being compared. This process results in huge amounts of data for each theme. For example, Glaser and Strauss (1965), in an original paper published before their work on developing grounded theory, looked at the process of dying by exploring hypotheses about 'awareness', 'expectedness' and 'rate of dying'. They collected their data from a premature baby unit and a neurosurgical ward, areas where 'patient awareness' is likely to be minimized. They then sampled an intensive care unit where 'awareness' was maximized and a cancer ward where 'awareness' was both maximized and minimized. They were then able to compare the themes emerging from the data to construct their theoretical framework. When new categories no longer emerged from the data (*theoretical saturation*) the process of data analysis was considered complete. The main objective of theoretical sampling is to minimize and maximize differences between groups.

A further example of this sort of process is the study by Traynor (1994) who compared the views and values of community nurses and their managers on the effects of changes in community care. However, the managers were interviewed and these were subsequently transcribed and coded (with one exception) whereas the nurses completed a questionnaire survey and their non-numerical comments at the end of their questionnaires (one-third of those returned) were then transcribed and coded. Although the author tries to establish the representativeness of his sample, the critical reader should be cautious about accepting the credibility of the conclusions since they are based on mixed comparative methods of data collection and analysis.

Analytic induction

This method of data analysis involves a systematic attempt to find evidence which contradicts a theoretical framework by looking at examples which differ in known ways from others. The theory is then modified until no other 'exceptions to the rule' can be found. The necessary steps are as follows:

- A tentative theoretical framework is prepared
- An alternative framework is constructed to account for the findings derived from the data
- Each of a small number of new cases, chosen to be different from the original sample (sometimes from the same setting, sometimes from a different one) is considered in the light of the competing frameworks with the object of deciding which provides the best 'fit'. If the findings cannot be accounted for by either framework, another is constructed and the whole cycle repeated.

In the selection of new cases, the researcher should explicitly seek to maximize the chances of discovering exceptions in order to test the hypothesis or framework. This is continued until all sources of likely negative evidence have been explored. A similar process is used for discourse analysis.

Although case studies are not really a distinctive method of data analysis, they are increasingly used in the study of health care systems and should be included in this section. For example, in a study of the impact of general management in the NHS, an investigator, when confronted by differing accounts from stakeholders, would either probe or return to interviews, to try and account for discrepancies with the theoretical framework. Case studies, in particular, should try to get an accurate picture by means of triangulation so that degrees of convergence and divergence can be carefully considered and included within a framework. The critical reader should evaluate published case studies with this in mind.

A similar process was used by Patterson (1995) in her study of how residents adjusted to life in a nursing home. Rather than try and fault her continuing analysis by finding new cases, she informally reviewed the interview data with the resident using the exact phrases as identified by them. Residents were then able to contradict or expand upon thoughts they might not have anticipated at the time of the interview.

Summary

As mentioned in the introduction to this section, more than is the case in quantitative research, interpretation is *always* involved in qualitative research and writing is thus a key part of data analysis. The questions the critical reader should therefore ask are:

- Is the process of data analysis transparent, comprehensive and clearly written? For example, has the writer considered their 'conceptual baggage'?
- Have the authors used an appropriate method for sorting and coding their data?
- Are sufficient data, in the form of examples and quotes from transcripts, included to justify the themes which have emerged to form the basis of the theoretical framework?

A final note on inductive and deductive reasoning

In general, quantitative data analysis (statistical inference) is based on deductive reasoning. This is the logical movement from the general to the particular and is the procedure behind classical logic. Examples of deductive reasoning may be found in the stories of

Sherlock Holmes. If, for example, he knows that green clay is only found in Basingstoke, and the suspected murderer has green clay on his shoes, then he *deduces* that the murderer has been in Basingstoke.

Qualitative data analysis is underpinned by inductive reasoning whereby specific findings are generalized to substantiate theories of, for example, human behaviour. This procedure is the basis of observational research and may best be understood as the logical movement from the particular to the general. An example of such reasoning might be a detailed case study observation of an autistic child's behaviour with his or her mother to support the theory that autistic children have difficulty with emotional expression.

These processes are considered in more detail in Chapter 4. Also, for an easy introduction to these ideas, the critical reader is referred to Medawar (1969).

Chapter conclusion

In her paper on the strengths and weaknesses of quantitative and qualitative research, Carr (1994) argues that if nursing scholars limit themselves to one method of enquiry, restrictions will be placed on the development of nursing knowledge. We hope that on completing this chapter, the diligent reader will have the necessary understanding, confidence and skills to evaluate both quantitative and qualitative methods of data analysis. Historically, nursing researchers have often confined themselves to qualitative research in the mistaken belief that somehow it is 'easier'. This – we hope the reader will agree – is not the case and equally systematic and rigorous appraisal of the published literature is necessary in both qualitative and quantitative research. Neither approach is superior to the other – they are two sides of the same coin and combining the strengths of both approaches in triangulation, if money and time permit, is a valuable means of discovering the truth about nursing. Moody *et al* (1988) reported in their analysis of a decade of nursing practice research that there was an increasing use of sophisticated research methodology. In preparing our contribution for this book, this is a trend which has become increasingly evident. We hope that our two chapters will support and encourage nurses to continue this process.

Exercise 7.2   Read the following article and answer the questions below:
Gullicks JN and Crase SJ (1993) Sibling behaviour with a newborn: parents' expectations and observations. *Journal of Obstetric, Gynecological and Neonatal Nursing* 22: 438–444.

- Which sort of data have the authors collected?
- How have these data been analyzed?
- Has an appropriate statistical test been used to compare the parents' expectations and observations?
- How confident are you on the basis of the analysis presented that, generally, parents expect more negative behaviour than they actually observe?
- On what do you base this confidence?

Exercise 7.3   Read the following article and answer the questions below:
Oleson M, Heading C, McGlynn Shadick K, Bistodeau J (1994) Quality of life in long-stay institutions in England: nurse and resident perceptions. *Journal of Advanced Nursing* 20: 23–32.

- Which sort of data have been collected by the authors?
- How have these data been analyzed?
- Is this approach appropriate to answer the research questions?
- Which themes emerged from the structured interviews?
- How were these categorized?
- To what extent are the nursing implications of the study supported by the analysis of the data collected?

Further reading   The main topics outlined in this chapter are covered in greater depth in these texts. Burns and Grove (1995) is particularly recommended for a comprehensive review of nursing research. Knapp (1985) is a good introduction to the use of statistics for novice researchers.

Burns N and Grove SK (1993) *The Practice of Nursing Research – Conduct, Critique and Utilization*. Philadelphia, PA: WB Saunders.

Burns N and Grove SK (1995) *Understanding Nursing Research*. Philadelphia, PA: WB Saunders.

Duff ME (1985) A research appraisal checklist for evaluating research reports. *Nursing and Health Care* 6(11): 539–547.

Fleming JW and Hayter J (1974) Reading research reports critically. *Nursing Outlook* 22: 172–175.

Hardey M and Mulhall A (eds) (1994) *Nursing Research Theory and Practice*. London: Chapman & Hall.

Huff D (1973) *How to Lie with Statistics*. Harmondsworth: Penguin.

Knapp RG (1985) *Basic Statistics for Nurses*, 2nd edn. Chichester: John Wiley.

The Research Awareness Programme: Module 10: *Evaluating a Research Report*. London: Distance Learning Centre, South Bank Polytechnic.

Ward MJ and Felter ME (1978) What guidelines should be followed in critically evaluating research reports? *Nursing Research* **27**: 120-126.

References

Armstrong D, Calnan M and Grace J (1990) *Research Methods for General Practitioners*. Oxford: Oxford University Press.

Berg A, Hansson UW and Hallborg IR (1994) Nurses' creativity, tedium and burnout during 1 year of clinical supervision and implementation of individually planned nursing care: comparisons between a ward for severely demented patients and a similar control ward. *Journal. of Advanced Nursing* **20**: 742–749.

Campbell MJ and Machin D (1990) *Medical Statistics – A Commonsense Approach*. Chichester: John Wiley.

Carr LT (1994) The strengths and weaknesses of quantitative and qualitative research: what method for nursing? *Journal of Advanced Nursing* **20**: 716–721.

Cohen J (1977) *Statistical Power Analysis for the Behavioural Sciences*. New York: Academic Press.

Dealey C (1994) Monitoring the pressure sore problem in a teaching hospital. *Journal of Advanced Nursing* **20**: 652–659.

Donovan J (1995) The process of analysis during a grounded theory study of men during their partners' pregnancies. *Journal of Advanced Nursing* **21**: 708–715.

Fagin L, Brown D, Bartlett H, Leary J and Carson J (1995) The Claybury community psychiatric nurse stress study: is it more stressful to work in hospital or the community? *Journal of Advanced Nursing* **22**: 347–358.

Gardner MJ and Altman DG (1989) *Statistics with Confidence, Confidence Intervals and Statistical Guidelines*. London: British Medical Journal Press.

Glaser BG and Strauss AL (1965) Temporal aspects of dying as a non-scheduled status passage. *Amer.J Social* **71**: 48–59.

Janke JR (1994) Development of the breastfeeding attrition prediction tool. *Nursing Research* **43**(2): 100–110.

Lauver D and Tak Y (1995) Optimism and coping with a breast cancer symptom. *Nursing Research* **44**(4): 202–207.

Medawar P (1969) *Induction and Intuition in Scientific Thought*. London: Methuen.

Moody LE (1988). Analysis of a decade of nursing practice research: 1977–1986. *Nursing Research* **37**(6): 374–379.

Palmer MH (1995) Nurses' knowledge and beliefs about continence interventions in long-term care. *Journal of Advanced Nursing* **21**: 1065–1072.

Patterson BJ (1995) The process of social support: adjusting to life in a nursing home. *Journal of Advanced Nursing* **21**: 682–689.

Sherman RE and Polit DF (1990) Statistical power in nursing research. *Nursing Research* **39**(6): 365–369.

Strauss A and Corbin J (1990) *Basics of Qualitative Research*. Thousand Oaks, CA: Sage.

Traynor M (1994) The views and values of community nurses and their managers: research in progress – one person's pain, another person's vision. *Journal of Advanced Nursing* **20**: 101–109.

Yamashita M (1995) Job satisfaction in Japanese nurses. *Journal of Advanced Nursing* **22**: 158–164.

8 Populations and samples: identifying the boundaries of research

Christine Ingleton

Introduction

Sampling considerations pervade all aspects of the research process. Yet in many nursing studies the sampling plan is the weakest part of the study. The correct match of the sampling procedures to the research aims and methods is an important consideration in assessing the trustworthiness or validity of the research findings. An appreciation of the process of sampling and the rationale underpinning sampling decisions is essential for researchers *and* consumers of research. An understanding of how sampling decisions may affect findings will also help in making more informed decisions about their applicability to clinical practice.

In this chapter I will first discuss why researchers base their work on samples. I will go on to examine ways in which researchers set boundaries in quantitative designs and then consider how boundaries are constructed in qualitative studies. It will become clear that qualitative and quantitative approaches address boundary setting differently, and judgments about the appropriateness and rigour of the sampling strategy in published research should be made with this in mind.

Key issues

- Populations and samples
- Sampling within quantitative designs
- Sampling within qualitative designs

Why do researchers need to identify samples?

Research in the health care setting usually involves the collection of data on a sample of people, rather than on the entire population of cases in which the researcher is interested (known as a census). Often, because of the number of people involved, the researcher does not have the resources to study the whole population. There are other reasons (see Box 8.1) why researchers may choose not to measure the whole population.

Box 8.1
Reasons for taking a sample

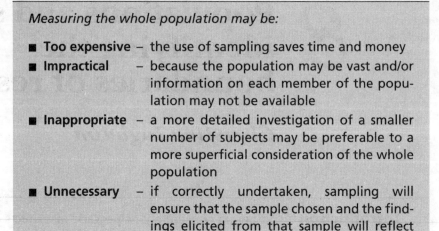

Measuring the whole population may be:

- **Too expensive** – the use of sampling saves time and money
- **Impractical** – because the population may be vast and/or information on each member of the population may not be available
- **Inappropriate** – a more detailed investigation of a smaller number of subjects may be preferable to a more superficial consideration of the whole population
- **Unnecessary** – if correctly undertaken, sampling will ensure that the sample chosen and the findings elicited from that sample will reflect the wider population

Types of sample

The methodological literature on sampling generally makes a distinction between **probability** (random) sampling and **non-probability** (non-random) sampling. The purpose of most quantitative research is to examine the distribution of previously identified phenomena within a population and/or to explore and test relationships between variables (Field and Morse 1985). Given this purpose, it is appropriate that probability sampling should be used whenever possible in order to permit an estimate of sampling error and a calculation of the degree of confidence with which findings may be generalized to a wider population.

Summary

There are a number of reasons why researchers do not operate censuses but instead choose to investigate a sample of the population of interest. Box 8.1 shows that some of these reasons are pragmatic (the researcher has no real choice) while others have more of a theoretical basis (there is no requirement that the views of a whole population are canvassed). Sampling decisions affect the value or credibility of research findings, particularly when the researcher attempts to extrapolate findings to a wider population than the one studied. The process of sampling and the rationale underpinning sampling decisions are therefore important issues to consider when critically analyzing published research with a view to its applicability to clinical practice.

Boundary setting in quantitative research

DePoy and Gitlin (1994) describe boundary setting in the quantitative domain as **deductive**. That is, the researcher begins with a notion of whom she or he wishes to study, and clearly defines the characteristics or attributes of that group. This is referred to as the **population**. The population for a study is typically reported as

Table 8.1
Examples of populations and samples

Population	Possible sample selection
All district nurses working in one region in the UK	100 district nurses selected for a study of job satisfaction
All deaths occurring in one city in the UK between 1995–1996	300 case notes selected by researcher to establish place of death
The pulse rate of a patient during a 24-hour period	Hourly measurements of patient's pulse rate recorded by staff
Nurse/patient interactions in a care of the elderly setting	Six patients observed and video-recorded during interactions with trained nurses at meal times, over three days.

being composed of two groups – the **target population** and the **accessible population**. The sample is drawn from the population, and is thus a subset of the defined population. Table 8.1 shows examples of populations and samples.

Probability sampling refers to techniques that are based on probability theory (see Polgar and Thomas (1993) for an in-depth discussion). The two central features of probability theory as applied to sampling are that:

- The researcher has access to every member of the population
- Every member or element of the population has an equal and non-zero chance of being selected for the sample (i.e. they must *not* have *no chance* of being selected).

The important point to remember is that the probability of each member or element being included in the sample is known and greater than zero. By knowing the size of the population and the degree of chance that each element may be selected, a researcher can calculate the sampling error. Sampling error refers to the estimated difference between data obtained from a random sample and the data that would be obtained if the entire population was measured. It indicates how representative the sample is of the population – an important criterion, given that the main purpose of quantitative research is to generalize to a wider population. However, every study will contain a degree of sampling error to the extent that results are never 100% representative of the population. Every sample will be slightly dissimilar from a subsequent sample drawn from the same population. There is no such thing as the 'perfect sample'.

Table 8.2 *Probability sampling – description, advantages and disadvantages*

Type of sample	Description	Advantages	Disadvantages
Simple random	■ Obtain sampling frame ■ Number members consecutively ■ Select sample through table of random numbers	■ Little knowledge of population required ■ Most unbiased of probability methods	■ Complete sampling frame essential ■ Time consuming ■ Expensive
Stratified	■ Divide into strata ■ Ascertain number of cases for each stratum ■ Randomly sample each subgroup	■ Assures certain characteristics of the population are represented ■ Increases probability of sample being representative by lowering sampling error	■ Requires complete sampling frame ■ Costly and time consuming to stratify lists ■ Statistics more complex
Proportionate	■ Sample is drawn so that each strata is equal to its proportion		
Disproportionate	■ Oversample a disproportionately small stratum to ensure they are represented and allow comparisons		
Systematic	■ Obtain sampling frame ■ Decide on sample size ■ Agree sampling interval ■ Select every (n)th element	■ Easy to select sample ■ Economical ■ Time saving and efficient	■ Bias in the form of non-randomness ■ After the first case is selected, population members do not have equal chance of selection
Cluster	■ Groups or 'clusters' are selected from population ■ Successive selections are made (region, district, hospital) ■ Random sampling from cluster	■ Economical ■ Useful when sampling frame unavailable. Characteristics of clusters can be estimated	■ Subjects may not accurately reflect characteristics of population and therefore generalization should be limited to the population of the clustering variable ■ Larger sampling error than other probability samples ■ Statistics are complex

There are a number of different ways of obtaining a probability sample. Four of the most common ways are discussed in this chapter:

- Simple random sampling
- Systematic sampling
- Stratified random sampling
- Cluster sampling.

An overview of these approaches and their advantages and disadvantages is shown in Table 8.2. Please note that the sampling techniques discussed under the headings of quantitative and qualitative sampling issues are concerned with the *identification* of respondents for studies. Later in the chapter I will consider other indications for sampling.

Simple random sampling

This method of probability sampling attempts to ensure that every person or every element in the population has an equal chance of being included in the study. The sample is deemed to be 'representative' and the findings generalizable. This method involves the selection, at random, of the required number of individuals for the sample from a list of the population (**sampling frame**). Once the sampling frame is obtained, individuals are assigned numbers consecutively. Then a random selection of the required number is made. Random numbers may be generated by using a lottery method (such as numbers being drawn out of a hat), random number tables or a computer. Many text books on statistics (e.g. Kirkwood 1988) contain random number tables. It is important to bear in mind that a researcher cannot select a simple random sample without a full and up-to-date list of the population. Plant and Foster (1993) used a random sample in their study of AIDS-related experience, knowledge, attitudes and beliefs amongst nurses in an area with a high rate of HIV infection (Box 8.2). The implications of this approach were that

Box 8.2
Example using random sampling

AIDS-related experience, knowledge, attitudes and beliefs amongst nurses in an area with a high rate of HIV infection

This study involved a cross-sectional survey of a **representative** sample of qualified nurses working in Lothian Region (**population**). Respondents were selected from current hospital staff lists (**sampling frame**) of medical, surgical and psychiatric nurses. Respondents were chosen for inclusion in the study using a **random number table (random sampling)**.

Sampling was organized to produce samples of 200 medical, 200 surgical and 200 psychiatric nurses at four levels of seniority.

Plant and Foster (1993)

the findings could be considered to be representative of nurses working in medical, surgical and psychiatric nursing in Lothian.

Systematic sampling

Simple random sampling can often be time consuming and laborious. Systematic sampling offers a simpler method of randomly selecting a sample. It involves the selection of every 'nth' case drawn from a sampling frame at fixed intervals, for example, every 'nth' patient on a waiting list for orthopaedic surgery or every 'nth' trained nurse on the ward 'off duty' list. However, for systematic sampling to fulfil the requirements of a probability sample, the population must be listed in a random order. To return to the example of ward off duty as a means of selecting a sample of nurses; if the population was listed in order of seniority starting with the sister, every 'nth' nurse selected would clearly not be random. Because of the non-random order of the 'off duty' list, bias would be introduced and, this in turn, would affect the external validity (generalizability) of the study. It is also important that the first element or member of the sample must be selected randomly. To do this, the researcher first divides the population (N) by the size of the desired sample (n) to obtain the sample interval width (k). The sampling interval is the distance between the elements selected for the sample. Supposing a researcher wishes to study a group of 50 practice nurses and knows from the sampling frame that there is a population of 500, the sampling interval would be as follows:

$$k = 500/50 = 10$$

Every tenth name on the list of practice nurses would be sampled. After the sampling interval has been set, the researcher would use a table of random numbers to obtain a starting point for the selection of the 50 subjects. As the population size in this case is 500 and a sample size of 50 is required, a number between 1 and 500 is randomly selected. If, for example, the number selected is 54, the practice nurse assigned number 54, 64, 74, and so forth would be included in the sample until 50 cases had been chosen.

Stratified random sampling

In stratified random sampling, the population is divided into smaller homogenous subgroups called strata, where members of the group share a particular characteristic (e.g. stratum A may be males and stratum B may be females). These characteristics are chosen for stratification based on the assumption that they will have an effect on the variables under study. The researcher then randomly samples within the strata. There are two ways of achieving this. The researcher may sample proportionately (in relation to the relative size of the stratum) or disproportionately. For example, if a patient population in a General Practice consisted of 10% Asians, 5% Afro-Caribbeans, and 85% Caucasians, then a proportional stratified sample of 100 patients, with ethnic background as the stratifying variable, would consist of 10, 5 and 85 patients from the respective sub-populations. Clearly it would be inappropriate to draw conclusions about the characteristics of Afro-Caribbeans based on only 5 cases. If comparisons are sought between strata of unequal membership size, as in this example, a disproportional sampling design would be appropriate. The sampling portions may be altered to ensure there is some representation of minority groups, even to the extent of including all members. Antonson and Robertson (1993) employed proportional stratified random sampling in their study of consumer-defined needs amenable to community nursing intervention (Box 8.3).

Box 8.3
Example using proportional stratified sampling

A study of consumer-defined needs amenable to community nursing intervention

This was a descriptive survey using postal questionnaires. The area surveyed constitutes one Scottish Health Board (**population**). The samples were selected by **proportional, stratified random sampling** using the Community Health Index.

Stratification variables were age (18–30, 31–43, 44–56, 57–69, 70 and over) and geographical area (urban, semi-rural, rural).

The sample size was determined by the need to allow for at least 25 members in the smallest stratum. A 50% response rate was estimated.

With these points in mind, a sample of 1770 was chosen, based on calculations to allow for:

- The population estimates within each stratum
- Estimated accuracy of sampling frame
- 5% standard error.

Details of non response were given in the report.

Antonson and Robertson (1993)

Cluster sampling

This involves dividing the population into a number of units, or clusters, each of which contains individuals with a range of characteristics. The clusters themselves are chosen on a random basis. To illustrate what is involved in cluster sampling, imagine that a researcher wishes to interview 100 nurse teachers in the UK. If the 100 names were chosen through a simple random sampling procedure, it is likely that the researcher would be confronted with the prospect of travelling around a vast geographically scattered sample in order to conduct the interviews. Clearly, this would not only be expensive and time consuming, it may also prove difficult or impossible to obtain a full list of the population (sampling frame). In cluster sampling, large groups or clusters make up the sampling units. If we imagine there are 100 nurse education centres in the UK, teachers within each site would be called a cluster. Ten sites or 'clusters' could be randomly selected and a random selection of ten teachers within each cluster could be taken. Because the sample is selected from clusters in two or more separate stages and involves sampling different geographical areas, this approach is sometimes known as multi-stage or area sampling. Malson et al (1996) used a multi-stage sampling technique to select study sites for in-depth case studies in a study of the impact of the NHS reforms on UK palliative care services.

Quota sampling

Although quota sampling is *not* a probability sample it shares some of the characteristics of stratified random sampling in that the first phase entails dividing the population into homogenous strata and selecting elements from each. The crucial difference lies in the procedure by which potential subjects from each stratum are secured. Whilst stratified random sampling involves a random sampling method of obtaining sample members, quota sampling obtains respondents through convenience samples.

Age, sex, designation or grade, religion, ethnicity, medical diagnosis, educational attainment and socioeconomic status are examples which are likely to be relevant stratifying variables in health care research. For example, if the researcher is interested in exploring whether the experience of managing an ileostomy is different for people depending on age and sex and a sample of 100 is desired, a quota of 25% elderly males, 25% elderly females, 25% young females and 25% young males may be set. This sampling strategy is considered inherently inferior in quantitative research as a way of guaranteeing a sample representative of the population (Sapsford and Abbott 1994) because it is not possible to calculate sampling error. Equally within a qualitative framework this sampling strategy is treated with caution since it selects a sample on the basis of predetermined criteria and hence reduces the inductive analytical power of naturalistic enquiry (Field and Morse 1985). However, in the absence of a full list of the population a quota sample at least ensures that various subgroups within the population are represented.

Summary

A 'sample' is the term given to any subset of a wider population under scrutiny. In quantitative studies the researcher will typically attempt to use a probability sample of some kind, to allow at least tentative generalization to a wider population. There are a number of ways in which probability samples can be drawn, each of which has its own particular strengths and weaknesses (see Table

8.2). Information on how a sample is identified is therefore of particular importance to the critical reader of quantitative research papers, as a failure to do this correctly can easily negate claims to 'generalizability' to any other population than the one under scrutiny.

Sampling in the qualitative domain

As described in previous chapters of this book, qualitative research seeks to explore and understand phenomena. Since the most appropriate and fruitful research subjects (or informants) may not be equally dispersed within a population, it is logical for researchers to make use of sampling techniques which allow them to identify those with the specific information they require. Also, since the basic purpose of qualitative inquiry is exploration and understanding, the researcher often does not know the boundaries of the research population at the outset. Accordingly, researchers often find that the most appropriate boundaries for the sample emerge during the process of data collection and analysis rather than being predetermined at the start.

De Poy and Gitlin (1994) describe the process of sampling within the qualitative domain as dynamic and inductive. The researcher often starts broadly and frequently samples all events and individuals within the sphere of interest. As fieldwork and interviewing progresses, the broad ideas, concepts and questions become more clearly defined and focused. Throughout this process the researcher is making decisions about who to interview and who and/or what to observe. The chosen sampling techniques need to be appropriate to the purpose of the study. The three main types of sampling are now considered:

■ Convenience
■ Purposive (including theoretical)
■ Snowball (network) sampling.

Convenience sampling

As the name implies, convenience sampling invites the most readily available people who meet the inclusion criteria to act as subjects in a study. The process of selecting participants is continued until the required sample size has been attained. This approach is also sometimes referred to as **volunteer**, **opportunistic** or **accidental sampling**. Researchers may perhaps rely on respondents already known to them or identify respondents through their membership in a group. For instance, a researcher interested in studying the experiences of women combining a nursing career with motherhood might begin by interviewing friends in this situation. He/she might also contact a self-help organisation such as the *Working Mothers' Association*, or advertise in the nursing press for respondents to contact them. Although there are limitations with this approach in terms of its ability to generalize to a wider population, it is sometimes the only feasible way of obtaining a sample. For example, it is not always possible (or indeed necessary) to identify the total population; problems may exist with respondent accessibility, time and money. There may also be ethical constraints. Ashworth and Hagan (1993) encountered some of these problems in a qualitative study of non-geriatric urinary incontinence sufferers (See Box 8.4).

Box 8.4
Example using convenience sampling

> *The meaning of incontinence: a qualitative study of non-geriatric urinary incontinence sufferers*
>
> This study examined the meaning of incontinence to 'non-geriatric' urinary incontinence sufferers and highlighted the difficulties in accessing a suitable sample.
>
> No sampling frame was available for such a group, and so interviewees were contacted through newspaper advertisements.
>
> In-depth qualitative interviews were conducted with 28 young or middle aged women who suffered urinary incontinence. The authors aimed at a sample:
>
> - Evenly divided between women aged 25–40 and 41–55
> - Made up of mothers with between one and four children
> - Divided between short-term (less than a year), mid-term (one to less than four years) and long-term duration
> - Composed of interviewees who had not sought professional help.
>
> An adequate sample was difficult to attract, giving weight to the idea that incontinence is a taboo subject. In this situation a convenience sample was the only option open to the researchers.

Ashworth and Hagan (1993)

It is useful to note that many studies undertaken by health professionals use convenience samples, even when the study is quantitative in orientation. This is particularly the case when research has been carried out in the pursuit of an academic qualification and so time and money have been at a premium. This does not *necessarily* negate the results of such studies. It does, however, place some doubt over their generalizability and this is something of which the critical reader should be aware.

Purposive sampling

Purposive sampling is also referred to as judgmental sampling and involves the 'hand-picking' of individuals by the researcher based on certain predefined criteria. As the name suggests, the researcher purposively chooses informants who are seen as able to add to, support or refute the developing theory in relation to the topic under investigation and thus provide the most relevant information in relation to the aims of the study. Initially the researcher may select a range of informants whose experience is broadly typical. Then as the study progresses, informants with more particular knowledge and experience are intentionally sought. For instance, if a researcher wished to conduct a study on experiences of pain in labour, he or she might begin by interviewing a cross section of women and then conduct more in-depth interviews with women who had experienced either a 'good' or 'bad' experience of pain relief during labour.

In a grounded theory approach to research (see Chapter 7, page 173), this type of sampling is known as **theoretical sampling** (Strauss and Corbin 1990). Theoretical sampling is the process of data collection for generating theory in which the researcher jointly collects, codes and analyzes data and decides what data to collect and who to collect it from, in order to develop his/her theory as it emerges. This type of sampling is based on the underlying assumption that the researcher has sufficient knowledge about the population of interest to choose specific subjects for the study. Melia (1987) used this approach to selecting a sample in her study of the socialization of student nurses. Mays and Pope (1995) provide an example of how theoretical sampling might work in relation to a study to explore how and why team work in primary health care is more or less successful in different general practices. In this hypothetical study theoretical sampling is proposed as the strategy of choice because some of the theoretically relevant characteristics of general practice affecting variations in team work, such as the frequency of opportunities for communication among team members and the local organization of services, are relevant to the research question. Though not statistically representative of general practices, such a sample is theoretically informed and relevant to the aim of the research, that is, to understand social processes. Purposive sampling is commonly used in nursing studies, and many examples exist in current published research. For example, Beedham and Wilson-Barnett (1993) used a combined strategy of both purposive and snowball sampling to evaluate the services for people with HIV/AIDS in an inner-city health authority, from a providers' perspective (Box 8.5). The main limitation of purposive sampling is that, since it relies on the researcher's knowledge of the population, bias may enter the selection process.

Box 8.5
*Example using
combined purposive
and snowball
sampling*

*Evaluation of services for people with HIV/AIDS in an inner city
health authority: perspective of key service providers*

This study used a cross-sectional design, the aim being to gather
largely qualitative data. The sample consisted of 47 key service
providers to people with HIV/AIDS in Camberwell. The key service providers comprised 16 representatives from hospital and
community health care teams, 7 from voluntary organisations
and 8 representatives of statutory and voluntary services for
intravenous drug abusers.

Respondents were selected both according to their ability to
provide useful and relevant information on the topics being
investigated and through **nomination** as 'experts' in the field by
other respondents.

The method therefore used the concepts of both **purposive sampling** and **snowball** or **network sampling**.

Beedham and Wilson-Barnett (1993)

*Snowball or
network sampling*

Another method of obtaining a convenience sample is through
snowball or network sampling. This method is also referred to as
nominated sampling. The researcher contacts one or two people 'in
the field' and once trust and rapport has been established, asks the
first respondent to nominate or introduce them to another person to
interview. In this way the sampling frame is built around social networks. This technique is particularly useful when the researcher is
regarded with suspicion by the population of interest. It is also a useful approach when there is difficulty in identifying members of the
population, for example when this is a clandestine group. As an illustration, suppose a researcher is interested in studying the health
needs of prostitutes or intravenous drug users, they might find it
impossible to access respondents other than through the use of a
snowball sample.

Summary

In qualitative research, the identification of a sample as representative as possible of the parent population is considered less of an
imperative than a sample which provides the information required
by the researcher. As a result, the qualitative researcher may not
identify the total population at the outset, not least because they
may not know what it is. Within such a system there is obviously
a concern about bias introduced by not *necessarily* using a sample which might provide a range of opinion. Three recognized
methods for sampling in the qualitative domain have been discussed in this section. The critical reader of qualitative research

papers must therefore ask themselves whether an unreasonable degree of bias has been introduced due to the requirement for the most relevant data to answer the research question. If the researcher has provided details of their sampling processes, this should not be difficult.

The critical reader also needs to be aware that it is not uncommon for researchers (particularly those new to research) to use non-probability sampling techniques in quantitative studies, yet attempt to generalize to wider populations, basically because they know no better. The editing and reviewing process leading up to publication is not so rigorous that such work is not published. A knowledge of how sampling affects the quality and range of the data collected, as well as the appropriateness of generalizing from that data, is therefore an imperative for anyone seeking to evaluate the rigour of a research project.

Sampling for other reasons

The different sampling techniques detailed so far have been concerned with identifying respondents or 'informants' for study. However, there are other aspects of sampling which are more concerned with ensuring that the researcher gains a 'truthful' or valid understanding of the phenomena being studied. These include:

- Time sampling
- Event sampling
- Setting sampling.

To some degree, these processes are relevant to research carried out in both the quantitative and qualitative domains.

Time sampling

Within any social organization, activities and events may alter and vary with time. Researchers have to consider the time dimensions in all field situations (Burgess 1991). Often it is necessary to sample activities and events that occur over a period of time, as well as activities or established routines that occur at particular hours in the day. Similarly, it might be appropriate to observe the research setting on different days of the week or even at different times of the year. Suppose a researcher was interested in exploring the experience of triage in an accident and emergency department. It would be likely that they would discover very different patterns of activity at different times of the week, for example, at weekends when patients do not have easy access to a GP. In time sampling, some rationale is used to select the time intervals during which data gathering takes place.

Event sampling

Within any research setting, the researcher typically has to make decisions about which events to observe. In order to obtain a comprehensive picture it may be necessary to sample discrete sets of events. These events have been described as the routine, the special and the untoward (Schatzman and Strauss 1973). For example, a study of liaison between community nurses and GPs may need to focus on:

■ Routine mechanisms for communication exchange (such as the weekly primary health care team meeting)
■ Special events when opportunistic liaison may take place (such as a one-off staff seminar)
■ Untoward or unplanned events (such as informal communications in car journeys when visiting patients).

McCann & McKenna (1993) used event sampling as a strategy to conduct an examination of touch between nurses and elderly patients in a continuing care setting in Northern Ireland (Box 8.6).

Both time sampling and event sampling can be random or non-random depending on the study aims and are often used in observational studies.

Box 8.6
Example using event sampling

> *An examination of touch between nurses and elderly patients in a continuing care setting in Northern Ireland*
>
> The aim of the study was to discover the amount and type of touch received by elderly patients from nurses, and to assess the elderly patients' perceptions of the touch given by nurses. The hospitalized elderly were chosen as the **target population** for the study as they were identified as a group particularly prone to sensory deprivation who receive the least amount of expressive touch. The **accessible population** was a group of elderly patients in a continuing care/rehabilitation ward in Northern Ireland.
>
> From the total number of 29 patients on the ward, 14 met the designated criteria of:
>
> ■ Being 65 years of age or more
> ■ Spending 2 weeks on ward prior to data collection
> ■ Having sufficient understanding to take part
> ■ Being orientated to time and place.
>
> **Event sampling** was deemed the most appropriate, as opposed to using a pre-set time frame. Observation data were collected over a period of 2 days, with a total of 16 hours being spent in observation. The subjects were chosen randomly. Direct non-participant observation was judged the best method for the observation of the 'touch episodes'.

McCann and McKenna (1993)

Sampling by
setting

It is important for researchers to select an appropriate setting for data collection as the situation has an effect upon the phenomena under study and the kind of data that can be gathered. For instance, if a researcher was attempting to describe relatives' involvement in patient care, it might be necessary to sample wards with different layouts and designs since the degree of privacy might be a factor influencing their decision to become involved in the care. Whether the researcher chooses to select one location (as in a single in-depth case study) or a number of locations (as in multiple case designs), decisions should be determined by the research aims and methodological framework underpinning the design (see Yin 1994 for a detailed discussion).

Qualitative studies are more likely to stress the setting and site of the research study. For example, ethnographic studies typically describe the informants, setting and context in great detail. The reason for this is that qualitative research is usually conducted in a naturalistic setting, and the study context in which the phenomenon of interest takes place is considered to be a part of the phenomenon itself (Field and Morse 1985). Field's (1989) study of nursing patients who were dying provides an excellent example of the importance of understanding contextual factors in order to understand phenomena.

I have so far concentrated on the reasons for selecting a sample and some of the ways in which that selection is made. After deciding on the approach, the next step is to decide on the sample size. Regardless of the research approach the issue of sample size is an important consideration, particularly as the optimum number of cases that should be included in the sample is one of the less well understood aspects of sampling.

Summary

To gain greater understanding of any phenomenon or concept involving human behaviour, it is often necessary to collect data from subjects at different times (time sampling), doing a range of different things (event sampling), in a range of settings. Evidence of these sampling processes is important if the results are to be considered valid and trustworthy.

What size of
sample?

One of the most commonly-held views by people new to research is that *the* most important thing is to have a large sample. Does sample size matter? And if it does, how do we decide whether a sample is big enough? There are no simple rules for determining the most appropriate sample size. Whilst a number of formulae are to be found in the literature (Armitage and Berry 1987) they do not produce conclusive answers. These formulae take into account factors, such as the level of confidence, which needs to be attained in the findings, the size of the population and the variability of the measures when they are applied to the study population (Atkinson 1991). Whilst decisions about sample size are often determined with scientific principles in mind, they have to be achieved within the practicalities of the real world. Broadly speaking, most researchers working within a positivist framework would agree that larger samples are more representative of the population than smaller samples. This is because the sampling error will decrease as the sample size increases. Whilst this is so, it must be remembered that a large sample cannot correct or compensate for a faulty sampling design or loosely formulated rationale. Equally, the suggestion that a larger sample is always better does not apply in studies where the type of sample is purposive or theoretical – quite the contrary, as too many informants could serve to cloud the issues and overcomplicate the complex process of analysis (Roberts and Ogden Burke 1989). For this reason, the number of informants is usually smaller than in quantitative studies. When deciding on a sample size a number of factors, both scientific and practical, need to be borne in mind:

■ Homogeneity of population
■ Orientation of the study
■ Type of analysis
■ Practical considerations.

Homogeneity of population

The homogeneity of the population also affects the sample size required. If individual subjects are very much alike in all variables other than the one being measured, a small sample may be sufficient. In other words, the more variability there is in the population, the larger the sample size indicated. If the researcher needs to be very precise in generalizing to the population based on sample data, a larger sample may be required to accurately represent the variability within the population and so add weight to their claims to generalizability.

Orientation of the study

The orientation of the study also has implications for the required sample size. If the research is qualitative in nature, then the sample size is guided by different rules than those for quantitative studies. When using a grounded theory approach, for example, the researcher continues asking questions until she or he is persuaded that a conceptual framework has emerged which is integrated and which explains the phenomena of interest, and that no new phenomena are emerging. In such studies the number of informants is not determined in advance as the researcher continues to collect data until no new information is forthcoming. This means that it is not possible to predict the required sample size at the outset. However, when presenting the final report, the researcher should describe and justify the final sample size. The critical reader should observe that this is in fact the case.

When probability sampling is used, it is possible to calculate the precise number of subjects needed by using a statistical procedure called **power analysis** (see Chapter 7, page 170). Henry (1990) gives an introduction to the topic, which is recommended if you wish to acquaint yourself with the theory and practice of this. However, it is a complex activity which usually requires the assistance of a statistician. It is not discussed further here.

Type of analysis   The type of analysis planned has a bearing on sample size, as does the number of strata or categories into which the data may be subdivided. If the intention is to tabulate information, respondents will need to be divided into different categories, for example, male and female. Figure 8.1 shows how the division of a relatively large sample of 84 people by only two variables (gender and team in which individuals work) can substantially reduce the sample size within each cell of a table. This has implications for analysis since a number of common statistical tests, such as the chi-squared test (χ^2), demand certain minimum cell frequencies.

Because qualitative data are more cumbersome and time consuming to manipulate and analyze, most qualitative studies are confined to a small sample. This does not mean that descriptions of the sampling strategy are any less important. Providing a clear and systematic account of the sampling strategy will allow readers to judge how trustworthy or rigorous the study is. Adequate sample size is generally determined through saturation (Glaser and Strauss 1967) and recurrent patterning, in which the researcher discovers that further participants give similar rather than dissimilar information.

Figure 8.1
Size of samples following division by two variables (gender and teams in which individuals work)

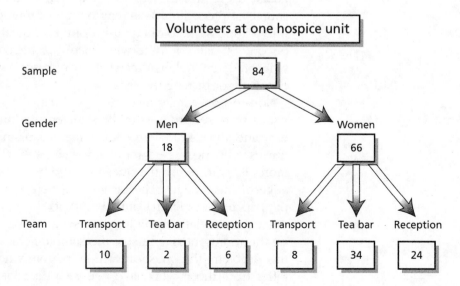

Practical considerations

Practical considerations, such as the length of time available to complete the study, the availability of respondents, and financial and human resources at the researcher's disposal, will invariably influence the size of the sample. Because of these constraints many nursing research studies are confined to small convenience samples. Even though these studies may be limited in terms of their ability to generalize to a wider population, they can generate valuable information if they are well planned and conclusions are consistent with the level of existing nursing knowledge.

Summary

It is clear that determining the sample size is an integral and complex part of any research study. The rationale used to determine an adequate size for the sample is linked to the homogeneity of the population, the purpose and design of the study and the type of analysis planned, as well as the practicalities of conducting research in the 'real world' of health care. Even if meticulous attention is given to the sampling plan, the *risk* of sample bias is always present and the reasons for this will now be discussed.

Sources of sampling bias

Whilst sampling error may occur by chance, sampling bias is something different, and although the terms are sometimes used interchangeably in the literature, the two concepts should be considered separately. Sampling bias is caused by the researcher and occurs when samples are not planned sufficiently carefully. A degree of bias will be present in all sampling strategies, either from procedural or personal reactivity. Procedural reactivity occurs if the procedures used distort or bias the data. These may include the time of day or year of data collection; the place the data were gathered; the language used; and the social circumstances of the subjects. Another source of procedural bias may be the sampling frame. Either it may prove impossible to obtain a list of the population or such a list may be out of date or otherwise incorrect. Personal reactivity occurs when the researcher affects the way responses are given, thereby distorting or biasing the data.

Non-response may also be a problem. For instance, if questionnaires were sent to a carefully selected random sample of nurses to examine their knowledge of primary nursing, it is possible that nurses who possessed more knowledge of these issues would be more likely to return the questionnaire than nurses with little knowledge of this subject. The basic issue here is that those who do not participate may differ from those who do. For this reason anything other than a relatively high response rate (over 65%) may cast doubts on the representativeness of the sample achieved. When faced with this problem, the question of how people who have not responded differ from those who have needs to be addressed. Robson (1993) suggests some ways in which researchers can tackle this crucial question. For example, in a postal survey it is possible to compare late returners of questionnaires with earlier ones, or those responding after one, or two, reminders with those responding without prompting. If the researcher knows some of the characteristics of the population it may be possible to check to see whether the sample obtained is reasonably typical of the population. In any survey where there is differential responding between categories (for example a low response rate from Afro-Caribbean males), a comparison can be made between their responses and those from other categories. However, there are no absolute solutions, only palliatives (Robson 1993).

Within a qualitative framework, the 'reluctant informant' can be likened to the non-responder in quantitative research. Some lack of response is inevitable but nevertheless a clear description of those refusing to participate in the study is important to the credibility of the research (Field and Morse 1985). Equally relevant is the use of the 'volunteer' as a potential research subject. Regardless of the type of sampling strategy, the ethics of health care research demand that subjects agree to participate in research voluntarily. Not all selected subjects will consent to participate, so there is a potential for bias.

Summary

Sampling bias occurs when a researcher fails to plan their sampling processes adequately. Having knowledge of how sampling *should* take place provides some protection for the critical reader of research. The important thing to remember is that bias will be present to some degree in any research project. The critical reader needs to be able to decide whether or not that bias can *reasonably* be seen to negate the conclusions and generalizations asserted from the findings.

Critiquing the sample

In many nursing investigations, the sampling plan is the weakest aspect of the study. You will usually find a section of the research report that describes the study sample, setting or site, population, or some combination of these terms, in varying degrees of depth. These research concepts are an integral component of the study and should be carefully and systematically made explicit by the researcher, regardless of the design or orientation of the research. Sampling is judged to be one important facet of the methodology and as such is generally presented in the 'methods' section of the report, although there may be a separate section on the sample. There are many examples of published guidelines for critiquing the sampling section of a research report (see for example, Burns and Grove 1993, Polit and Hungler 1991). These guidelines are generally comprehensive but some list up to 16 criteria for critiquing the sampling plan, rendering them impractical and unwieldy to apply in everyday practice. Five key criteria by which to critique the sampling plan are shown in Box 8.7. The following discussion will focus on these criteria.

Box 8.7
*Critiquing the
sampling plan*

- Is the population (target and accessible) and study setting clearly described?
- Does the type of sample fit with the overall purpose of the study and type of design?
- Is the sample size underpinned by a sound methodological and theoretical rationale which is clearly explained and justified?
- Are all known and probable sources of bias made explicit and minimized? Can you identify others which are not?
- Are the findings, conclusions and generalizations (if made) appropriate and consistent with the sampling strategy used?

Initially the parameters or characteristics of the study population and/or setting should be specified. This should include a description of the population and how it was identified and should state both the inclusion and exclusion criteria for the study.

Next, the sampling plan's appropriateness to the research design should be evaluated. When critiquing qualitative research designs, you should apply criteria related to sampling strategies that are relevant for the particular type of qualitative study. As we have seen, these are generally inductive and purposive. Equally, when critiquing quantitative research designs, you should apply criteria related to sampling strategies that are consistent with the type of design. These, as we have observed above, are commonly deductive. Lack of adherence to the principles of random selection in the case of quantitative designs jeopardizes the representativeness of the sample and thus the external validity of the study.

You will then be seeking to ensure that the sample size is appropriate within the external constraints imposed (e.g. ethical, financial, time). A clear theoretical and methodological rationale for the sample size should be given. In the case of quantitative studies, confirmation is needed that the assistance of a statistician has been sought, and that a power analysis has been undertaken if the study is evaluating an intervention. Pointing out both the attrition rate and non-response rate and examining the effects on the findings are also imperative to recognizing any limitations posed by the size of the sample. In qualitative designs, evidence that there are sufficient informants to describe and explain the phenomena (but not too numerous to obscure the issues) needs to be considered.

You will then need to consider if the researcher has made known any possible sources of bias, and what steps have been taken to minimize that bias. As we have seen, the strength of the probability sample resides in the reduction of sampling error and sampling bias to a known minimum. Inaccessible populations, unavailability of chosen sample, incomplete sampling frames and high attrition rates compound sampling biases. In qualitative studies researchers must maintain a delicate balance between using themselves as research instruments and ensuring that their views do not bias, lead, or inhibit the participants (Robinson and Thorne 1988). For this reason it is imperative that the researcher makes explicit her/his background and credentials.

Finally, and perhaps most important, are the issues of consistency of findings and conclusions with the sampling strategy used. In other words, how restrained is the researcher about the inferences and conclusions drawn from the data and is there recognition of the limitations of the study (bearing in mind that there is no such thing as the 'perfect sample')? In the case of quantitative studies, how reliable (consistent), valid (true) and therefore generalizable are the findings from the sample to the population? For qualitative studies, these criteria can be considered as analogous to transferability, credibility, confirmability and truth value (see Leininger 1985). These issues are also discussed in Chapter 6. In the real world of health research it may not be feasible or indeed appropriate to fulfil all these criteria. Possibly more relevant is that you remain alert to claims that cannot be substantiated.

Chapter conclusion

In this chapter we have seen that sampling considerations are central to the research process no matter what research strategy or investigatory technique is used. Each sampling strategy has different advantages and limitations, so each is best suited to a specific type of study aim and design. In many nursing studies, the sampling plan is the weakest facet of the study design. The sampling plan therefore warrants particular scrutiny because if it is flawed in some way, the findings and conclusions may be misleading. For this reason it is important that research consumers have an understanding of both the process of sampling and the rationale behind the sampling plan. They will then be able to make sound judgments on the rigour of the research and the applicability of the findings to health care practice.

Exercise 8.1

Consider how each of the following sampling techniques might introduce bias into a study design:

- Convenience sampling
- Purposive sampling
- Stratified random sampling
- Quota sampling.

Further reading Atkinson I (1992) Survey design and sampling. In Cormack D (ed) *The Research Process in Nursing*. Oxford: Blackwell Scientific Publications.

The discussion focuses primarily on sampling in survey research and emphasizes sampling in the quantitative domain.

Burgess RG (ed) (1991) *Elements of Sampling in Field Research. Field Research: a Sourcebook and Field Manual*. London: Routledge.

Contains a series of chapters on sampling in field research. This text takes the form of a book of readings which bring together styles of field research used principally by researchers in sociology and anthropology.

DePoy E and Gitlin L (1994) *Introduction to Research: Multiple Strategies for Health and Human Services*. St Louis, MO: Mosby.

See Chapter 12 for a comprehensive account of boundary setting and sampling and domain selection. Equal attention is given to sampling in both quantitative and qualitative designs. Well illustrated with examples from practice.

Hammersley M and Atkinson P (1989) *Ethnography: Principles in Practice*. London: Routledge.

See Chapter 2 for a detailed consideration of sampling in ethnographic research. Sampling within cases, time, people, and context are considered.

Strauss A and Corbin J (1990) *Basics of Qualitative Research: Grounded Theory Procedures and Techniques*. Newbury Park, DC: Sage.

The eleventh chapter provides a useful, systematic and practical account of theoretical sampling with reference to grounded theory.

Yin RK (1994) *Case Study Research: Design and Methods,* 2nd edn. Applied Social Research Methods Series, Volume 5. Thousand Oaks CA: Sage.

Chapter 2 provides a detailed appraisal of sampling logic in case study research and evaluation.

References

Antonson M and Robertson C (1993) A study of consumer defined needs amenable to community nursing intervention. *Journal of Advanced Nursing* **18**: 1617–1625.

Armitage P and Berry G (1987) *Statistical Methods in Medical Research*, 2nd edn. Oxford: Blackwell Scientific Publications.

Ashworth P and Hagan M (1993) The meaning of incontinence: a qualitative study of non-geriatric urinary incontinence sufferers. *Journal of Advanced Nursing* **18**: 1415–1423.

Atkinson I (1991) Survey and Sampling. In Cormack D (ed) *The Research Process in Nursing*. Oxford: Blackwell Scientific Publications.

Beedham H and Wilson-Barnett J (1993) Evaluation of services for people with HIV/AIDS in an inner-city health authority: perspective of key service providers. *Journal of Advanced Nursing* **18**: 69–79.

Burgess RG (ed) (1991) *Elements of Sampling in Field Research. Field Research: a Sourcebook and Field Manual*. London: Routledge.

Burns N and Grove SK (1993) *The Practice of Nursing Research: Conduct, Critique and Utilization*, 2nd edn. Philadelphia, PA: WB Saunders.

Depoy E and Gitlin L (1994) *Introduction to Research: Multiple Strategies for Health and Human Services*. St Louis, MO: Mosby.

Field PA and Morse JM (1985) *Nursing Research: The Application of Qualitative Approaches*. London: Croom Helm.

Field D (1989) *Nursing the Dying*. London: Tavistock/Routledge.

Glaser and Strass (1967). *The Discovery of Grounded Theory:* strategies for qualitative research. Chicago: AVC.

Henry GT (1990) *Practical Sampling*. Newbury Park, DC and London: Sage.

Kirkwood BR (1988) *Essentials of Medical Statistics*. Oxford: Blackwell Scientific Publications.

Leininger MM (ed) (1985) Qualitative Research Methods in Nursing. Orlando, FL: Grune & Stratton.

McKann K and McKenna H (1993) An examination of touch between nurses and elderly patients in a continuing care setting. *Journal of Advanced Nursing* **18**: 838–846.

Malson H, Clark D, Small N and Mallett K (1996) Impact of the NHS reforms on UK Palliative Care Services. *European Journal of Palliative Care* **3**(2) 68–71.

Mays N and Pope C (1995) Rigour and qualitative research. *British Medical Journal* **331**: 109–112.

Melia K (1987) *Learning and Working*. London: Tavistock.

Plant M and Foster J (1993) AIDS-related experience, knowledge, attitudes and beliefs amongst nurses in an area with a high rate of HIV infection. *Journal of Advanced Nursing* **18**: 80–88.

Polgar S and Thomas S (1993) *Introduction to Research in the Health Sciences*, 2nd edn. Melbourne: Churchill Livingstone.

Polit DF and Hungler B (1991) *Nursing Research: Principles and Methods*, 4th edn. Philadelphia, PA: Lippincott.

Roberts CA and Ogden Burke S (1989) *Nursing Research: A Quantitative and Qualitative Approach*. Boston: Jones and Bartlett.

Robinson CA and Thorne SE (1988) Dilemmas of ethics and validity in qualitative nursing research. *The Canadian Journal of Nursing Research* **20**: 65–76.

Robson C (1993) *Real World Research: A Resource for Social Scientists and Practitioner Researchers*. Oxford: Blackwell Scientific Publications.

Sapsford R and Abbott P (1994) *Research Methods for Nurses and the Caring Professions*. Buckingham: Open University Press.

Schatzman L and Strauss AL (1973) *Field Research: Strategies for a Natural Sociology*. Englewood Cliffs, NJ: Prentice Hall.

Strauss A and Corbin T (1990) *Basics of Qualitative Research: Grounded Theory Procedures and Techniques*. Newbury Park, DC: Sage.

Yin RK (1994) *Case Study Research: Design and Methods*, 2nd edn. Applied Social Research Methods Series, Vol 5. Thousand Oaks, CA: Sage.

9 Critiquing ethical issues in published research

Liz Matthews, Angela Venables

Introduction

Health care research raises many questions about what is right or wrong, good or bad, what is acceptable or not acceptable. With advances in health care technology, doctors and professionals in allied fields can aid conception, manipulate the human gene pool and breed animals with transgenic qualities (Carlin 1995) thus providing the possibility of a brave new world where disease is conquered, people live longer and suffer less. Although such pursuits may in themselves appear worthy, the route taken to solve such problems can at times be perceived by the general public to be unacceptable, thus raising the question 'should we do this?' rather than 'can we do this?'

The question 'should we do this?' has been debated at length in the media about the use of animal organs such as pigs' kidneys in human transplantation. Certainly by allowing such research, lives may be saved or improved by increasing the number of organs available for transplant. However, some groups in society find this solution unacceptable from a religious or moral perspective. The question 'can we do this?' is essentially concerned with identifying and solving the potential and actual consequential risks of such procedures and the scientific problems associated with the process. For instance, if we transplant the organs of an animal into a human, will this result in the possibility of transferring potentially dangerous bacteria or viruses from one species (pigs) to another (man)? If we do, what are the possible long-term implications for that individual and indeed society?

In general terms, health care research is perceived as being an overall good, providing benefits for society at large. However, the history of health care research illustrates how the pursuit of such an overall 'good' can be abused and manipulated by a minority of researchers. Detailed examples of such abuses are described by Beecher (1966), Pappworth (1968) and Pence (1990). The abuses of research participants have resulted in the formation of international and national guidelines designed to reduce this risk (see Appendix). However, the question remains – do readers of research need to consider whether the findings of 'unethical' studies should be used at all

See Appendix: *British guidelines on ethics and research*, page 229 when forming a body of scientific knowledge? Opinion appears to be divided on this point. One argument is that since data from such studies is available we should use it, no matter what circumstances were used to collect it. The other argument is that by accepting such data we in some way condone the action of the researchers who obtained it in questionable circumstances.

The introduction of local research ethics committees (LRECs) across the United Kingdom (DoH 1991) has provided a screening system by which ethically questionable studies requiring access to patients and clients of health services can be sifted out before they start. This may lead the critical reader of research to surmise that published research is ethical because of the degree of scrutiny it has endured during the process from its original inception to its publication. However, a number of authors identify diversity of practice in the approval process for research which may result in the same study being approved by the LREC in one district health authority but not in another. While (1995), for example, describes the variation she experienced when gaining approval for a multicentred study focusing on the needs and provision of care to children who might be expected to die during childhood. Oakley (1992) highlights similar problems in the USA during the process of gaining approval for a multicentred study of social support and motherhood. The screening processes provided by LRECs are therefore fallible and the assumption that all published research is ethically sound is questionable, given the degree of variation and subjective appraisal of LRECs during the approval process. Consequently the critical reader of research needs a basic understanding of ethical principles and their application to health care research in order to evaluate the ethical implications of studies.

The challenge for health workers

The critical reader of research requires sufficient knowledge of ethical principles to be able to decide for him or herself whether a research project has been carried out in an ethical manner. This requires some insight into ethical theories which can inform and solve the ethical dilemmas associated with research. This chapter describes one particular ethical framework which will aid the reader of published research to draw their own conclusions about the integrity of a study. This is the Four Principles and Scope of Application approach advanced by Beauchamp and Childress (1989) and Gillon (1994). Each of the four ethical principles is discussed in relation to different research designs, highlighting the inherent ethical implications. Issues are highlighted concerning each principle, which can then be applied to hypothetical research examples at the end of the chapter. A fundamental point to recognize is that a research project which is completely sound in ethical terms is very hard to achieve and so is very hard to find. The aim must be to establish that the researcher has done all in their power to protect the rights of their research subjects, balanced against the need for rigour in the processes followed.

Key issues

■ The ethical nature of research
■ Research and promoting respect for autonomy
■ Beneficence and non-maleficence and research
■ Justice and research
■ Critical appraisal of the ethical issues in research reports

Ethical principles transcend research approaches

There are many issues to consider in an evaluation of the ethical component of published research. Variations in research approaches mean that quantitative designs may raise ethical difficulties not apparent in qualitative designs and vice versa. However, similar questions should be asked about ethical issues in research, irrespective of the approaches used during the research process.

Unfortunately, it may be difficult to consider the ethical issues within published work, as information on ethical considerations tends to focus on how the researcher overcame ethical problems which they themselves identified. The information needed to establish whether the researcher systematically considered *all* potential difficulties and took appropriate action to enable them to act ethically is often inadequate or even missing.

To be able to evaluate the ethical aspects of research, the critical reader needs to decide whether the researcher has considered all the ethical dilemmas which can be associated with the project. A straightforward approach to this task is provided by the Four Principles plus Scope of Application approach advocated by Beauchamp and Childress (1989) and Gillon (1994). This framework provides a 'simple, accessible and culturally neutral approach' (Gillon 1994) to inform the evaluation of the ethical dimensions of research reports.

The Four Principles plus Scope of Application approach

The Four Principles plus Scope of Application approach is a complete moral theory in itself encompassing the application of various rules or principles that should be upheld. Beauchamp and Childress (1989) and Gillon (1994) claim that whatever our personal philosophy, politics, religion, moral theory or life stance, we will find no difficulty in committing ourselves to four *prima facie* (absolute) moral principles (Gillon 1994). *Prima facie* refers to those principles which ought to be upheld in any situation. Should any one of those principles be breached, clear justification for that action must be provided if an act is to be perceived as morally justifiable. The remaining principles must also be upheld.

The four *prima facie* moral principles are:

- Respect for autonomy (the obligation to respect the decision-making capacities of autonomous people)
- Beneficence (the obligation to provide benefits and balance these benefits against risks)
- Non-maleficence (the obligation to avoid causing harm)
- Justice (the obligation of fairness in the distribution of benefits and risks).

The approach does not provide a method for ranking these principles in order of importance but it can help health care workers make decisions about moral issues when critically appraising published research. As a result, this model provides a set of moral commitments, a common moral language and a common set of moral issues (Gillon 1994)

The following discussion examines the four principles along with their scope of application when reading published research. Autonomy and justice are considered separately. Beneficence and non-maleficence are discussed together for ease of explanation and brevity.

Autonomy

Respect for persons incorporates at least two fundamental ethical considerations in research, namely:

- *respect for autonomy – which requires that those who are capable of deliberation about their personal choices should be allowed to exercise their capacity for self determination; and*
- *the protection of persons with impaired or diminished autonomy, which requires that those who are dependent or vulnerable be afforded security against abuse.*

(Council for International Organizations in Collaboration with World Health Organization 1993: 10)

The need for research subjects to have a choice about whether or not they participate in a research study is a fundamental obligation in relation to respect for autonomy (Beauchamp and Childress 1989) and this is a question that should be asked in any research critique. However, it is debatable whether, in the context of research, choice or consent can be ever be fully informed in practice. Silverman (1989) argues that the obligation to uphold the primacy of informed consent to participate in research studies should be no different to the notion of the patient who consents for any health care intervention.

However, there are differences in practical terms between gaining consent for treatment to gaining consent to participate in a research study.

Consent to treatment differs from consent to participate in research

Consent to treatment indicates that a patient is accessing that treatment for their own benefit. For example, they may undergo diagnostic tests because of symptoms they have experienced, or treatment to alleviate symptoms or cure disease. Whatever the reason, the patient has something to gain from consenting (Association of Community Health Councils (ACHC) 1990).

Consent to participate in research is different, in the sense that the researcher usually wants something from the patient. The purpose of the consent approach is also different in that researchers need the research subjects to participate and so need to provide the relevant information to enable them to reach an informed decision (ACHC 1990). This is important as it may mean that they agree to participate in clinical trials where outcomes are uncertain; for example, to test new drug regimens, to identify adverse effects, or evaluate new treatments to determine their effectiveness. In qualitative research projects they may be asked to explore sensitive and emotive topic areas such as feelings about a partner's sudden death, or experiences of a life-threatening disease (Cowles 1988, Ramos 1989).

Whatever the reason, a research subject is to some degree being used as a 'means to an end'. In practical terms the result is that tighter controls are applied to the process of gaining consent from individuals who are participating in research studies, when compared with the processes of gaining consent from people to participate in health care interventions.

There are a number of issues to be considered when evaluating the autonomy of research subjects. These can be broadly categorized along the following dimensions identified by Faden and Beauchamp (1986):

- Disclosure and non-disclosure of information
- Understanding
- Voluntariness.

We consider it necessary to explore the notion of veracity (truth-telling) under the heading of disclosure and non-disclosure of information, as a cornerstone of the relationship between the professional and the patient/client is the existence of trust. Such trust is dependent upon the idea that professionals will tell the truth. Bok (1984) identifies that health care professionals are the only group afforded the privilege of withholding information from their patients, as the motive behind such an action could be justified as being in the patient's best interests. In research, if we cannot rely on the truthfulness of the researcher, we cannot rely upon the body of knowledge generated by that research, which in turn underpins clinical practice.

The concept of 'broad consent'

Legally, the gaining of broad consent is necessary in both treatment and research situations (NHSME 1990), in that the individual needs to be aware that they:

- Have the choice to refuse to participate
- Can withdraw from treatment or the study at any particular stage which they (rather than the clinician or researcher) identify
- Can refuse or withdraw without fear of any form of retribution or punishment.

Broad consent also implies an autonomous deliberate judgment on the basis of sufficient and comprehensible information (Neuberger 1992). In health research, fairly tight controls mean that the researcher must demonstrate to an independent body (the LREC) the process of gaining consent to participate in a research study before the study begins. This allows scrutiny of the process to determine whether respect for persons will be upheld.

In practical terms this means that a researcher must produce and use a consent form (Neuberger 1992). The consent form should ensure that potential subjects know that they are participating in a research study as opposed to a normal treatment (NHSME 1990), are over the age of 18 years (Dimond 1990) and have the capacity to understand the information given to them (Faden and Beauchamp 1986). The researcher must also provide a written protocol which specifies in advance both the individual characteristics required within the sample group to be studied and what, in precise terms, will happen to each participant during the study (ACHC 1990). Every published research report should include a clear description of the way in which subjects have consented to participate. There should also be an indication that the study was approved by an independent review body (usually the LREC), as this indicates that the process of gaining consent has been scrutinized.

Disclosure/non-disclosure of information

A research report should indicate that approval was gained from an independent review body (LREC) and that consent to participate was gained from each respondent. In itself this would indicate that the respondents were made aware of the fact that they were part of a research study. However, as a critical reader it is important to consider whether the researcher has disclosed the information necessary to enable subjects to make an informed choice. For example, to encourage participation a researcher might selectively control information given to potential subjects. To a certain degree this can be justified by the application of the doctrine of therapeutic privilege – to disclose all the known risks may induce too much anxiety or distress for the respondent. Thus, a researcher may be allowed to determine what is in the respondent's interests to know concerning reasonable risks (NHSME 1990).

Another justification for the selective withholding of information is that the purpose of the study may be to identify unknown risks. In such cases the risk is assumed not to be expected and therefore need not be disclosed. This aspect will be discussed later in this chapter.

See *Beneficence and non-maleficence*, page 214

When considering the selective disclosure of information, some research methods are more vulnerable than others in relation to the manipulation of information. These methods include experimental treatments such as previously untried surgical procedures (e.g. various forms of organ transplantation, Pence 1990), epidemiological studies which monitor the natural progress of diseases such as the Tuskagee Study (Burns and Grove 1993) and the cervical dysplasia study described by Paul (1988), as well as comparative studies of treatment within randomized controlled trials, such as the management of screening detected ductal carcinoma in situ as discussed by Thornton (1993).

In such research the type of information given by the researcher to the respondent may be biased towards the positive aspects of the study, with the negative aspects underemphasized (Pence 1990). Ideally, written *and* verbal information should be provided to ensure that a balanced explanation is given. Since all written information for participants in a study should be evaluated in advance by the LREC, there is some degree of control of selective disclosure of information. A further safeguard would be for an independent observer to be present during the consent interview. This person may be a relative, a health care worker, in research involving children or persons with mental health or learning difficulties, or a legal guardian (Neuberger 1992, Dimond 1990, Mencap 1989). The critical reader should be alert to evidence of the presence or absence of such mechanisms in research reports.

Another indicator of good practice is that consent is obtained from the respondent before their enrolment within the study. This allows the respondent time to reflect on the information given. A minimum reflection time of 24 hours should be allowed by the researcher to give the person time to think about and formulate questions they may wish to raise about the study and their participation in it (Pence 1990).

Selective non-disclosure

Veracity and disclosure/non-disclosure of information is also associated with the imparting of filtered information by the researcher to the respondent. In such instances, consideration must be given to whether planned, intentional non-disclosure of information to research participants is ever acceptable. Some examples of the types of research design which may consider this acceptable are randomized controlled trials, trials involving the use of placebos, and 'blind' experiments where deception is considered acceptable (even necessary) in an attempt to compensate for, or reduce, possible bias. Similarly, in social and behavioural research complete disclosure of information may jeopardize the study in that the participants may alter their behaviour to that which they think the researcher requires. This is often referred to as a socially desirable response (Burns and Grove 1993, Polit and Hungler 1989). The important question for an individual study is how acceptable is the degree of non-disclosure?

In randomized clinical trials there is no justification for failing to disclose that the research design includes the use of placebos or a non-treatment group. Similarly, there is no justification for failing to disclose the method of assignment to an arm of such a trial (Neuberger 1992, Beauchamp and Childress 1989). This is because it is only with such information that research respondents can give consent to participate which is truly informed. However, this only supplies them with the information needed to decide whether or not to participate. It is not necessary to inform them of the arm of the trial to which they have been assigned (Neuberger 1992), for example control or therapy.

Beauchamp and Childress (1989: 99) identify that deception may be acceptable in research if the following criteria are adhered to:

- Deception is essential in order to obtain important information
- No substantial risk is attached
- Other moral principles are not violated such as autonomy or beneficence/non-maleficence
- Subjects are informed that deception is part of the study before they consent to participate.

When deception is used, the risks to the respondent should be minimal and outweighed by the expected benefits. One of the classic psychological experiments which has been heavily criticised for the degree of deception used by the researcher is Stanley Milgramme's study of obedience (Faden and Beauchamp 1986). To reduce the social response bias Milgramme deliberately lied to the respondents about the aim of the research study. Respondents were informed that the study was to explore the respondent's ability to recall information during times of stress when in fact the study was designed to explore the respondents' willingness to comply to authority. The consequences of Milgramme's action to deceive have meant that the findings from this study are open to constant criticism from his peers, at least from an ethical perspective.

Understanding   In the context of negotiating consent to participate in research, it is necessary to consider not only the extent of disclosure of information, but also whether that information was understood by the potential research subject. In a classic article, Beecher (1966) concludes that ordinary patients will not knowingly risk their health or their life merely for the sake of science. In studies associated with high and/or substantial risks, one indication that respondents may not have understood the significance of those risks is a high rate of agreement to participate. When this occurs it may suggest that understanding was insufficient to support the notion of informed consent, or that these risks were not disclosed – otherwise it is likely that fewer people would have agreed to participate.

At this point, it is important to acknowledge that the assessment of the respondent's degree of understanding is as difficult in research as it is in clinical practice. Improved information sheets and good communication skills may not necessarily mean that all patients understand what is said to them (Neuberger 1992). Certain individuals and within-sample populations are particularly vulnerable in this respect. Vulnerable populations include:

- Ethnic minority groups (especially where English is a second language)
- Children (especially neonates)
- Individuals with mental health problems
- Individuals with learning difficulties
- Individuals from lower socioeconomic groups[1].

A person's capacity to understand the information given to them is linked to their level of cognitive competence (Faden and Beauchamp 1986). With regard to broad consent, competence becomes a gatekeeper. In other words, if individuals are regarded as incompetent, they cannot give broad consent. In health care practice, the decision as to who is competent or not competent is determined by the physician. In research, it is often the case that the decision about who is competent or not competent to give consent to participate in research is determined by the researcher (Faden and Beauchamp 1986) under the guidance of the relevant research ethics committee. This can result in ethical as well as legal problems for more vulnerable respondents, such as children and people with mental health problems or learning difficulties. For individuals with mental illness, it is considered unethical to presume they do not have the capacity to make a competent decision (Royal College of Psychiatrists 1990) and therefore are unable to give consent to participate. In this instance the doctrine of respect for persons is applied. However, in

---

1. Years in education is recognized as a more reliable indicator of understanding than social stratification (Dalla-Vorgia et al 1992).

cases of non-therapeutic research, one must consider whether those people who are deemed to have a reduced capacity to make a competent decision should be participating in any case – a point which applies to individuals from any vulnerable group.

In this instance therapeutic research is defined as that which will in some way have expected but not assured benefits for the individual respondent. This may mean an improvement in their quality of life in either a physical or a psychological sense.

Eighteen years of age is used as a chronological indicator of maturity for competence to broad consent to participate in research studies (Dimond 1990). However, guidelines from the British Paediatric Association (1992) indicate that a child from the age of seven years may make a competent decision about whether to participate in a research study. From an ethical perspective, researchers should involve the parent or legal guardian of a child in the consent process. However, it is considered unethical for the parents' views to override that of the child if the child does not want to participate (British Paediatric Association 1992). Since most children want to please their parents, the difficulties with this issue remain complex. Such issues have resulted in discussions as to whether children should participate in non-therapeutic research studies at all (Neuberger 1992, Dimond 1990).

Voluntariness

When respondents participate in a research study, there is an assumption that they are doing so of their own free will and are not coerced into the process by force or threat or by monetary or material gain (Pence 1990). In some instances, healthy volunteers may be paid a nominal sum of money (for instance when testing a new vaccine) in early clinical trials. However, any monetary gain must be seen as that which would *not* greatly influence their decision to participate. It should be noted that coercion to participate may be implied by psychological perception rather than physical threat or material gain. The respondent may believe that by participating in the research they may have their chances of a positive health outcome enhanced (Neuberger 1992, Pence 1990) or at least avoid the negative implications of being viewed as uncooperative.

The relationship between the researcher and the respondent can be of particular importance in certain areas of enquiry. In educational research for instance, projects may involve accessing a 'convenient' sample of respondents who are enrolled on an educational programme managed by the researcher. As a result there may be a fear of reprisal if prospective respondents do not participate and this may influence their decision to take part in the study. In turn this may influence the nature of the respondents and hence the data obtained within the study. For example, respondents wishing to find favour with the lecturer may be the ones who volunteer and who may give socially desirable answers to any questions asked (Hughes 1990).

Some issues associated with voluntariness can be difficult to overcome within the context of a particular study, given the nature of the study and the characteristics of the respondents. For example, studies which test new drugs or treatments which may reduce mortality and morbidity can influence the voluntariness of participants. Patients may feel that the only way to access a particular drug or treatment is to volunteer to participate in a research study (Walley and Barton 1995). This may mean that a researcher is overwhelmed by volunteers wishing to participate. In such studies clear criteria need to be identified with regard to who will or will not be selected and why. This allows the researcher to demonstrate that groups or individuals have been selected fairly and that they are not favouring one individual or group over another. This issue will be discussed later in the chapter.

See *Justice*, page 218

The characteristics of some individuals may mean that they have unrealistic expectations about the benefits of participating in a study. For example, they may wish to participate with the false hope of a cure or may be so desperate to improve the quality of their lives that they underestimate the risks involved with participation. To reduce this possibility, researchers must be able to demonstrate that they have not misled participants. This can be achieved by providing clear information sheets identifying the risks and benefits and involving a third party in the consenting process.

Summary

When evaluating published research in relation to the principle of autonomy, consideration should be given to the idea of broad consent, the degree of information disclosed to the research participants and whether the individuals or groups involved were likely to have understood the information given. If there was selective non-disclosure of information, it is important to consider whether this was justifiable. The relationship between the researcher and the respondent should also be considered to determine whether this could have affected the voluntariness of the respondent.

Beneficence and non-maleficence

In the context of research, beneficence and non-maleficence refer to the ethical obligation to maximize benefits and to minimize harm.

This principle gives rise to norms requiring that the risks of research be reasonable in the light of expected benefits, that the research design be sound, and that the investigators be compe-

tent both to conduct the research and to safeguard the welfare of the research subjects. Beneficence further proscribes the deliberate infliction of harm on persons; this aspect of beneficence is expressed as a separate principle – non-maleficence (to do no harm)'

(Council for International Organizations in Collaboration with World Health Organization 1993: 10)

In this section we consider the issues of risk/benefit ratios and inclusion/exclusion criteria as they are generally perceived – in terms of societal benefit.

The risk–benefit ratio

The terms beneficence and non-maleficence are used to describe the idea of maximizing benefits and minimizing harm (Beauchamp and Childress 1989). In research these terms are often applied in what is known as the risk–benefit ratio. Research ethics committees seek to evaluate risks and benefits by considering the balance of overall benefit that may be accrued to society by the outcome of the research. This involves an evaluation of the associated risks for individual respondents and, to a lesser degree, the risks to society in general. Within health care, the intention of research is generally perceived in terms of societal benefit – the outcome of any study should increase medical, nursing or social knowledge in some way. Advancing the expertise and knowledge base of these disciplines may directly or indirectly improve health care delivery and health care outcomes. However, it is unlikely to benefit individual respondents participating in the research. This is especially so in non-therapeutic (descriptive) research.

In practical terms the main problem when considering the risk–benefit ratio of a study is the subjectivity in deciding what is defined as a minimal risk to that of a substantial risk. Baum *et al* (1989) define minimal risk as the level of risk that would normally occur within the individual's own social environment. In other words, risks which would be comparable to the treatment regimen the individual would be prescribed in 'normal' circumstances. Substantial risk, on the other hand, would be defined as that which could cause death or hospital admission, or dramatically alter the individual's quality of life (ACHC 1990) when this would not normally be expected.

Risk can also be associated with the degree of pain experienced by a subject, or, as in psychological studies, the degree of distress. Qualitative studies which seek to explore and describe respondents' feelings or experiences of illness or bereavement may also cause distress. In such cases psychological harm may be caused, as the researcher may ask probing questions which force respondents to confront areas of personal trauma they would rather not revisit.

Cowles (1988) reflects on this issue in discussing her research which involved interviews with adult relatives of homicide victims during the first four months following the murder. She suggests that ethical issues commonly considered by individual researchers and ethics committees may not be enough to evaluate the moral appropriateness of the research, which tends to be compared against the risks and benefits associated with scientific values. More practical concerns need to be considered, such as the degree of emotional response and the impact this may have on both the researcher and subject. It should also be acknowledged that such research can be viewed as helpful or even therapeutic by some research subjects. For example, Crookes (1996) found that a number of the bereaved nurses he interviewed in a study of personal bereavement in nurses were grateful for the opportunity to tell their story. For some it was the first time they had been given the chance to do so.

Strategies for maintaining objectivity and making decisions about what information may be too personal to use as data, need to be identified before the study begins, as well as during the study. Certainly in studies requiring observational data collection, the researcher needs to establish when they would intervene if it appeared that the situation was in danger of harming the subject in some way. Ramos (1989) suggests that in this instance the researcher becomes the subject's advocate, in that they are acting in their interests by protecting them from harm.

The researcher's obligation is to respect the privacy of participants and uphold confidentiality. This aspect is exemplified by the notion of promise-keeping between the researcher and the participant. However, it is important for the researcher to consider in advance any aspects of the study which may mean that they (the researcher) would need to breach confidentiality in order to protect members of the public. For example, although the researcher must be able to assure the participant that information is confidential, what if the participant discloses information that, if not acted upon, may endanger other individuals? In such instances, clear boundaries must be established between the researcher and the participant and the action that would be taken if sensitive situations arise should be made explicit.

In epidemiological research, the risks associated with observing patterns or the nature of a disease process mean that criteria for withdrawing respondents from a study should be identified before the study begins. The research question may consider the natural course of a disease such as syphilis (Tuskagee study, Pence 1990), or cervical dysplagia (Paul 1988). In such circumstances, it is important to determine in advance the percentage or number of respondents needed to progress to a given point in the disease process in order to answer the question posed by the research.

Inclusion and exclusion criteria

When reading published papers it is important to consider whether the author has taken into account the up-to-date knowledge base associated with a particular research question. This should be addressed within the literature review and in turn should establish the criteria for exclusion and withdrawal of the respondents involved in the study, as well as justifying the continuing inclusion of subjects within the study. Criteria for inclusion and exclusion of research respondents are also relevant when considering the risks and benefits associated with clinical trials and randomization as already discussed.

Neuberger (1992) discusses the problems of patients understanding the concept of randomization. This method of selection may be perceived as unfair if the trial is considered to have great benefits to the individuals involved in the 'experimental' group. Individuals may wish only to participate in those areas of the study that they perceive to be in their interests. Consent to participate in randomized controlled trials can therefore be problematic from both the researcher's and respondent's perspectives. Neuberger (1992) identifies a variety of models that have been proposed to make the process of randomization easier to explain and administer (see Table 9.1).

Table 9.1
Models for randomizing subjects in experimental studies

Model	Disadvantage
Patients could be pre-randomized and then asked to consent to one arm of the trial only	Misleads patient as they may not fully understand that they are participating in a trial
Patients could be pre-randomized and not told	Unethical unless there are exceptional circumstances. It is difficult to imagine what those circumstances might be
Patients could be given an information sheet which explains that taking part in the trial is likely to be of benefit to patients	May be dishonest because the whole point of a trial is that no-one knows which treatment group the patient is in

(Neuberger 1992, reproduced by permission)

There is no ideal model for gaining consent to participation in a randomized controlled trial. However, this design is generally considered ethically sound because randomization is the only fair way to distribute the risks and benefits of the study fairly across the sample group.

Summary

Beneficence and non-maleficence refer to the imperative to do good and to do no harm. When evaluating published research with regard to these principles a number of questions should be considered, including:

■ What was the risk–benefit ratio (i.e. was the risk to participants acceptable in that it was minimal or congruent with normal treatments)?
■ Was any risk equally distributed across the sample?
■ Were there mechanisms to protect the privacy and confidentiality of individual participants?
■ Were inclusion and exclusion criteria discussed fully with potential research subjects?

Justice

In the context of research, justice refers to:

'... *the ethical obligation to treat each person in accordance with what is morally right and proper – to give each person what is due to him or her'*
(Council for International Organizations in Collaboration with World Health Organization 1993: 10)

Gillon (1994) claims that:

'justice is synonymous with fairness and can be summarized as the moral obligation to act on the basis of fair adjudication between competing claims'

(Gillon 1994)

This section covers:

■ Distributive justice (via randomization)
■ Vulnerability of research subjects
■ Scientific fraud
■ Publication bias.

Distributive justice

In research ethics, the principle of justice refers primarily to ensuring that the benefits and burdens of participation are equally distributed across the sample group. The idea of justice also requires that there should be some indication of 'fairness' in the selection of the sample group identified. This will indicate the degree of vulnerability associated with the sample group. Some groups in society are more vulnerable to possible manipulation by the researcher than others. This may be because of impaired or diminished ability to understand what is expected of them (as in persons with mental health or learning difficulties), or because they do not understand what is being said to them (for example people who do not speak English as a first language). Other groups of individuals are more vulnerable to manipulation due to the nature of their occupation (such as armed service personnel and students). They may participate in research because of the fear of reprisal such as losing their job, reduced chances of promotion, or perhaps exam failure. One should look out for evidence of all these issues when reading and evaluating research papers.

Randomization

The process of randomization is perceived as the fairest way of achieving distributive justice. It is noteworthy therefore that in certain cases randomization is advocated not only to adhere to theories of probability (see Chapters 5 and 7) but also for ethical reasons. Distribution of risk is a narrow interpretation of the concept of justice because for some researchers *need* may be of equal importance (Warnock 1994). Imagine that some form of drug has shown astonishing results in clinical trials, in that anyone who takes it within 48 hours of having a heart attack appears to have a substantial chance of total recovery. Is it then appropriate that individuals who have had a heart attack have the possibility of being randomized into a control arm, receive a placebo and thus reduce the possibility that they will recover totally? Similarly, if respondents are chronically sick with no hope of a cure but there is a treatment that will alleviate their suffering in some way, is it fair that the treatment is withheld in the pursuit of the objectivity which randomized controlled trials afford? Certainly in these examples, distributive justice (as in randomization) should be seen as secondary to the needs of respondents. In these instances the vulnerable nature of the sample group must be considered in the context of the type of research design posed to address the question. It may be more appropriate from the perspective of need that the design of such trials afford a degree of treatment for *all*, rather than merely *some* respondents.

Vulnerability of subjects

Some groups are particularly vulnerable with respect to the principle of justice or fair treatment within research studies. It has been suggested, for example, that women are vulnerable because of their general acceptance of the medicalization of their health (Turner 1987) especially in studies relating to reproduction. In reviewing a study of cervical dysplasia, Paul (1988) suggested that women may ask fewer questions about their progress whilst involved in a study.

Children may be more vulnerable because of their restricted autonomy in choosing to participate in research studies, the decision being made by the parent or legal guardian for children under the age of seven years (Neuberger 1992) and often for much older children (see earlier discussion, page 213).

Whatever the reason, the nature of the sample group will provide some indication of their degree of vulnerability to manipulation by the researcher and the reader should be keenly aware of this. When reading published research, the critical reader should look for criteria for inclusion and exclusion of individuals from the study, along with a clear rationale for such choices.

An example of a study where a vulnerable group was apparently not protected is the Tuskagee Study. This study began in 1932 and concluded in 1972 (Pence 1990). A sample group of black respondents in a southern state of the USA were recruited with the intention of examining the progress of syphilis in male respondents, to determine the degree of mortality and morbidity associated with the disease (Pence 1990, Burns and Grove 1993). Since syphilis can affect any individual across the whole breadth of socioeconomic backgrounds, the obvious question raised is why were only black respondents chosen to participate in the study? The answer appears to be bound up in the fact that the black population of the state were mainly uneducated and poor, and therefore particularly vulnerable to manipulation.

Fraud or deliberate deception

In research, deliberate deception is fundamentally wrong in that the researcher intentionally manipulates or even invents data to suit their own ends. Burns and Grove (1993) describe such activities as scientific fraud. They define this as:

> *'fabrication, falsification, plagiarism or other practices that seriously deviate from those that are commonly accepted by the scientific community for proposing, conducting or reporting research'*
>
> (Burns and Grove 1993: 113)

Unfortunately, as Neuberger (1992) identifies, research ethics committees have no legal jurisdiction in the matter of continuous monitoring of studies once approval has been granted. Much of the responsibility therefore lies with the individual researcher or research team.

The critical reader may be able to discern some aspects of scientific fraud, by virtue of having advanced knowledge in areas such as research design and data analysis, or perhaps the specific area of research. However, there is no foolproof way of establishing whether a scientific fraud has been committed from reading a research report. To protect against the publication of questionable research, articles submitted for publication in refereed journals are vetted by experts before acceptance for publication. However, no amount of 'critical analysis' can entirely circumvent such deception.

If fraud is suspected, the author may be asked to produce raw data for scrutiny; for example, research journals, interview recordings, and completed questionnaires. If they are unable to do so the research would not be published and an investigation might be carried out by the relevant professional body. In the USA independent regulatory bodies monitor the possibility of research fraud and have the authority to prosecute in such cases. However, no such body exists in the UK and the professional groups involved in health care are responsible for regulating their own research practice. In some cases, medical practitioners found guilty of research fraud have been removed from the medical register (Miller 1997).

Publication bias

Publication bias refers to the general trend of positive bias in published research material. Readers of research must always consider that for every research study which is published, another unpublished study may exist. This in part is due to a reluctance to publish studies that are inconclusive or do not demonstrate significant results. A true overall picture of the current state of knowledge may therefore be difficult to determine.

There are compensatory mechanisms in some areas of research to ameliorate positive publication bias. For example, pharmaceutical companies must provide LRECs with an assurance that *all* results will be published, whatever the findings, before the study is approved. However, there are various ways in which studies can be published without their necessarily being disseminated through scientific journals, for example, in company publications. For papers reporting studies involving meta-analysis (see Chapter 10) authors need to demonstrate a balance of studies from which the data is drawn for analysis and this should include published and unpublished sources.

Summary

When evaluating published research and the principle of justice, consideration should be given to the following:

- Whether the sample population is vulnerable to manipulation by the researcher
- Whether the limitations of the study are clearly identified and discussed
- Whether the population sample was selected fairly
- Whether the sample was appropriate to answer the research question.

The justness of the published research should also be considered in relation to the degree to which the findings can be seen to be supported by the the data and whether the research report or publication has been subject to external scrutiny (i.e. refereed).

Chapter conclusion

Evaluating ethical issues in published research can be a difficult task for the reader. The purpose of this chapter is to provide an ethical framework that can be used to identify the ethical problems associated with different research approaches. An ethical framework provides 'clues' on what to look for when reading published research and this may make the evaluation less daunting. The framework also provides the reader with a structure upon which to base moral judgments. The principles inherent within the framework are common to all ethical theories and underpin professional codes of conduct. When using the framework, it is important that consideration is given to each of the four principles. This allows all areas of research practice (such as sampling techniques, reducing risks and maximizing benefits) to be examined.

The application of the principles identified within the ethical framework may give the reader a more critical insight into the 'world' of the research participant, enabling them in some way to put themselves into the research participants' shoes to consider what is or is not acceptable. Unfortunately, history has provided us with examples of how research participants may be manipulated and abused by researchers. In response to such examples, tighter controls are now applied to the process of research, through the establishment of local research ethics committees. This may lead us to assume that published research need not be critically examined for ethical weaknesses. However, published research is not necessarily good research and should not be accepted at face value. It is for this reason that an understanding of how to evaluate the ethical nature of published research is required.

Exercises

The Four Principles plus Scope approach affords a structured ethical framework by which readers of published research can make decisions about the ethical strengths and weaknesses of any particular study. The principles identified are common to all ethical theories and are intended to guide the reader through the dilemmas associated with research practice. In considering those principles and the scope of application, areas of good practice can be highlighted in published work. The examples presented here are intended to give the reader the opportunity to observe the practical use of the Four Principles plus Scope approach to evaluate the ethical dimension of three different research studies.

These examples are hypothetical. Using the Four Principles plus Scope framework, the reader can consider the possible ethical problems associated with the examples. Identifying the ethical issues under the headings: respect for autonomy, beneficence, non-maleficence, justice and veracity, consider ways in which the ethical nature of the study could have been improved. Authors' notes are offered for each example.

Example 1

This example is a study which will determine whether gynaecology ward nurses provide sufficient support for women undergoing termination of pregnancy.

Design
The study was by retrospective questionnaire which examined the participants' perception of their whole experience whilst in hospital, and their perception of the support offered by ward staff. The questionnaire was sent to all women who underwent a termination of pregnancy in June of 1997. Participants were selected by randomly identifying names from theatre records and addresses from medical notes. To ensure adequate return rates of the questionnaire a second form was sent, followed up by a telephone call requesting completion.

Example 2

This example is a study of the airway management skills of recovery nurses during the patient's recovery phase from general anaesthesia post surgery.

Consent was gained from the clinical management team of the teaching hospital and approval was given by the relevant research ethics committee.

Design
During the patient's recovery phase from general anaesthesia a convenience sample of recovery nurses were studied to observe their airway management skills. Data were collected using activity sampling by non-participant observation methods during a 12-hour shift on five consecutive days.

Example 3

This example is a study of a new drug for patients with AIDS who were intolerant of AZT, the new standard treatment.

The study was multicentred, consent was gained from all participants, and approval was sought from the relevant research ethics committees.

Trial design

Double-blind randomized controlled trial. The trial consisted of three arms, patients were randomized onto one arm of the trial only.

Figure 9.2
Study protocol

Arm 1 = 0_1 X 0_2
                                High dose
                            Drug intervention

Arm 2 = 0_1 X 0_2
                                Low dose
                            Drug intervention

Arm 3 = 0_1 X 0_2
                                Placebo
                        Non-treatment group

Key: 0_1 = pre-treatment measurement
      0_2 = post-treatment measurement
      X = treatment

Adapted from Neuberger (1992: 38)

Discussion of exercises

Example 1

Autonomy

It is difficult to determine whether broad consent to participate in this study could be achieved. Certainly, retrospective consent is a difficult concept to uphold from an ethical perspective in research as it is in clinical practice. The nature of retrospective consent means that moral judgments as to whether or not it is an acceptable way to afford the individual any choice to participate is wholly dependent upon the individual's specific experience of their termination of pregnancy. You would therefore be more inclined to agree to participate retrospectively if you had particularly strong negative or positive experiences. This in itself would introduce a degree of bias within the data collection methods.

Good practice would also indicate that consent to participate in research should be a prospective act to enable the participant the choice of participating or not. One could argue that by the very act of filling in and returning the questionnaire the participants 'consented' to the study. However, given the degree of pressure placed on the participants by the researcher to comply in returning the questionnaire, one could say that a degree of coercion was apparent in this example which may not be deemed reasonable.

In regard to maintaining the patients' privacy within the autonomy principle, the difficulty arises as to whether or not the participant is afforded that right. Some women choose to have terminations without their partner's or family's knowledge. However, if a postal questionnaire arrives at the participant's home without their prior knowledge it may be opened and read by other members of the household, thus increasing the risk of breaching privacy and confidentiality.

Beneficence/non-maleficence   As with any sensitive topic area, the possible harm caused by asking the participants about their termination experience should be considered. For instance, what strategies has the researcher put into place which will enable the participants to seek further help or counselling if they should wish it? Certainly, if the termination was performed for congenital abnormalities of the fetus, then the needs of the participant may be different from those who chose to have the termination for social or economic reasons. Different support systems would be necessary. The time given for completion of the questionnaire can also be an issue. For example, is it emotionally more distressing to answer such questions shortly after the event, or should a period of time lapse in order to allow the participant to come to terms with the procedure?

Follow-up telephone conversations are also difficult to justify in this instance, given the possibility that confidentiality may be breached for those women who do not wish their partner or family to know about their termination.

Justice   When selecting a sample of participants for a study of this nature, exclusion criteria need to be clearly identified. Women's reasons for deciding to have a termination are varied. Terminations of pregnancy carry a variety of physical risks associated with the type of procedure and the length of the pregnancy. It may be that those pregnancies which are terminated after 24 weeks' gestation have more traumatic results from a physical and emotional perspective for the participant, when compared with terminations carried out before eight weeks' gestation.

Staff who assist the women through these experiences may also be more likely to emotionally support those participants who are deemed to be having the termination for the 'right' rather than 'wrong' reasons. Clear limits need to be predetermined about the nature of the sample group to be studied.

Example 1: conclusion   It would appear that in this example the principles of autonomy, beneficence/non-maleficence and justice were all threatened. Little thought had been given to the participants' rights to privacy and confidentiality within the principle of autonomy. Retrospective consent to participate in this example is inadequate from a purely ethical perspective. In regard to benefit and harm there is no evidence of strategies put in place by the researcher to minimize risk. Similarly, within the justice principle exclusion criteria were not formulated to ensure fairness either in the interpretation of the results or selection of the sample group. Perhaps a more appropriate research method in this instance would be:

- Prospective consent for confidential interview away from the participant's home
- A selected sample group dependent on type and stage of termination
- Consideration of the timing of the interview
- Support strategies available for the participant if needed.

Example 2   *Autonomy*

There are two main problems about consent to participate in this example. The first is whether or not the nurses who will be observed during this study had the choice to refuse to participate. Although the management team had given consent to the researcher to access the facilities and the group of workers, this does not necessarily mean that the individual nurses involved were approached to give their consent to be observed during their working practice.

To observe the nurses during their working practice the researcher will also need to observe the patient during their recovery from general anaesthesia. It could be argued that implied consent was given by patients because they chose to access a teaching hospital for their surgery. But does implied consent in this instance equate to the principle of broad consent? Certainly the opportunity to refuse to participate is not apparent.

Beneficence/non-maleficence

The main concern with this example is that of minimizing risk. In this example the researcher needs to identify what determines safe practice and how they will react if they see unsafe practice occurring, before the study begins. The researcher should identify clear parameters which are made known to the groups of nurses being observed about when the researcher would intervene. In a sense, the researcher becomes an advocate for the patient who is unable to act for him or herself due to the nature of their physical condition following anaesthesia. The consequential risks of poor airway management skills by nurses may mean that the patient experiences respiratory distress. If the researcher can foresee that risks to the patient are likely to occur, they have an obligation to intervene, even if the nurse managing the patient's airway has not perceived the situation to be threatening to the patient.

The implications of this project are potentially difficult for the researcher disseminating the study's findings. If nurses are not safe to practise, the researcher has an obligation to inform the management team of that unit. By doing so they would be protecting the patients' interests and thus upholding codes of professional conduct. However, the implications for those nurses could be potentially harmful. It would be unacceptable to say that nurses were safe when they were not. Similarly, nurses who are safe may wish to be identified as such, so issues such as privacy and confidentiality are of importance. The dilemma for the researcher is how to balance those issues and retain trust whilst upholding confidentiality.

Support strategies agreed by all the groups involved must be identified before the study begins. For example, education and training may be seen as a positive support strategy which will benefit the nurses, the patients and the organization. The dilemma for the researcher is reduced, and trust between the researcher and all groups is maintained.

Justice   Clear criteria for the selection of the sample group of nurses and their patients need to be identified. Similarly, contextual criteria for the ways in which nurses are allocated specific types of patients to manage post anaesthesia should be considered. For example, nurses vary in their degree of skill. Some nurses will be novices, particularly if they are new to a particular specialty, some will be developing skills, and some will be experts. The level of skill will depend on a number of factors, such as years of experience, observational perception and the way in which individuals apply their knowledge base to a given situation.

Similarly, the needs of the individual patient will affect the ways in which their airway is managed after anaesthesia. Some patients may be intubated, some may have laryngeal masks, whilst some may have guedal airways, so the needs of the patient will differ. Other factors will influence the risk of possible airway compromise such as anatomical abnormalities, the site and nature of the patient's surgery and any underlying medical condition. It would therefore be unfair and potentially hazardous to the patient if novices were allocated to patient groups who were thought to be potentially at high risk of respiratory compromise during their recovery. In this example the distribution of need with regard to the allocation of appropriately skilled nurses to particularly vulnerable patients needs to be identified.

Example 2: conclusion   In this example the principles of beneficence/non-maleficence are of primary importance for minimizing risks to individual patients. The researcher has an obligation to the nurses who will be observed in their practice to uphold the promise of confidentiality, yet be able to balance this requirement between the needs of the nurses, the organization and the patient within the principles of veracity and justice.

Clear lines of dissemination of the study's findings would reduce some of the dilemma but would not overcome the difficulties of consent.

A more appropriate design for this study may be that the methods for data collection are focused in another way. For instance, observation of skills through skills laboratories would reduce the risk to patients. Nurses can then self-assess, aided possibly by computer software packages. Education and training can become part of the study, thus ensuring positive action.

Example 3   Autonomy

Broad consent was gained from each participant, and approval was given by the relevant research ethics committees. However, whether the participants had any real personal choice as to whether or not they agreed to take part in this trial is debatable. For example, the sample group were intolerant of the only known standard treatment. Their only hope of receiving any treatment which might improve their quality of life was to enter this trial. By doing so, they would have the chance of receiving the new treatment. Voluntariness within the principle of autonomy becomes threatened in this instance.

Beneficence/non-maleficence

The perceived risk to the participants accessing this trial was that they may be assigned to the placebo arm, thus receiving no treatment at all. Scientifically this would appear to be the most effective way to evaluate the outcome of the new treatment objectively. However, it is not unreasonable to imagine that all participants would want some form of the new treatment. It may be more ethical to distribute the benefits of participation in the study by removing the placebo arm, thus establishing a trial which affords all patients the drug in some form. In this instance it may be appropriate to accept that the distribution of benefit (receiving some treatment) supersedes the scientific objective of having a control group (no treatment) for comparison of outcome.

If this trial continued with the placebo arm, all participants would have to be informed of that fact. To deceive the participants by not informing them that a non-treatment group would be included in the design would be unethical about the disclosure of risks and benefits. However, to inform the participant of the risk of receiving no treatment may mean that the patients re-randomize themselves. In other words, they may distribute benefits (receiving treatment) by sharing out the drugs amongst themselves outside the clinic after they have been allocated by the researcher.

Justice

Distribution is fairly achieved in regard to the process of randomization. All participants would have an equal chance of distribution to the placebo arm of the trial. Therefore risk is fairly distributed without influence of bias. However, this example illustrates the complex nature of justice in research practice as discussed by Warnock (1994) in that distributive justice may supersede the needs of the participants. The desperate need of the participants to have some form of treatment would seem the fairest option from a humanitarian perspective, even if it threatens the scientific validity of the results. The feelings and hopes of the participants should not be overlooked in the pursuit of validity.

Example 3: conclusion   It would appear that to ensure fair distribution of benefit over risk a more appropriate design for this trial would be one which has no placebo arm. Thus all participants receive some form of the new treatment. Although this design is less scientific in terms of internal validity, it upholds the needs of the participants in terms of justice, beneficence and non-maleficence. The principle of autonomy is still problematic in relation to the degree of personal choice the patient has about enrolling in this study. The desperate nature of their condition may mean that their hopes for some form of treatment which might result in an improvement in their condition limits voluntariness. A more ethically sound design in this instance would be:

Figure 9.3

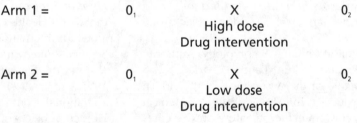

Arm 1 = 0_1 X 0_2
                        High dose
                        Drug intervention

Arm 2 = 0_1 X 0_2
                        Low dose
                        Drug intervention

Key: 0_1 = pre-treatment measurement
      0_2 = post-treatment measurement
      X = treatment

Appendix: British guidelines on ethics in research

Allen and Hanbury *Guidelines for Clinical Trials – Compensation for Patients*. SALMP/AH91/D89, 20 Dec 1991.

Association of the British Pharmaceutical Industry *Good Clinical (Research) Practice*. ABPI, December 1992.

Association of the British Pharmaceutical Industry *Guidelines for Phase IV Clinical Trials*. ABPI, September 1993.

Association of the British Pharmaceutical Industry *Relationships between the Medical Profession and the Pharmaceutical Industry*. ABPI, June 1994.

Association of Independent Clinical Research Contractors *Guidelines for Research Ethics Committees*. AICRC, June 1992.

British Medical Association *Improving the Network of Local Ethical Research Committees and the Establishment of a National Ethical Research Committee*. BMA Council Resolution 8/1/86, printed as Appendix V of *Philosophy & Practice of Medical Ethics*, Unwin Brothers, Surrey, 1988, pp123–127.

British Medical Association *'Research'*. In:

Philosophy & Practice of Medical Ethics. Unwin Brothers, Surrey, 1988, pp75–77.

British Paediatric Association, Ethics Advisory Committee *Guidelines for the Ethical Conduct of Medical Research Involving Children*. BPA, August 1992.

British Psychological Society *Ethical Principles for Conducting Research with Human Participants*. In British Psychological Society, Code of Conduct, Ethical Principles and Guidelines, September 1993.

British Sociological Association *Statement of Ethical Practice*. BSA, 1993.

Broad RD (ICI) *Review of Good Laboratory Practices in the UK and Europe*. In Wells F (ed) (1990) *Medicines: Good Practice Guidelines*. Belfast: Queens University. pp 11–13.

Clothier Committee *Report of the Committee on the Ethics of Gene Therapy*. CM 1788, 1992.

Department of Health *Local Research Ethics Committees* (The Department of Health Guidelines). DoH, 1991.

Human Fertilisation and Embryology Act 1990 In: Morgan D and Lee RG (1991) Blackstone's *Guide to the Human Fertilisation and Embryology Act 1990*. London: Blackstone Press, pp186–225.

Human Fertilisation and Embryology Authority *Code of Practice*. HFEA, London, 1991.

Joint Committee of the Association of the British Pharmaceutical Industry, British Medical Association, Committee on Safety of Medicines and Royal College of General Practitioners *Guidelines on Postmarking Surveillance*. In Wells F (ed) (1990) *Medicines: Good Practice Guidelines*. Belfast: Queens University, pp 125–127.

Medical Research Council *The Ethical Conduct of Research on Children*. MRC, London, 1991.

Medical Research Council *The Ethical Conduct of Research on the Mentally Incapacitated*. MRC, London, 1991.

Medicines Commission *Advice to Health Ministers on Healthy Volunteer Studies*. Department of Health and Social Services, June 1987.

Royal College of Physicians, Faculty of Operational Medicine *Guidance on Ethics for Occupational Physicians*. RCP, London, 3rd edn, 1986.

Royal College of Physicians *Guidelines on the Practice of Ethics in Medical Research involving Human Subjects*. RCP, London, 2nd edn, 1986.

Royal College of Nursing *Ethics Related to Research in Nursing*. Harrow: Scutari Publications, 1993.

Royal College of Psychiatrists (1990) Guidelines for research ethics committees on psychiatric research involving human subjects. *Psychiatric Bulletin* **14**: 48–52.

United Kingdom Central Council for Nursing, Midwifery and Health Visiting *Acquired Immune Deficiency Syndrome and Human Immuno-deficiency Virus Infection (AIDS and HIV Infection)* and *Anonymous Testing for the Prevalence of the Human Immuno-deficiency Virus (HIV)*. UKCC, March, 1994.

International guidelines on ethics in research

Council for International Organizations of Medical Sciences *International Ethical Guidelines for Biomedical Research Involving Human Subjects* (Revised version of the 1982 *Proposed Guidelines for Biomedical Research Involving Human Subjects*). CIOMS in collaboration with the World Health Organization, 1993.

Council for International Organizations of Medical Sciences *International Guidelines for Ethical Review of Epidemiological Studies*. CIOMS, 1991.

The National Commission for the Protection of Human Subjects of Biomedical and Behavioral Research *The Belmont Report: Ethical Principles and Guidelines for the Protection of Human Subjects of Research*. Office for Protection from Research Risks, April 1979.

Committee for Proprietary Medicinal Products (CPMP) Working Party on Efficacy of Medicinal Products in the European Community *Notes for Guidance: Good Clinical Practice for Trials on Medicinal Products in the European Community*. CPMP 111/3976/88-EN, 1990.

Danish Ministry of Health *Research Involving Human Subjects: Ethics and Law* (proposed legislation). Copenhagen, 1989, pp89–96.

Department of Health and Human Services *Rules and Regulations 45 CFR 46*. In Levine RJ (1986) *Ethics and Regulation of Clinical Research*, Baltimore and Munich: Urban and Schwarzenberg, 2nd edn, 1986, pp393–412.

Medical Research Council of Canada *Guidelines on Research Involving Human Subjects*. MRCC, 1987.

World Medical Assembly *Declaration of Helsinki* Amended 1989. In Department of Health *Local Research Ethics Committees*. DoH, 1991.

References

Association of Community Health Councils Working Party on Local Ethics Committees (1990) *Information Resource Pack for Lay Members of Local Research Ethics Committees*. London: Community Health Council.

Baum M, Zikha J and Houghton J (1989) Ethics of clinical research: lessons for the future. *British Medical Journal* **229**(7): 251–253.

Beauchamp TL and & Childress JF (1989) *Principles of Biomedical Ethics*, 3rd edn. Oxford: Oxford University Press.

Beecher H (1966) Ethics and clinical research. *New England Journal of Medicine* **274**(24): 1354–1360.

Bok S (1984) *Secrets: on the Ethics of Concealment and Revelation*. London: Oxford University Press.

British Paediatric Association (1992) Ethics Advisory Committee: *Guidelines for the Ethical Conduct of Medical Research Using Children*. London: BPA.

Burns N and Grove S (1993) *The Practice of Nursing Research: Conduct, Critique and Utilisation*, 2nd edn. Philadelphia, PA: WB Saunders.

Carlin (1995) US/*Genetic engineering: religious leaders take on scientists who play God*. Independent on Sunday 4 June: 16.

Council for International Organisations of Medical Sciences (CIOMS) in collaboration with the WHO (1993) *International Ethical Guidelines for Biomedical Research Involving Human Subjects*. Geneva: CIOMS.

Cowles K (1988) Issues in qualitative research on sensitive topics. *Western Journal of Nursing Research* **10**(2): 163–179.

Crookes PA (1996) *Personal Bereavement in Registered General Nurses* Unpublished PhD thesis. Hull: University of Hull.

Dalla-Vorgia P, Katsaiyanni K, Garanis TN, Drogari P, Kaitselinis A (1992) Attitudes of a Mediterranean population to the truthtelling issue. *Journal of Medical Ethics* **18**: 67–74.

Department of Health 1991. Local research ethics committees. London: DoH.

Dimond BC (1990) *Legal Aspects of Nursing*. Prentice Hall: London.

Faden R and Beauchamp TL (1986) *A History and Theory of Informed Consent*. Oxford: Oxford University Press.

Gillon R (1994) Medical ethics: four principles plus attention to scope. *British Medical Journal* **309**: 184–188.

Hughes P (1990) Evaluating the impact of continual professional education (ENB 941). *Nurse Education Today* **10**: 428–436.

MENCAP (1989) *Competency and Consent to Medical Treatment*: A report of the working party on the legal, medical and ethical issues of mental handicap convened by MENCAP. London: MENCAP.

Miller B (1997) Honesty on trial. *Nursing Times* **93**(35): 10–11.

Neuberger J (1992) *Ethics and Health Care: The Role of Research Ethics Committees in the United Kingdom*. London: King's Fund Institute.

National Health Service Management Executive (NHSME) (1990) *Consent to Treatment Guidelines*. London: HMSO.

Oakley A (1992) *Social Support and Motherhood*. Oxford: Blackwell.

Pappworth MH (1968) *Human Guinea Pigs*. Beacon: Boston.

Paul C (1988) The New Zealand cervical cancer study: could it happen again? *British Medical Journal* **297**: 533–538.

Pence GE (1990) *Classic Cases in Medical Ethics*. London: McGraw-Hill.

Polit DF and Hungler BP (1989) *Essentials of Nursing Research: Methods, Appraisal and Utilization*, 2nd edn. London: Lippincott.

Ramos MC (1989) Some ethical implications of qualitative research. *Research in Nursing and Health* **12**: 57–63.

Royal College of Psychiatrists (1990) Guidelines for Research. Ethics Committees on Psychiatric Research involving Human Subjects. *Psychiatric Bulletin* **14**: 48–61.

Silverman WA (1989) The myth of informed consent: in daily practice and clinical trials *Journal of Medical Ethics* **15**: 6–11.

Thornton H (1993) Whose interests: patients' or researchers'? *Bulletin of Medical Ethics* XX: 13–19.

Turner BS (1987) *Medical Power and Social Knowledge*. London: Sage Publications.

Walley T and Barton S (1995) A purchaser perspective of managing new drugs: Interferon Beta as a case study. *British Medical Journal* **311**: 796–799.

Warnock M (1994) Comments: Principles of Health Care Ethics. *British Medical Journal* **38**: 988–989.

While AE (1995) Ethics Committees: impediments to research or guardians of ethical standards? *British Medical Journal* **311**: 661.

10 Reviewing and interpreting research: identifying implications for practice

Sue Davies

Introduction

Where is the knowledge we have lost in information?
(From *Choruses From the Rock*, a poem by T S Eliot)

One of the most difficult tasks for anyone wanting to ensure that their practice is research-based is synthesizing the evidence from a mass of literature into clear indicators for practice. Most of us have, at some time or other, sat beside a pile of research papers and articles with pen poised thinking 'where do I begin?' The purpose of this chapter is to provide some practical suggestions for extracting the relevant information from the literature, organizing that information and presenting it in a way that clearly identifies the implications for practice, education and further research.

At points within the chapter, reference is made to a literature review carried out as part of a research project funded by the English National Board for Nursing, Midwifery and Health Visiting with which I was recently involved (Davies *et al* 1997a). The project aimed to evaluate the extent to which educational programmes in nursing enable nurses to promote the autonomy and independence of older people in their care. As well as identifying the focus and methods for the study, the review suggested a range of nursing interventions for promoting patient/client autonomy and independence, and so also provided indicators for nursing practice. Some of the tools and techniques which we used for reviewing this large body of literature are included within this chapter in the hope that readers will be able to modify and adapt our approach to suit their own purposes.

Key issues

- The importance of critical reviews of literature
- Types of literature review, systematic review and meta-analysis
- Purposes of a literature review
- Stages in the literature review process
- Structuring and writing a review

Synthesis: a complex skill

If the current emphasis on self-directed professional education is to be successful in enhancing the quality of health care, practitioners need to develop the habit of critically evaluating and integrating literature early in their careers. Research modules on nursing programmes across the country, and indeed this book, have been developed with this aim in mind. Unfortunately however, most published reviews of nursing literature present a largely narrative description rather than a critical evaluation of existing material and there are few good examples to act as a guide. In a useful article, Nicky Cullum (1994) has summarized the pitfalls commonly found in published literature reviews. These are shown in Box 10.1.

Box 10.1
Common pitfalls in published literature reviews

- Reviews often fail to identify strengths and weaknesses in the primary research
- Reviewers usually only use a subset of the available research and fail to make explicit the criteria for inclusion of material
- Reviewers usually only refer to published research, the publication of which is biased in favour of that which demonstrates statistically significant findings
- Reviewers usually report so little of the methodology used in reviewing that it is impossible for the reader to judge the validity of the review
- The review often fails to address the rigour with which the existing knowledge base has been constructed.

Cullum (1994)

In recent years, there are signs that the review of published and unpublished research literature is developing a methodology in its own right (Roe 1994), raising the hope that the limitations identified by Cullum may become a thing of the past. With the establishment of centres for the systematic review and dissemination of research evidence, such as the NHS Centre for Reviews and Dissemination in York and the Cochrane Collaboration, research synthesis is being recognized as a rigorous and scientific process. In order to appreciate how reviews in nursing might contribute to nursing knowledge and practice, it is important to recognize the range of possible approaches to reviewing material and these will now be discussed.

Types of review

Reviews of research-based evidence and other literature can be broadly divided under three headings:

- Literature review
- Systematic review
- Meta-analysis.

The more general term **literature review** is used to describe the process of synthesizing the results and conclusions of a number of publications on a given topic. This type of review will incorporate all types of literature relating to the topic, not just those based upon empirical research. **Systematic review** refers to the process of comprehensively identifying all the research on a given topic and synthesizing the findings. Systematic reviews are normally based on research which meets strict inclusion criteria such as random allocation to experimental and control groups. Examples of published systematic reviews include Brooker *et al's* review of the effectiveness of community mental health nursing interventions in the UK (Brooker *et al* 1996) and Cullum *et al's* review of interventions for reducing the incidence of pressure sores (Cullum *et al* 1995).

In recent years, there has been a growing interest in the process of combining empirical evidence from studies conducted in a similar way. This process, known as **meta-analysis**, involves transforming the findings of reviewed studies to a common metric and then using statistical tests to determine whether there are overall effects, subsample effects and associations among attributes of studies and particular findings (Ganong 1987). In other words, the review incorporates a specific statistical technique to assemble the results of several studies into a single estimate. As the number of studies relevant to nursing which have adopted an experimental design

Box 10.2
An example of meta-analysis

Waddell (1992) reports a meta-analysis of 34 published and unpublished studies designed to test the hypothesis that continuing professional education has a positive effect on nursing practice. Studies were selected using the following criteria:

- The intervention consisted of a programme of Continuing Nurse Education
- The effect of the treatment was assessed by examining practice-related behaviours or chart audits which documented practice
- There were sufficient data to compute an effect size.

On the basis of the review, Waddell suggests that we can have greater confidence in the assumption that continuing education has an impact on practice. However, more than one third of the studies failed to report the reliability and validity of the instruments used to measure the effects of education on practice. In the absence of information on the validity and reliability of tools to measure practice, Waddell's conclusion should be viewed with caution.

increases, the number of meta-analyses of substantive bodies of literature is also likely to increase. One example is Waddell's (1992) meta-analysis of the effects of continuing professional education on practice (Box 10.2).

The remainder of this chapter will focus on the development of the more comprehensive type of literature review, which is likely to incorporate a range of types of material and evidence. For a more in-depth discussion of systematic reviews and meta-analysis, the interested reader is referred to Chalmers and Altman (1995) and Droogan and Song (1996).

Purposes of a literature review

The broad aim of any literature review is to synthesize the critical evaluation of existing work on a topic. More specifically, a literature review should perform the following functions:

- Identify the context in which the problem or topic is being explored
- Outline what is known about a topic
- Identify and define concepts and variables of relevance to the topic
- Review the methods used to study the topic
- Identify theoretical and conceptual frameworks within which the topic can be explored
- Suggest appropriate indicators for practice, education and further research.

These functions may be covered in different proportions depending on the overall purpose and focus of the review. For example, a literature review prepared for a course assignment is likely to focus more on the findings of the review and implications for practice. In comparison, a literature review conducted as a stage in a research process which needs to provide the foundation for empirical work, is likely to place more emphasis on the definition of concepts and variables. However, a good review will perform all the functions listed to a greater or lesser extent and each will now be considered in more detail.

Identify the context in which the problem or topic is being explored

Whatever the focus of the review, it is essential that the reviewer identifies the rationale underpinning their efforts. They should identify reasons for why it is important to undertake the review at this time and for how it will contribute to an understanding of the topic. It is likely that this will necessitate a consideration of the professional and political factors, including government policies, influencing developments relating to the subject area. It may also be appropriate for the author to indicate their personal motivation for undertaking the review.

Outline what is known about the topic

It is perhaps a truism that science is a cumulative enterprise (Becker 1986). Certainly, research needs to build upon existing work if knowledge, and as a consequence practice, are to move forward. In contrast to the physical sciences, single studies in the social and behavioural sciences rarely provide definitive answers to research questions. Rather, progress is accomplished through the identification of trends from the synthesis of findings from a number of studies. A review of the literature needs to indicate the current 'state of the art' in relation to the topic being investigated.

Identify and define relevant concepts and variables

In identifying what is already known about a topic, it is important to define key concepts and variables. For example, a review of research to evaluate the implementation of primary nursing would need to indicate how primary nursing had been defined and described by the authors of relevant research reports. It may be that key concepts have been measured in different ways by different researchers, leading to apparently contradictory findings.

Review the methods used to study the topic see Chapter 5

The main consideration is whether the research methods were sufficiently rigorous to produce valid information. The methods of study will also provide an indication of the type of information produced and the level of knowledge created by the body of literature to date.

Identify theoretical and conceptual frameworks within which the topic can be explored

A literature review should identify the current state of knowledge with reference to theory development in relation to the topic under consideration. This will involve the identification and critique of conceptual and theoretical frameworks which have provided the basis for empirical study (see Chapter 4). It is important that any literature review on a particular topic identifies assumptions upon which the body of literature has been developed as these may influence the applicability of the findings of the review.

Identify appropriate indicators for practice, education and further research

Hunt (1981) suggests that research in nursing provides three types of practice indicator: what nurses should do, what nurses should try and indicators of practices and procedures for which there is no sound basis. By identifying the level of knowledge in relation to the topic under consideration (see Chapter 5), critical readers can determine which type of indicator is produced by the body of literature under review. Implications for education and gaps in knowledge suggesting the need for further research should also be identified.

Summary

The ability to synthesize information from the critical evaluation of research reports on a given topic is an important skill for all engaged in health care practice. There are a number of approaches to reviewing literature including systematic review and meta-analysis as well as the more all-encompassing review which will also include non-empirical literature. The choice of approach depends on the purpose of the review. Functions of the literature review include summarizing the current state of knowledge in relation to a given topic, defining key concepts and variables, examining the conceptual and theoretical frameworks which have been used to study the topic, reviewing methods to indicate the existing level of knowledge in relation to the topic and identifying implications for practice, education and research.

Literature reviews have the potential to inform health care practice in a whole host of ways. However, in order to make an impact, reviews need to demonstrate a systematic and logical method. The rest of this chapter will be devoted to describing the stages in this process in more detail. First, the arguments for adopting an organized approach will be revisited.

A methodology for reviewing literature

The importance of a systematic approach

The process of identifying and retrieving literature relevant to a particular topic has been comprehensively discussed in Chapter 3. However, it is worth reiterating here that whatever the purpose of the review, it is essential that the approach to collecting, organizing and reviewing material is as systematic as possible. Ganong (1987) suggests that the approach to reviewing a research-based body of literature needs to be as systematic as an empirical research process. Unfortunately, few published literature reviews meet the standards of primary research (Lederman 1992).

Stages in the review process

Jackson (1980) proposes that the methodology of literature reviewing involves six stages:

1. Selecting the hypotheses or questions for the review
2. Sampling the research to be reviewed
3. Representing the characteristics of the studies and their findings
4. Analyzing the findings
5. Interpreting the results
6. Reporting the review.

The analysis of material can also be divided into three stages:

1. Classifying material
2. Identifying themes and concepts
3. Theoretical and methodological critique.

Before considering each of these steps in more detail, it is important to think about the best way of recording information for the review. Some of these points are also covered in Chapter 3.

Recording information

Perhaps the most fundamental rule is to avoid recording references or useful quotes on bits of paper that can easily be lost or separated. Once again the key is to be systematic in your approach. In a useful paper on how to survive writing a thesis, Johanson (1985) compares the virtual impossibility of writing a literature review from pages of notes and photocopies of articles with the ease of writing using an organized system which has extracted the relevant information.

With the ready availability of computer technology, an important decision facing the would-be literature reviewer is whether to record information on a computer database or to use a manual system. A number of packages are now available to assist in the process of recording and retrieving information for a literature review. These bibliographic tools can take the chore out of adding references to a review and most now allow sophisticated manipulation of information (*Endnote, Reference Manager* and *Idealist* are examples). However, data entry for all these packages can be time-consuming, particularly for anyone unfamiliar with their use. In making a decision about the most appropriate system the following points are worth taking into account.

The size of the database

If the database is going to be very large it is probably worth investing the effort into computerizing the information, particularly if data can be copied across to the text file for word-processing.

The level of manipulation required

If the records will require frequent and highly sophisticated manipulation that cannot easily be done manually, then use of a package such as Idealist may be preferable.

The main source of references

If the literature search is being carried out mainly via online databases and information can be downloaded and incorporated into the review database, this may be the most efficient way to store information.

Use of a computerized database for storing the information extracted during the review process does have a number of disadvantages. Access to computer terminals may be limited, for example. Many computers are not portable enough to be taken into a library, therefore information will need to be transcribed twice. It may be necessary to rely on printouts to compare entries since only one record is displayed at a time. It is also worth bearing in mind that computer disks can be corrupted and hard disks do occasionally crash! However, it is also possible to lose manual records.

If using a computer package, it is essential to maintain a back-up which is stored separately from the main computer. In my own department a corrupted disk is currently the most popular excuse for students' late submission of course work! Whichever system is used, it should be kept as simple as possible, otherwise recording references becomes time-consuming and tedious.

Finally, it is important to organize photocopies of items within the database, for example by numbering each item and cross-referencing, either to cards or to each computerized entry. It is extremely frustrating to be in the final stages of writing and having to search for an elusive item in order to check a quote or page number.

Classifying material

One of the first steps in reviewing a collection of literature is to categorize the information contained within individual papers and articles. Polit and Hungler (1991) have provided a very useful classification based upon five types of information. These are:

- Facts, statistics and research findings
- Theoretical discussion
- Research methods and procedures
- Opinions and viewpoints
- Anecdotes and clinical descriptions.

Different types of information can contribute to a literature review in different ways. However, a research-based review should focus mainly upon information in the first three categories listed above. Opinions and anecdotes can be used to illustrate points and are also useful in suggesting concepts and ideas for new research.

A second useful step in classifying material is to rate each item according to its value and relevance to the focus of the review. For example, a research report which has investigated a similar area of study might be awarded three points whereas a paper of only marginal relevance to the topic under investigation might be awarded only one point. This type of rating approach helps to identify quickly those papers which will contribute most significantly to the review.

It is also useful to classify each item of literature in relation to the field of study, particularly for reviews where a consideration of a broad body of literature is indicated. For example, when reviewing the literature relating to practice supervision for nursing students, White *et al* (1993) examined information relating to social work and teacher education as well as nursing literature.

Exercise 10.1

- Choose a topic relevant to your own practice
- Identify at least ten references related to the topic using any resources to which you have access (e.g. CD-ROM, abstracting indexes).
- Using the abstract for each item, attempt to classify the items using Polit and Hungler's classification system.

Identifying themes: developing a theme matrix

It is important to identify themes and concepts within the literature in order to determine the appropriate structure for the review. These should emerge from the literature rather than being imposed by the reviewer. In fact some authors have suggested that synthesizing material for a literature review can benefit from an approach similar to content analysis used in qualitative research (Nolan *et al* 1997). An easy way to approach this process is to read through each item and identify the major themes or issues covered within the paper. A list of themes can then be developed and these can be condensed into broader themes once all the material for review has been considered.

A simple method for identifying themes is to record information on a theme matrix (Table 10.1). This consists of two axes with numbered items on the vertical axis and categories/themes on the horizontal axis. Items can be classified according to categories relevant to the review and themes identified, simply extending the x-axis as new themes emerge. The cells of the matrix can be used to incorporate additional information or reminders about the way in which each theme features within the paper. Once all the literature has been categorized in this way, themes can be condensed into broader categories as appropriate. Computerized databases can help in this process.

Exercise 10.2

■ Develop a theme matrix on the basis of the ten papers identified in the previous exercise
■ What are the major themes?
■ How could these help you to synthesize the material you have collected?

Critical analysis

Having classified the material for review and identified the major themes within the body of literature as a whole, the reviewer is ready to begin a more detailed critical analysis of the material. Critical review of literature broadly involves two aspects: theoretical critique and methodological critique. Theoretical critique is perhaps the most difficult and most commonly neglected aspect of literature review and will be dealt with first.

Theoretical critique

In Chapter 4, Lorraine Ellis and Patrick Crookes describe how theoretical and conceptual frameworks contribute to a research study. Most readers of this volume could be forgiven for imagining that much applied research in nursing and health care is not informed by theory at all: a good deal of published research appears to evaluate a procedure or explore a need in a simple 'fact-gathering' way and then present the findings (Sapsford 1994). However, facts are always underpinned by theory – they do not exist in isolation. Furthermore, it has been suggested (Gilbert 1993) that research is only useful if it

Table 10.1 An example of an extract from theme matrix: Promoting autonomy and independence among older people

| Classification | | | | | | | | Themes | | | | |
Author and date	No	Ty	Or	Fi	Us	Multidisciplinary teamwork	Professional autonomy	Routinized care	Nurse–patient relationship	Professional education
Waters K 1994	1	1	GB	Re	***	X Therapist/ nurse		X Default mechanism		X Role in rehab
Reed J 1994	2	1	GB	AC CC	***	X Differences in settings	X Nurse as gatekeeper Competition			X Values Medical model
Faucett et al 1990	3	1/2	US	CC	**			X Orem influence on practice	X Participation	X
Evers H 1984	4	1	GB	CC	***	X Hierarchy Medical model	X Effect on practice	X Patient careers		X
Miller A 1985	5	1	GB	AC Re CC	***			X Individualized care affects outcomes	X Primary nursing	X
Raatikainen R 1991	6	1	Fn	Co	*			X Self-activeness	X Participation Esteem	

Key to classification

No – Number of paper
Or – Country of origin
Ty – Type
1 Facts, statistics, research findings
2 Theory or interpretation
3 Methodology
4 Opinions, beliefs, points of view
5 Anecdotes, clinical impressions, narrations of incidents

Fi – Field of study
AC – Acute care
CC – Continuing care
Co – Community care
Re – Rehabilitation

Us – Usefulness
*** High
** Moderate
* Low

X – Major theme

contributes to generalizable laws and principles that can be applied in a range of situations and circumstances in order to predict events. Nevertheless, the identification and development of theoretical and conceptual frameworks in much published nursing research is limited.

In Chapter 4 the various ways in which theoretical and conceptual frameworks and assumptions contribute to research design was outlined. However, as the authors point out, it is not uncommon for researchers to fail to make these assumptions explicit when writing research reports. This may be the first challenge for the reviewer: to identify the assumptions and theoretical ideas upon which the study has been developed. The second challenge is to question these assumptions and consider alternative theoretical explanations for the phenomena under investigation. This point is illustrated by the experiences of the ENB project research team referred to in the Introduction when we were searching for a tool to measure nurses' attitudes to older people as a way of 'measuring' the impact of an educational programme (Davies *et al* 1997).

The research team originally intended to make use of existing scales to measure nurses' attitudes and knowledge and to make minor adjustments to previously developed tools for observation. Our review of the literature identified a number of questionnaires and schedules for observing nursing practice which we could have used. However, when we began to think about the theoretical assumptions underpinning the development and use of these tools, we decided they were not appropriate to our study. We found that the most commonly used attitude scales such as the Kogan Old People Scale (Kogan 1961) and Palmore's Facts on Ageing scale (Palmore 1977) were developed to determine negative stereotypes and inaccurate knowledge about older people *within the general population*. We decided it would be inappropriate to use these questionnaires to measure nurses' attitudes to the older people *in their care*. In other words, the scales were too general to be relevant to the specific focus of our study.

Furthermore, the assumptions underpinning the use of these scales are based upon a linear model of the impact of education on nursing practice, that is, that education influences attitudes to older people in society which influence nursing practice. As a research team, we felt that that such a model was too simplistic to represent the relationship between education and practice accurately and ignored the multiple factors which influence this relationship. These factors are illustrated in the conceptual framework adapted from Wright (1988) and included as Figure 4.2 (page 102) in this book. The research team accepted this framework as a more accurate representation of the way in which education influences nursing practice and decided that a more useful focus within the context of the study would be to determine attitudes towards behaviour essential to the nursing care of older people. In the absence of appropriate existing scales, the research team developed a questionnaire and observation schedule specifically for the purpose of the study.

A further example of theoretical critique is provided by Abbott and Sapsford's work on mothers of children with learning difficulties (Abbott and Sapsford 1992). The aim of the research was to describe the extent to which caring for a child with learning difficulties altered the mothers' lives. Sixteen mothers were interviewed on two separate occasions one year apart. In a subsequent paper, Sapsford (1994) identifies the theoretical perspectives which underpinned the work. These were:

■ A feminist perspective which suggests that mothering is not an innate activity but something which is hard work and does not necessarily come naturally to women
■ The myth of community care: a perspective which separates the rhetoric of community from the reality of inadequate services and lack of support.

Both these perspectives were used to guide the interviews which were conversational, tape-recorded and transcribed. It is possible to critique these perspectives – as a critical consumer of research it is essential to do this since these assumptions are likely to have influenced the whole course of the study. Theories can be tentatively accepted if there is a substantial body of evidence demonstrating their legitimacy. However, it is the researcher's responsibility to present this evidence in support of their own theoretical perspective. Most importantly perhaps, as a practitioner, you should 'beware the dominant ideology' which could 'blinker' you to alternative theoretical perspectives which might offer greater illumination of the topic under review.

Exercise 10.3	■ Select two of the papers from the first exercise for more detailed study
	■ Try to identify the conceptual or theoretical framework on which each study is based
	■ Has the researcher presented sufficient evidence in support of the theoretical assumptions underpinning the study?
	■ Does the theoretical or conceptual basis of the study suggest ideological assumptions which may have influenced the findings?

Methodological critique

Most readers of this chapter will probably have had experience of critiquing individual research reports, particularly since the research critique appears to be a common assessment strategy for research modules on both pre- and postregistration educational programmes in nursing and health care. It is important that nurses and other health carers are encouraged to develop skills in critiquing research reports as this 'critical' culture has long been absent in the 'softer' caring disciplines. However, the value of a detailed review of one research paper for informing practice is questionable since it is unlikely to be appropriate to change nursing practice on the evidence of one study. Detailed checklists for critiquing individual research reports also become somewhat redundant in the context of reviewing a large body of literature.

Numerous checklists for reviewing individual research reports are available. However, in order to review a *body* of literature, a more pragmatic approach is required. In a very useful book on writing for social scientists, Cuba (1993) suggests that the following information should be extracted for each item in the review:

- A complete bibliographic reference
- The major questions posed in the study
- The method of investigation
- The major variables/concepts of interest and their operational definition
- The study population and sample
- The findings
- The authors' conclusions.

The methodological critique for each item can then be framed around the following questions adapted from Depoy and Gitlin (1994) in conjunction with material presented in earlier chapters of this book:

- What is the existing level of knowledge in relation to the topic and the population of interest? (see Chapters 1, 3, 4, 5)
- Does the research design used within the study reflect the existing level of knowledge and are the resultant findings at the level of exploration, description or prediction (Chapters 4, 5)?
- Consider the research strategy or design used in each study (Chapter 5):
  – Is it appropriate for the existing level of knowledge?
  – Is it appropriate to answer the question? (Chapters 5, 6, 7, 8, 9)
- Is there compatibility between procedures, findings and conclusions? (Chapters 6, 7, 9)
- Consider the boundaries of each study – what level of knowledge exists for the population and setting you are interested in? (Chapter 8)

Once this information has been extracted for each item and entered into the database (see Figure 3.4) a useful next step is to develop a methodological matrix for each theme (Table 10.2). This approach

See Figure 3.4, page 71

Table 10.2 *An example of a methodological matrix*
Promoting autonomy and independence among older people *(extract from methodological review for Concept: 'Routinised care')*

Author, Date, Number	Level of knowledge	Focus Boundaries of study	Methods – critique	Findings – compatibility
Waters 1994 1	Description/explanation	Styles of nursing in a rehabilitation setting 31 patients 2 rehab wards 1 hospital Purposive sample	Continuous non-participant observation ?? validity of observation schedule not established	Institutional practices impinge on patient experiences Rehab role poorly understood
Miller 1985 5	Association/prediction	Relationship between methods of care organization and patient outcomes Purposive/population/criteria 168 patients in 5 wards: acute, rehab, continuing care	Experimental design Outcome measure: patient dependency ?? limited measure	Individualized care reduces dependency for patients in hospital for more than one month
Faucett et al 1990 2	Exploration/association	Effects of implementing self-care model Convenience sample 50 residents in each of two nursing home care units	Quasi-experiment (no randomization) Documentary analysis (care plans) Interviews with nursing staff ?? design of documentation may influence record of care	Interviews identify impact on practice – not confirmed by documentation of care Recommend longitudinal study

enables easy comparison of studies relating to similar themes and issues. A similar approach can be used to extract the relevant information from non-empirical sources and suggested criteria are included in Box 10.3.

Box 10.3
Guiding questions for evaluating non-research sources

- What way of knowing and level of knowledge are presented?
- Was the work presented clearly, unambiguously and consistently?
- What is the purpose of the work? Implicit? Stated?
- How does the purpose influence the knowledge discussed in the work?
- What is the scope and/or application of the paper?
- What support exists for the claims being made in the source?
- What debates, new ideas, and trends are presented in the work?
- What are the strengths and weaknesses of the work?
- What research queries, or questions, emerge from the work?

DePoy and Gitlin (1994: 74)

Summary

The key to a successful literature review is a systematic approach. Items should be classified and relevant information extracted and stored in a database. The development of theme and method matrices is one approach to the classification and categorization of information.

Putting it all together

There is no strict 'recipe' for writing a literature review and the most appropriate format will often be determined by the literature under consideration. However, there are some general points which will help to ensure that the review remains focused and succeeds in identifying clear research-based indicators for practice, education and further research where these exist.

Aims and objectives

An important first step is to identify clear aims and objectives for the review. These should be written down and incorporated into the introduction. It is particularly important to return regularly to the aims in order to make sure that the review doesn't lose focus, so it is useful to keep them close by throughout the process of writing.

Structured plan

It is also important to have a plan since a good review requires structure and organization. The appropriate structure will usually emerge from a consideration of the main themes within the literature, which can then form sub-headings. It is important to use sub-headings within the written review in order to guide the reader around the main themes and issues. Several levels of heading can be used to provide a clear indication of the structure of the review if necessary. For example, our review of the literature on the promotion of autonomy and independence for older people was divided under three major sub-headings (Davies *et al* 1997b). These were:

1. Characteristics of autonomy, independence and dependence

This section considered definitions of the key concepts.

2. Autonomy and independence: why are these important concepts for nursing?

This section attempted to demonstrate the relevance of the key concepts for older people and hence for nursing practice.

3. How can nurses promote patient/client autonomy and independence?

This section, which formed the bulk of the review, considered nursing interventions and organizational factors for which there was empirical evidence to suggest an association with enhanced autonomy and independence for older people receiving nursing care. This broad theme was further sub-divided under four headings to reflect the main categories of intervention which emerged from the literature. These were:

- Systems of care delivery which promote comprehensive individualized assessment
- Attempts to encourage patients/clients to participate in decisions about their care
- Patterns of communication which avoid exerting power and control over patients/clients
- Attempts to modify the environment to promote autonomy and independence and minimize risk.

Drawing on these themes, the authors were able to identify some general principles for caregiving which can enable nurses to promote self-determination and independence for older people in their care.

Within each section of the review it is important to emphasize relatedness and keep the reader aware of the way in which the literature under discussion is related to your topic. Try to avoid presenting a sequential list of studies and their characteristics; rather compare and contrast studies to identify commonalities and contradictions. Where contradictions are found, try to identify possible explanations such as the use of a different conceptual framework. This is where the synthesis of findings and evidence starts to take shape.

Structure   As mentioned previously, there is no right or wrong way to structure the review. The following outline is intended merely as a guide to ensure that all relevant information is included. As with any research-based paper, it is essential that the review has a clear introduction, a middle section where the main arguments are developed, and a concise summary. Within these broad parameters, the final structure of the review will be determined by the nature of the topic, in particular the themes which have emerged from the consideration of the literature.

Introduction   This should provide a brief overview, stating the focus of the review and defining limits such as time period covered and data-bases searched. It is important to describe the methods for undertaking the review, including criteria for the selection of items. Ideally, all relevant literature will be reviewed but it is usually necessary to base a review upon a sample of the literature or to select on the basis of predetermined criteria. The introduction should also outline the structure of the review including the main themes and sub-headings.

Critical review of specific themes and concepts   Integrative reviews should present sufficient detail to allow the reader to assess the appropriateness of the review procedures as well as threats to the validity of the review findings (Jackson 1980). In other words, it is important to include enough information about the studies reviewed to allow readers to examine the evidence and draw their own conclusions. Important characteristics to report include:

- Sample size
- Characteristics of respondents
- Methods for assigning subjects to groups
- Measurement of dependent and independent variables
- Sample attrition
- Method of data analysis
- Theory or conceptual framework used.

One of the clearest and simplest ways to represent characteristics of the primary research is through the construction of tables or matrices. The use of tables allows the reviewer to present the reader with a considerable amount of raw data. The narrative can then focus upon a systematic examination, summary and discussion of major findings and conclusions. A good example is provided by Caris Verhallen *et al* (1997) in a review of literature on nurses' communication with older people.

Within this section, you should discuss in some detail those studies which are most relevant to the aims of the review. Studies using similar methodologies or with similar findings should be compared to identify similarities and differences. Other studies can be grouped together where the evidence suggests similar conclusions. Don't feel that all the material reviewed needs to be mentioned. In particular, avoid forcing a reference into a review if it does not seem to fit.

Summary   This section should include a précis of both theoretical and methodological critiques as well as identifying the main findings of the review. Essentially, the summary should represent a synthesis of existing literature indicating the state of current knowledge about the topic under investigation. It is particularly important to identify clear indicators for practice, education and further research based upon the evaluation of existing evidence. Gaps in current knowledge and areas of research inactivity should be noted. Although it is essential that the review represents the important points and issues *emerging from the literature* rather than your own opinion, this section requires critical judgment about the extensiveness and dependability of information on a topic. However, the reviewer should present facts and findings in the 'tentative language that befits scientific enquiry' (Polit and Hungler 1991). Finally, the summary should identify the implications of the findings of the review for the provision of health care and for further research. Here it is important to bear in mind the concept of 'level of knowledge' (Chapter 5). The predominant methodologies used to research the topic and the level of knowledge created will provide an important indication of the ways in which the findings of the review can be used. The summary of the literature review for the autonomy project follows.

Example   **Summary and critique of literature review for ENB project (Davies *et al* 1997b)**

Because of the varied dimensions of the topic, a wide range of research approaches have been used to investigate both the process and outcome of nursing interventions aimed at promoting autonomy and independence for the older client/patient. Given these varied approaches, and the range of settings in which research has been conducted, it is difficult to compare and contrast individual studies in order to generate clear indicators for nursing practice. In effect, the body of research literature indicates rather more of 'what nurses could try' rather than 'what nurses should do' (Hunt 1981). In particular, there is little information to inform decisions related to the balance between minimizing risk and promoting patient/client autonomy. However, this is essentially an ethical debate which can perhaps only be informed to a limited extent by empirical work. In justifying and defending standards of care that meet basic humanitarian principles (Ebrahim et al 1994), nurses frequently need to rely upon non-empirical knowledge and understanding (Carper 1978).

Most research related to the topic has been carried out in long-term care settings and it may not always be appropriate to extrapolate from one care setting to another. Empirical evidence which identifies factors associated with the quality of care for patients in acute, rehabilitation and community settings (other than nursing homes) is limited. Moreover, research which has sought the views of older people themselves has focused upon those without a significant degree of cognitive impairment. Whilst it is likely that the principles of caregiving which have emerged from this review are as relevant to working with older people who are less 'active', the means of achieving them requires special consideration. There is some evidence, for example, that innovative approaches to user involvement can ensure that the views of very frail older people contribute to service development (Barnes and Walker 1996). However, there is an obvious need for further research, particularly in relation to identifying the views of service users themselves.

In spite of these methodological limitations, the body of literature provides some pointers for nursing practice. A consistent theme is the need to ensure that nursing care is tailored to individual needs if patients and clients are to achieve optimal levels of autonomy and independence. Individualized assessment and care planning underpin many of the strategies associated with the promotion of autonomy, independence and high quality care within the literature. Systems for care delivery which support patient-centred practice such as primary nursing and nurse-led team care have also been associated with higher levels of self-determination and patient satisfaction, although the evidence to date has emerged from a series of small-scale studies.

The evidence in relation to interpersonal strategies which encourage patient choice and participation in decision-making is more persuasive. In particular it appears that the ability to make even quite small decisions about day-to-day activities can have a significant impact on an older person's sense of control. A wealth of research conducted in a wide range of care settings has demonstrated the importance of adequate information in promoting patient recovery and this should form a fundamental principle of care delivery. The consequences of eliciting feedback from a patient in relation to care given is less well documented but some evidence suggests that identifying the patient/client's perspective should be a basic principle of care. In particular, there is evidence to suggest that there is often a disparity between nurses' perceptions and the perceptions of older people themselves in relation to priorities for caregiving.

Other strategies which recognize the patient as a person with individual needs include identifying the extent to which a patient or client wishes to be involved in care planning and delivery, demonstrating reciprocity within the nurse-patient relationship and attempting wherever possible to promote patients' privacy and dignity. However, nurses should also be alert to the socializing effects of institutions and organizations which may influence patients' expectations of their relationships with health-care professionals. Organizational barriers to change, such as fixed mealtimes within an institution or a lack of aids and equipment, may also act as a constraint upon patient choice and autonomy. Perhaps one of the most effective actions that nurses could take to promote greater autonomy and independence for older patients and clients would be to campaign for greater flexibility in these areas.

A note of caution is sounded in a useful review of the literature on patient empowerment (Elliott and Turrell 1996). While supporting the general ideal, the authors highlight several important tensions for nurses attempting to empower patients. These include advocating 'active' patients while allowing for patient individuality, acknowledging patients' right to decide but accepting the practical constraints on their freedom to choose, ensuring informed choice without creating information overload and providing individualized care without invading the patient's privacy. These tensions suggest the need for advanced interpersonal skills in order to maintain an appropriate balance between promoting autonomy and maintaining independence.

This review suggests a need for further research to establish patient and client outcomes in relation to specific nursing interventions aimed at promoting autonomy and independence. However, in the absence of firm predictive evidence, we would argue that there is sufficient descriptive research to suggest that the principles identified within this review should provide a basis for nurse education and practice at the present time. These are:

- Offering choice in relation to day-to-day activities
- Giving information about care
- Eliciting feedback on care given
- Encouraging participation in care planning
- Promoting independence in the activities of daily living
- Facilitating privacy and dignity
- Demonstrating reciprocity.

Some points about style

As with any piece of writing, it is important to ensure that a literature review is written in a clear and readable style and is structured to maintain the reader's interest. It is also important to maintain a balanced approach. Structured checklists for critiquing research reports can make reviewers very cynical about the literature by encouraging

Box 10.4
How not to include references!

Researchers (Findings and Lookin 1990; Seeker, Findings, Lookin & Arena, 1991; Wiseman, Searcher & Findings, 1992) often know a lot about their subject by the time they complete a study (Finis, Enders, Dunn, Over & Caput 1990; Terminus, Complete, Enders, Dunn & Last, 1989). For instance Findings and Lookin (1990) and Seeker et al (1991) believe it is difficult, if not impossible, to sum up that much information. Oodles, Much and Complex (1922) documented this in their seminal work, which was replicated by More, Less and Somme (1942). Social influence (Complete, Overmuch & Somme, 1952; Push, Pull & Shake, 1967), anxiety (Worried, Shook & Rattled 1987), and weariness (Tired, Worn & Shot, 1978) all play a role in the problem of condensing findings. Lost, Worried, Shook and Rattled (1988) confirmed these results. Given the plethora of information (Complete, Overmuch & More, 1952; Push, Pull and Heave, 1967; Worried, Shook and Catalysis, 1987), we definitely have sufficient evidence to indicate immediate action is necessary.

Downs (1994)

Box 10.5
Criteria for evaluating literature reviews

Introduction

- Is the rationale stated clearly so that the relevance of the review is determined quickly?
- Is the rationale important (significant)?
- Is the purpose of the review stated clearly?
- *Is the policy context for the review clearly identified?*

Methodology

- Were the criteria for the selection of references clearly identified?
- Did the author(s) critically assess the studies included in the review?
- *Are the limits of the review clearly identified (in terms of time period covered, databases searched)?*

Discussion or conclusions

- Did the author(s) integrate the selected references or merely restate the individual findings and conclusions?
- Were the conclusions supported by the references reviewed?

Application

- What information have you learned from this article that can be applied to practice?

Klausner and Green (1991)

a focus on weaknesses and limitations of a study rather than strengths. However, good research is very difficult to achieve and there is a danger that structured checklists may be over-critical. A balanced view is required which acknowledges the validity of current knowledge in addition to any limitations.

Downs (1994) highlights the issue of balance in relation to citation of references within a review of the literature (Box 10.4). She suggests that some statements are so obvious that they do not need to be supported with references. General comments can be used to introduce a paragraph without an accompanying string of citations. Authors can then be referred to one by one in the subsequent paragraph and the context of the opening statement is made clear. Downs suggests that it is generally unnecessary to cite more than four references to support previously established relationships. You should use the most recent and credible work as evidence. A literature review dominated by a laundry list of citations is boring reading and signals the author's inability to synthesize the content (Downs 1994). It is also important to be concise and to summarize. In other words: review the literature – don't reproduce it!

Klausner and Green (1991) suggest a series of criteria for evaluating literature reviews which can be helpful in attempting to construct your own review. An adapted version is included as Box 10.5.

Summary

As with any academic paper, a literature review should be clearly structured. The introduction should identify the focus and rationale for the review as well as the methods and boundaries. The main body of the review should be structured according to the key themes to emerge from the literature examined. Within each section, individual studies can then be compared and contrasted to identify consistent and contradictory findings. The final section should summarize the key points to emerge from the theoretical and methodological critique of individual items and identify implications of the review for practice, education and further research.

Exercise 10.4

Using one of the literature reviews listed at the end of this chapter, apply the criteria in Box 10.5 to critique the review. Alternatively, apply the criteria to a literature review which you have written yourself. How could the review be improved?

Putting reviews into practice

Issues relating to the use of research to inform practice are covered in detail in Chapters 11 and 12. However, an interesting suggestion for ensuring that systematic reviews inform nursing practice described by Swanson *et al* (1990) is worth mentioning here. The authors describe a research teaching strategy whereby nursing students are attached to nurses in a practice setting and collaborate to review the literature relating to a clinically defined problem. The resulting information is then shared with the practice team. Such initiatives can ensure that the work invested in reviewing the literature on a particular topic or problem has a direct impact on practice.

Chapter conclusion

With the current emphasis on evidence-based practice, the ability to review and synthesize the available literature on a particular topic is an essential skill for all those involved in health care. This chapter has outlined a systematic, step-by-step approach to literature review which should enable 'beginning' reviewers to overcome the first hurdle of knowing where to start. By following the steps outlined here, the critical reviewer should be able to produce a concise summary of the literature which evaluates both the theoretical basis of knowledge in a particular topic area and the methods used to generate that knowledge. Appropriate indicators for practice, education and research can then be identified in the light of the strengths and limitations of the body of literature reviewed. The next step is to ensure that these indicators are translated into action where appropriate and this particular challenge forms the focus of the final two chapters of this book.

Further reading

Articles and chapters about writing literature reviews
Cuba L (1993) *A Short Guide to Writing about Social Science.* New York: Harper Collins.
Cullum N (1994) Critical reviews of the literature. In Hardey M and Mulhall A (eds) *Nursing Research: Theory and Practice.* London: Chapman & Hall.
Locke (1993) *Proposals that work: a guide for planning dissertations and grant proposals.* London: Sage.

Examples of literature reviews
When writing a review for the first time it can be helpful to look at published examples and some useful reviews are listed here. Bear in mind, though, the limitations of many published reviews identified by Cullum (Box 10.1, page 234).

Bain L (1996) Preceptorship: a review of the literature. *Journal of Advanced Nursing* **24**(1): 104–107.

Barriball K, While A and Norman I (1992) Continuing professional education for qualified nurses: a review of the literature. *Journal of Advanced Nursing* **17**(9): 1129–1140.

Bergen A (1991) Nurses caring for the terminally ill in the community: a review of the literature. *International Journal of Nursing Studies* **28**(1): 89–101.

Caris Verhallen W, Kerkstra A and Bensing J (1997) The role of communication in nursing care for older people: a review of the literature. *Journal of Advanced Nursing* **25**: 915–933.

Davies S, Laker S and Ellis L (1997) Promoting autonomy and independence for older people within nursing practice: a review of the literature review. *Journal of Advanced Nursing* **26**(2): 408–417.

Goodman C (1986) Research on the informal carer: a selected literature review. *Journal of Advanced Nursing* **11**: 705–712.

Kelly M and May D (1982) Good and bad patients: a review of the literature and a theoretical critique. *Journal of Advanced Nursing* **7**: 147–156.

Webb C and Askham J (1987) Nurses' knowledge and attitudes about sexuality in health care – a review of the literature. *Nurse Education Today* **7**: 75–87.

References

Abbott P and Sapsford R (1992) Leaving it to mum: 'Community care' for mentally handicapped children. In Abbott P and Sapsford R (eds) *Research into Practice: A Reader for Nurses and the Caring Professions*. Buckingham: Open University Press.

Barnes M and Walker M (1996) Consumerism versus empowerment; a principled approach to the involvement of older service users. *Policy and Politics* **24**(4): 375–393.

Becker H (1986) Writing for social scientists: how to start and finish your thesis, book, or article. Chicago, University of Chicago Press.

Brooker C, Repper J and Booth A (1996) *The Effectiveness of Community Mental Health Nursing: a Review*. Sheffield: Sheffield Centre for Health and Related Research.

Caris Verhallen W, Kerkstra A and Bensing J (1997) The role of communication in nursing care for older people: a review of the literature. *Journal of Advanced Nursing* **25**(5): 915–933.

Carper BA (1978) Fundamental patterns of knowing in nursing. *Advances in Nursing Science* **1**(1): 13–23.

Chalmers I and Altman D (1995) *Systematic Reviews*. London: BMJ Publishing.

Cuba L (1993) *A Short Guide to Writing about Social Science*, 2nd edn. New York: Harper Collins.

Cullum N (1994) Critical reviews of the literature. In Hardey M and Mulhall A (eds) *Nursing Research: Theory and Practice*. London: Chapman & Hall.

Cullum N, Dickson R and Eastwood A (1995) The prevention and treatment of pressure sores: how effective are pressure-relieving interventions and risk assessment for the prevention and treatment of pressure sores? *Effective Health Care Bulletin* **2**(1).

Davies S, Ellis L, Laker S, *et al* (1997a) *Evaluation of pre- and post-registration education for the care of older people*. Final report to the English National Board for Nursing, Midwifery and Health Visiting. Sheffield: University of Sheffield.

Davies S, Laker S and Ellis L (1997b) Promoting autonomy and independence for older people within nursing practice: a literature review. *Journal of Advanced Nursing* **26**(2): 408–417.

DePoy E and Gitlin L (1993*) Introduction to Research: Multiple Strategies for Health and Human Services*. St Louis, MO: Mosby.

Downs FS (1994) Information Processing. *Nursing Research* **43**(6): 323.

Droogan J and Song F (1996) The process and importance of systematic reviews. *Nurse Researcher* **4**(1): 15–26.

Ebrahim S, Wallis C, Brittis S, Harwood R and Graham N (1994) Long term care for elderly people. *Quality in Health Care* **2**(3): 198–203.

Elliott M, Turrell A (1996) Understanding the conflicts of patient empowerment. *Nursing Standard* **10**(45): 43–47.

Evers H (1984) *Patients' Experiences and the Social Relations of Patient Care in Geriatric Wards*. Unpublished PhD thesis, Coventry: University of Warwick.

Faucett J, Ellis V, Underwood P, Naqvi A and Wilson D (1990) The effect of Orem's self-care model on nursing care in a nursing home setting. *Journal of Advanced Nursing* **15**(6): 659–666.

Ganong LH (1987) Integrative reviews of nursing research. *Research in Nursing and Health* **10**: 1–11.

Gilbert N (1993) Research, theory and method. In Gilbert N (ed) *Researching Social Life*. London: Sage.

Hunt J (1981) Indicators for nursing practice: the use of research findings, *Journal of Advanced Nursing* **12**(1), 101–110.

Jackson GB (1980) Methods for integrative reviews. *Review of Educational Research* **50**: 438–460.

Johanson L (1985) Ten hints for thesis survival. *Nursing Outlook* **33**(4): 206, 208.

Klausner LH and Green TG (1991) An instructional method for teaching literature evaluation. *Journal of Continuing Education in the Health Professions* **11**(4): 331–339.

Kogan N (1961) Attitudes towards old people: the development of a scale and examination of correlates. *Journal of Abnormal and Social Psychology* **62**: 44–54.

Lederman R (1992) Reviews of research literature: meta-analysis for synthesising. *American Journal of Maternal and Child Nursing* **17**(3): 157.

Miller A (1985) Nurse–patient dependency: is it iatrogenic? *Journal of Advanced Nursing* **10**: 63–9.

Nolan M, Nolan J and Booth A (1997) *Preparation for Multi-Professional/Multi-Agency Health Care Practice: The Nursing Contribution to Rehabilitation within the Multi-Disciplinary Team. Literature Review and Curriculum Analysis*. Final Report to the English National Board for Nursing, Midwifery and Health Visiting, London.

Palmore E (1977) Facts on aging. A short quiz. *The Gerontologist* **21**: 115–116.

Polit DF and Hungler BP (1991) *Nursing Research: Principles and Methods*. Philadelphia, PA: Lippincott.

Raatikainen R (1991) Self-activeness and the need for help in domiciliary care. *Journal of Advanced Nursing* **16**(10): 1150–1157.

Reed J (1994) Phenomenology without phenomena: a discussion of the use of phenomenology to examine expertise in long term care of elderly patients. *Journal of Advanced Nursing* **19**(2), 336–41.

Roe B (1994) Undertaking a critical review of the literature. *Nurse Researcher* **1**(1): 35–46.

Sapsford R (1994) Making sense of the literature. *Nurse Researcher* **1**(1): 23–30.

Swanson J, Easterling P, Costa L and Creamer-Bauer C (1990) Student-staff collaboration in identifying nursing problems and reviewing the literature. *Western Journal of Nursing Research* **12**(2): 262–266.

Waddell D (1992) The effects of continuing education on nursing practice: a meta-analysis. *Journal of Continuing Education in Nursing* **23**(4): 164–168.

Waters K (1994) Getting dressed in the early

morning: styles of staff/patient interaction on rehabilitation wards for elderly people. *Journal of Advanced Nursing* **19**(2), 239–248.

White E, Riley E, Davies S and Twinn S (1993) *A detailed study of the relationship between teaching, support, supervision and role modelling in clinical areas, within the context of Project 2000 courses.* Report for the English National Board for Nursing, Midwifery and Health Visiting, London.

Wright (1988) A reconceptualisation of the 'negative staff attitudes and poor care in nursing homes assumption'. *The Gerontologist* **28**(6): 813–820.

11 Factors which may inhibit the utilization of research findings in practice – and some solutions

Ann McDonnell

Introduction

The importance of basing health interventions on sound research findings wherever possible is an important goal in today's health service. It is difficult to overestimate the significance of this issue in terms of health gain, cost effectiveness, consumer preference and – last but not least – in terms of professional development.

The case for an evidence-based health service is undeniable and has been made throughout this book. Previous chapters have focused on the nature of research-based knowledge, the context of research and on the retrieval and analysis of existing research. Once equipped with the skills to understand and accomplish these complex *intellectual* challenges, you may feel it unnecessary to dwell on a chapter that considers the practicalities of *using* research. Surely when one has 'fathomed it out', the next step is relatively straightforward? Unfortunately, there is a growing body of opinion, supported in some areas by sound evidence, to suggest that research findings are often *not* used in practice and, consequently, potential improvements in the standard and quality of patient care are not being realized. This problem pervades all areas of health care practice although its significance has been most widely addressed in the fields of medicine and nursing.

The existence of a gap between research and practice in the field of health care has long been recognized. Peters (1992) notes that Lord Rothschild, speaking in 1968 to the World Health Organization, stated:

> *'If for the next 20 years, no further research were to be carried out, if there were a moratorium in research, the application of what is already known, of what has already been discovered, would result in widespread improvement in world health'*
>
> (Peters 1992: 68)

Peters argues that this contention still holds true within today's health service and that research utilization should be a crucial organizational goal.

In Chapter 2 Sue Read discusses the context of nursing and health care research and describes the evolution of the NHS Research and Development Strategy which addresses the dual challenge of maximizing the benefits of science and technology for health care and applying research rigour to the problems confronting health services (DoH 1993a). However, as Professor Peckham indicates in the same report, the ultimate return on any research investment depends on the *impact* of the research in practice. This issue will form the focus of this chapter, which will consider the factors which may inhibit the utilization of research in practice and propose some possible solutions to the problem.

Key issues

- Do nurses use research?
- Barriers to research utilization
- Possible solutions for overcoming the research–practice gap

Given the wealth of published material about research utilization in nursing and midwifery and current interest within the profession, the emphasis throughout this chapter will be primarily on nursing and midwifery contexts although reference will be made to other health professions where appropriate.

Preliminary points

It is first necessary to acknowledge the following important points:

- Not all nursing practice *can* be based on research, due to:
  - the current state of knowledge in relation to nursing practice and
  - the nature of nursing practice
- Not all research is *directly* usable in nursing practice
- Inappropriate use of research findings is just as problematic as not using the research we should.

Not all nursing practice can be based on research

The current state of knowledge in relation to nursing practice

It is a fallacy to assume that nurses fail to achieve the 'holy grail' of research-based practice merely because they do not use available research. Rather there is a *dearth* of valid research which is appropriate for application in practice. Much nursing research has been devoted to managerial and educational issues rather than nursing practice *per se*. Wilson-Barnett *et al* (1990) point out that although the proportion of clinically relevant studies is increasing, most involve description rather than evaluation of care. Consequently, we are not yet in a position as nurses or midwives where all the care we deliver *can* be based on robust scientific evidence.

Nurses have been accused of carrying out shotgun research – one-off studies in many different areas of interest (Hinshaw and Heinrich 1990). This pattern of sporadic research may have prevented us from developing any depth of knowledge about practice (Closs and Cheater 1994). Such a pattern may derive from the context of many nursing research studies in the UK which are carried out in order to fulfil the requirements of degree programmes rather than within the context of funded research.

In addition, some fields of nursing practice may be particularly under-researched. Luker and Kenrick (1992) discuss this in relation to community nursing and argue that most studies relating to 'technical' practices have been conducted in hospital environments, with little indication as to their transferability to the community setting.

The nature of nursing practice

The nature and complexity of nursing practice renders many aspects inaccessible to the research process. Baier (1988) makes these points in relation to the chronically mentally ill where research is extremely difficult to conduct, both for ethical reasons and because outcome criteria are hard to define. In many practice situations, nursing interventions can never be *purely* research-based because they are so complex and individualized. For example, whilst giving preoperative information to reduce post-operative pain and anxiety has a sound research base, the needs of a woman before mastectomy can only be met by a nurse who delivers care based on an *amalgam* of knowledge. Research-based knowledge or 'science' represents only one constituent in this blend. Equally important are other sources of knowledge such as empathy and personal knowledge which form part of what Carper (1978) describes as 'aesthetics' or the 'art of nursing'. Mike Nolan and Ulla Lundh discuss these issues more widely in Chapter 1 and note that science represents only one way of 'knowing' in health care.

Not all research is directly usable in nursing practice

Health care research does not always result in changes in practice, or provide what Williamson (1992) refers to as an 'off-the-peg' solution to a problem. Often the value of a research study is that it redefines the question, or alters our perceptions and causes us to reflect.

Many writers (for example Stetler and DiMaggio 1991, Rodgers 1994) refer to *'levels of utilisation'*. Following a literature search and a consultation exercise with 41 nurses, Rodgers (1994) concluded that research may be of:

- Direct use – explanatory and predictive findings immediately applicable to practice
- Indirect use – enlightening, extending understanding of practice
- Methodological use – e.g. measurement scales, outcome measures or tools that may be used in practice.

Exercise 11.1	*Try and think of an example of each level of research utilization*

Try and think of an example of each level of research utilization
You have probably been able to do this quickly for at least one of the levels, in relation to your own area of practice. Let us consider the field of practice nursing and the role of the practice nurse in the prevention of cardiovascular disease (CVD) and stroke. Examples in this context might include:

- **Direct** – a review of the evidence in the area of cholesterol screening (Anglia and Oxford RHA 1994) has indicated that population screening is contraindicated and that only those with other risk factors such as a family history of CVD should be screened
- **Indirect** – awareness of the substantive body of evidence that CVD and stroke are associated with a number of risk factors such as family history, hypertension, smoking, high plasma cholesterol, etc. (e.g. DoH 1993b, Trent RHA 1993)
- **Methodological** – the use of a risk assessment tool, e.g. the Dundee Risk Disk which has been shown to increase the accuracy of CVD risk assessment (Tunstall-Pedoe 1991)

Inappropriate use of research findings is just as problematic as not using the research we should

We may all have been tempted at times to change practice as a result of reading a single study without careful and critical consideration of issues such as its quality, generalizability, applicability to our own clinical setting and the existence of further supporting research. Let's consider a hypothetical example: a study comparing the effectiveness of acupuncture with more conventional methods of pain relief for women in labour is published in a well-known midwifery journal. The author reports that the women who received acupuncture reported lower levels of pain at every stage of labour. However, on closer reading, it becomes clear that only ten women from the same hospital were studied and the women in the acupuncture group were older and excluded primigravidae. The danger of using this study as a basis for recommending acupuncture as the analgesia of choice to *all* women in labour without further rigorous research on a larger scale, in a variety of settings, with a range of clearly defined outcome measures (and including an economic evaluation!), is clear.

Summary	Whilst the case for 'evidence-based health care' is undeniable, the use of research evidence in nursing practice can never provide all the answers. Our research base is patchy and we require other 'ways of knowing' in order to provide effective and appropriate patient care. Furthermore, given the potential hazards of misusing

research (see Chapter 1), the skills and tools for interpreting and evaluating research discussed in previous chapters are vital requirements for every nurse.

Do nurses use research?

Within the nursing literature, there is a wealth of anecdotal evidence suggesting that nurses fail to use research widely within their practice (e.g. Hunt 1981, Walsh and Ford 1989). However, on delving a little deeper into the literature on research utilization in nursing, it becomes apparent that there has been surprisingly little research in this area. Much of the existing evidence is also North American in origin and may therefore have limited relevance for the UK.

Although it is not the purpose of this chapter to provide a comprehensive review of the literature on research utilization by nurses, a brief outline is included in order to illustrate the paucity of our knowledge in this important area.

American studies

A number of studies have been carried out in the USA (Ketefian 1975, Kirchoff 1982, Kreuger 1982, Brett 1987, Champion and Leach 1989, Coyle and Sokop 1990, Stetler and DiMaggio 1991, Bostrom and Suter 1993, Rizzuto et al 1994). These report on the use of research by nurses in a variety of settings such as critical care units (CCUs) (Kirchoff 1982) and community hospitals (Ketefian 1975). The studies examine the level of research-based practice in relation to a wide variety of nursing interventions including oral temperature taking (Ketefian 1975), mutual goal setting (Kreuger 1982), IV cannula change and preoperative relaxation training (Brett 1987).

These studies demonstrate considerable variation in reported levels of research utilization. In Brett's (1987) study, 10 out of 14 research-based innovations were implemented by a majority of the nurses surveyed 'at least sometimes', although the level of adoption varied according to the practice concerned. In contrast, only 16% of the nurses surveyed by Bostrom and Suter (1993) reported making a research-based practice change during the previous six months.

Whilst it is clear that there is some evidence to indicate that nurses do not always base their practice on research findings, relatively little work has been done to date and the available evidence is limited in a number of important respects. Some studies used small, convenience samples, e.g. Ketefian (1975) (n = 87), Champion and Leach (1989) (n = 59), Stetler and DiMaggio (1989) (n = 24). Of those studies which selected respondents randomly, one was a small study (Coyle and Sokop 1990) (n = 20) and many had response rates of less than 60% (Kreuger 1982, Coyle and Sokop 1990, Bostrom and Suter 1993, Rizzuto *et al* 1994). In view of these limitations, the generalization of these findings to the majority of American nurses is inappropriate.

UK studies   The UK research in this field consists mostly of small studies of hospital nurses (Murray 1988, Webb and Mackenzie 1993, Lacey 1994, Hull 1995). Consequently, indications which suggest that research is not always applied in practice cannot be generalized beyond the respondents in each study.

It would not be surprising to find that many nurses often feel downhearted at the widespread concern and weight of opinion within the profession concerning their lack of research application. It may therefore be helpful to point out at this juncture that nurses are not alone! Failure to implement research into practice is a problem throughout the health service rather than a problem unique to nurses. Occupational therapists, physiotherapists, speech therapists and doctors all acknowledge problems in this area (Antman 1992, DoH 1992, DoH 1994). The Advisory Group on Health Technology Assessment, for example, note the unnecessary and damaging delays in the introduction of technologies such as tamoxifen and chemotherapy for early breast cancer and antiplatelet therapy in cardiovascular disease (DoH 1992). Given the generic nature of the problem, putting research into practice has become the focus for multidisciplinary interest both nationally and internationally.

Summary   Clearly, there is a need for more research to determine the extent of research utilization in a variety of fields of nursing in the UK. There are obvious problems associated with trying to measure activities such as research utilization (which may be a conscious or unconscious process). However, this work is crucial – without it we will be unable to assess the effectiveness of any strategy to promote evidence-based care.

Barriers to research utilization   *Do we really know why some nurses don't use research findings?*

Potential reasons for the 'research–practice gap' abound within the nursing literature, with a host of explanations ranging from the simple to the complex. Notable studies which have attempted to explore barriers to research use include American studies by Kreuger (1982), Brett (1987), Champion and Leach (1989), Coyle and Sokop (1990), Funk et al (1991), Bostrum and Suter (1993) and Rizzuto *et al* (1994); and UK studies by Luker and Kenrick (1992), Lacey (1994); and Rodgers (1994). However, there are considerable limitations in our current knowledge in this area in spite of this growing body of research. Some reasons for this will now be outlined.

Comparatively little research has been done on this complex topic and again, much of the literature in this area is North American in origin. Some studies focus *exclusively* on research utilization, e.g.

Kreuger (1982), Brett (1987), Champion and Leach (1989), Coyle and Sokop (1990), Funk et al (1991), Luker and Kenrick (1992), Lacey (1994) and Rodgers (1994). Others, e.g. Rizutto *et al* (1994) and Hicks (1995), address the conduct of research and the utilization of research findings within the broad remit of 'attitudes towards research' which may neglect aspects of what is essentially a very complex issue.

Of the studies which do focus on research utilization, the issue is addressed mainly from the perspective of individual practitioners. Although organizational factors are often discussed, few studies attempt to address the reasons why some practice settings have a *climate* which supports research utilization, and others do not.

Much of the literature focuses on hospital-based practitioners in particular settings and may not be relevant to other settings, for example the community (Brett 1987, Champion and Leach 1989, Coyle and Sokop 1990, Lacey 1994 and Rodgers 1994). Most studies rely on self-reported use of research as a measure of research in use, e.g. Kreuger (1982), Brett (1987), Champion and Leach (1989), Coyle and Sokop (1990), Funk *et al* (1991), Bostrum and Suter (1993) and Rizzuto *et al* (1994).

In summary, our current knowledge is sketchy and there is clearly a need for more research in this area, as proposed by the Taskforce on the Strategy for Research in Nursing, Midwifery and Health Visiting (DoH 1993c). Meanwhile, on the basis of the limited research to date and on the wealth of published anecdotal material, a number of possible barriers to research utilization can be identified.

Exercise 11.2	What do you think are the main barriers to research use? Before reading on, list as many as you can think of.

In the exercise above, you have probably identified a variety of barriers which relate to your own experience or that of your colleagues. You may find some of these included below.

Possible barriers may be considered under three headings:

- Barriers related to the accessibility of research
- Barriers related to the individual
- Barriers related to the setting.

Barriers related to the accessibility of research

Many of the barriers alluded to in the literature relate to the difficulties nurses face in either obtaining research reports or being able to interpret them sufficiently to make a decision on their potential value in practice. These problems are summarized below.

Research is not published

Many research studies are conducted to fulfil the requirements of academic courses and may never be submitted for publication. Hicks (1995) surveyed 500 UK nurses selected randomly through 50 senior nurse managers (with a 46% response rate). The results suggested a reluctance to submit research findings for publication due to a pronounced lack of confidence. This so-called 'grey' literature may include important contributions to nursing and midwifery knowledge.

Research findings are often disseminated through conferences or workshops that clinical nurses may not attend

Opportunities to attend conferences where up-to-date research is presented and discussed are likely to be few and far between for those at the 'coal-face' of nursing practice. It can also be quite intimidating for practitioners who lack confidence in their own awareness of research to question researchers in these fora and this may limit the value of such encounters.

Lack of access to library facilities

For many clinical nurses access to research may be severely limited by a lack of library facilities. Nurses interviewed by Rodgers (1994), for example, cited the location of the library or its inconvenient opening hours as barriers to research utilization. In a recent study of practice nurses, we found that 25% of a sample of more than 1000 practice nurses did not have easy access to library facilities (McDonnell *et al* 1997).

Research is often published in journals that clinical nurses don't read

Many research studies are published in academic research-based journals rather than in the more popular professional journals such as *Nursing Times* or *Nursing Standard*. Evidence suggests that clinical nurses are less likely to read research journals (Webb and Mackenzie 1993). The Research Assessment Exercise (to which academic departments of nursing are subject as part of the quality assurance system in higher education) compounds this situation. Researchers are given more credit for publishing in academic rather than professional journals and this gives researchers little incentive to publish their findings for a wider nursing audience.

Language used and user friendliness of research reports

The barrier presented by the use of language and terms that clinicians find hard to grapple with, coupled with a style which is seldom 'user friendly' is well known. This factor was identified as a potential barrier by nurses in studies by Webb and Mackenzie (1993) and Rodgers (1994).

Lack of user friendly research that has already been critiqued and its implications discussed

Based on my own experience of teaching research appreciation, I know that the task of trying to tease out the implications for practice from a piece of published research is daunting for many nurses. Critical appraisal of research findings demands considerable knowledge about the research process and complex intellectual skills. It is also a very time-consuming business. Armitage (1990) describes the activities of a small working group in Wales established to facilitate research utilization in practice. The group identified lack of critical reading skills as a major obstacle. A further illustration is provided by Hunt (1987) who conducted an action research study involving nurse teachers, ward sisters and nurse managers in the process of identifying nursing problems, evaluating and synthesizing relevant literature and applying the research in practice. The nurse teachers also found great difficulty in critiquing research reports.

Limited availability of research reviews

The difficulties associated with evaluating a **cumulative** body of research evidence are immense (Gould 1986, McIntosh 1995). The obstacle posed by this potential overload of information is cited in studies by Hunt (1987) and Rodgers (1994). When attempting to practice evidence-based nursing in relation to a particular patient problem, the clinician may be faced with a baffling range of research studies with findings which may even contradict each other – a daunting task for even the most determined practitioner. The complex and time-consuming nature of the process of synthesizing and evaluating large bodies of research is clearly beyond the remit of many practitioners, purely on a practical level.

Barriers related to the individual

Nurses don't read research

This view is often cited as one of the barriers to research utilization in nursing (e.g. Hunt 1981) and some studies have indeed indicated that many nurses may not read professional journals (Myco 1980, Webb and Mackenzie 1993). A significant link between reading research and reported research utilization was demonstrated in a study by Brett (1987), and in a number of studies nurses have identified professional journals as one of their sources of research awareness (Kreuger 1982, Stetler and DiMaggio 1989, Coyle and Sokop 1990, Rodgers 1994). The significance of professional reading habits may therefore be considerable in terms of research implementation.

Negative attitudes towards research

Nurses are often viewed as having negative attitudes towards research, although studies in this area indicate the complexities of the issues involved and by no means support such a clear-cut assertion. Champion and Leach (1989) and Lacey (1994), in studies with small samples of nurses, found some evidence of positive attitudes to research amongst qualified nurses, while Bostrom et al (1989) found that attitudes varied according to a number of factors including educational qualifications. It might be expected that a positive attitude towards research would act as a precursor to research utilization and this link has been demonstrated in studies by Champion and Leach

(1989) and Rizutto *et al* (1994). However, the possibility of individual practitioners of all disciplines rejecting research findings which do not concur with their own beliefs or experiences is all too real.

Nurses don't know how to use research

Once nurses have dealt with the tricky business of critical analysis, there remains the problem of how to implement the findings. As Closs and Cheater (1994) point out, criteria for research utilization are not well developed. Consequently, on what basis can we judge a body of research suitable for use in practice? If the research is suitable for use, what is the most appropriate way to *implement* the findings? These issues present problems for the aspiring research consumer.

Individual self-confidence

Many authors have identified lack of self-confidence as a barrier to research utilization. In a study by Pearcey (1995), 93% (n = 398) of the nurses surveyed felt a lack of confidence in their research skills – notably in their ability to read critically. Lack of self-confidence may also mean a reluctance to embrace change, resulting in the perpetuation of the rituals and rigid rules which guide much nursing practice, as suggested by Mander (1988). The nurses in Rodgers' study (1994) also mentioned fear of risk taking associated with trying out new ideas and a lack of faith in their own judgment. McIntosh (1995) raises another important aspect of this complex problem when she reminds us that if we derive a sense of personal worth from the work we do, it becomes very difficult to acknowledge that the way in which the work is done is less than ideal. It may pose an even more devastating threat to a professional whose *raison d'être* is to care for others, if the care she or he has been delivering over a period of years is shown not only to be less than ideal but positively harmful. Acceptance of research findings may not only challenge self-confidence, but may in some cases threaten self-esteem.

Barriers related to the setting

Within the nursing literature, many writers allude to contextual barriers to research implementation within nursing settings. These are discussed briefly below.

Lack of time for reading and working in busy areas

Community nurses interviewed by Luker and Kenrick (1992) described lack of time and pressure of work as important factors in determining their involvement in research. Similarly, hospital nurses interviewed by Rodgers (1994) cite lack of time for reading as a barrier. Given the demands of critical appraisal already discussed, the relevance of this issue for clinical nurses and midwives is clear.

Organizational barriers to change

The challenges of introducing change within a large organization are easy to underestimate. Hunt (1987) provides us with a salutary reminder of these issues in her report of an action research study aimed at introducing research-based care in two areas of nursing practice – mouth care and pre-operative fasting. Changing mouth care practices, for example, involved 'cumbersome and time-consuming' negotiations with the central sterile supplies department (CSSD) to cancel mouth packs and with the supplies department to supply soft, small toothbrushes to individual ward areas. Changing the management of preoperative fasting required the involvement and cooperation of many groups including operating staff, housekeeping staff, as well as day and night nursing staff. It can therefore be seen that 'winning hearts and minds' in order to change practice is only half the battle. The practicalities of change can also present major hurdles.

Lack of authority to change procedures

Perceived lack of authority is often cited as a significant barrier to research utilization and was identified by nurses in studies by Funk *et al* (1991) and Lacey (1994). For example, a junior staff nurse may wish to abandon the use of antiseptic baths preoperatively but may see the power to do so resting with the ward manager.

Perceived lack of co-operation from managers or other professional groups

Lack of support from managers is cited in studies by Luker and Kenrick (1992), Rodgers (1994) and Lacey (1994). Clinicians may understandably need considerable managerial support when attempting to put research into practice. In a ward area, for example, lack of support from the charge nurse or clinical nurse manager may prove an impossible barrier to overcome.

Doctors are also presented as potential 'barriers' to research utilization by nurses (Rodgers 1994, Lacey 1994). Similarly, 44% of community nurses interviewed by Luker and Kenrick (1995) listed consultants' instructions as a constraint to their implementation of research-based practice in the treatment of leg ulcers.

Sleep (1992) cites 'medical dominance' as a force mitigating against using research-based knowledge in midwifery and McIntosh (1995) cites Sneddon (1992) who described the experience of a group of staff nurses working in palliative care whose attempts to utilize research-based knowledge on pain management were not welcomed by their medical colleagues.

Exercise 11.3

Think about a practice setting in which you have recently worked.

■ How many of the barriers listed here existed within this setting?
■ Can you think of any other barriers to research implementation which operate in your area?

Summary

Potential barriers to research utilization have been presented here under three headings for the sake of clarity. However, reality is infinitely more complicated than this. Real-life problems seldom fit into neat boxes and often defy classification. The barriers which may operate at any one time in your organization are likely to represent an amalgam of some (or even all!) of these. You have probably added a few more to the list. Williamson (1992) points out that barriers will always vary from place to place and from time to time. Health care practice is always based on shifting sands.

Recourse to the literature, although it can help our understanding, can seldom provide 'off the shelf' solutions to the problems that we are facing. The complexity of individual cases is further increased when we try to weigh up the relative strengths of different types of barriers. In a study of the influence of different kinds of variables on innovations in hospitals, Kimberley and Evanisko (1981) found that organizational level variables were better predictors of innovation than individual or contextual variables. Funk et al (1991) surveyed a stratified sample of 1989 nurses (40% response rate) from the American Nurses Association roster using a tool designed to explore barriers to using research findings. The two greatest barriers identified were organizational. Unfortunately, little UK research has been carried out which looks at the combined effects of different barriers and we remain largely ignorant of many of the processes which may be in operation.

Possible solutions

Whilst this section is not intended as a 'pick and mix' of instant solutions, it does attempt to pull together a number of initiatives and approaches which might prove useful. Some sections describe resources which are already available, while others describe initiatives which have been tried only on a limited basis. Some of these initiatives can be attempted by individual nurses and midwives, while others will need the collaboration of a group of people. Others could be incorporated into the research strategy of a particular trust or region.

Again, for the sake of clarity, possible solutions are presented under a series of headings:

- Initiatives to improve the accessibility of research
- Initiatives to overcome individual barriers
- Initiatives to overcome barriers related to the setting.

Initiatives to improve the accessibility of research

A number of initiatives aim to synthesize research findings.

Systematic reviews

Within the UK, two major centres have a remit to produce and commission systematic reviews of research findings. The Cochrane Collaboration is an international organization which involves the collaboration of researchers representing many health care disciplines, including nursing. At the UK Cochrane Centre, a review of randomized controlled trials in nursing has recently been completed by Dr Nicky Cullum. *The Cochrane Database of Systematic Reviews* is available on CD-ROM in many libraries and clinical areas. The *Pregnancy and Childbirth* database is already complete and is an invaluable resource to those working in the fields of midwifery and obstetrics, whilst work in other fields is ongoing. The NHS Centre for Reviews and Dissemination at the University of York, established in 1994, also commissions systematic research reviews as well as being involved in establishing mechanisms for disseminating research findings.

While it must be acknowledged that the production of systematic reviews in relation to nursing research is a relatively recent development, their potential to inform health care practice is immense. The sheer practicalities of synthesizing large volumes of information of varying quality and deciding on the implications for practice present insurmountable problems for many practitioners. Through the increased availability of rigorously conducted systematic reviews, one of the major barriers to research implementation may be overcome in the future.

Clinical guidelines
initiative

Many health professions use research-based guidelines or protocols to ensure that clinical practice is not only safe, but is also both clinically effective and cost effective. Within nursing, the NHS Executive is currently involved in developing guidelines for a range of clinical practices including pressure area care and the management of lymphoedema following breast surgery. In 1995, the Royal College of Nursing announced a strategy to disseminate, implement and evaluate national clinical guidelines. Sheldon *et al* (1994) review some of the work in this area and conclude that there is strong evidence that well-implemented guidelines can change practice. However, they also point out that the extent to which guidelines are valid, and lead to improvements in patient outcomes at acceptable costs, depends on the rigour of the processes of reviewing, synthesizing and incorporating information into guidelines.

Research-based
manuals and other
publications

A number of texts attempt specifically to apply research to practice situations, e.g. Wilson-Barnett and Batehup (1988), Royal Marsden Hospital (1992), Bulechek and McCloskey (1992), and these are discussed in the Further Reading for this chapter. This does not represent an exhaustive list of all research-based clinical texts, but it is worth highlighting that the strengths of publications such as these lie in the attempt to apply research to real-life nursing and midwifery contexts.

A number of regular newsheets are produced which also attempt to pull together research findings in relation to particular health care issues. These include *Bandolier* and the *Effective Health Care Bulletin*. Your own library may well receive these publications as well as local research newsletters which may contain useful research summaries. In addition, two journals focus on evidence-based nursing: *Clinical Effectiveness in Nursing* and *Evidence-based nursing*.

Initiatives aimed at making information easier to access

The NHS R&D Information Systems Strategy has resulted in the development of The National Research Register on CD-ROM – a suite of databases about current research projects of interest to the NHS. An increasing number of useful databases are available on CD-ROM at health service libraries, such as *MIRIAD*, the midwifery research database, which aims to help midwives to identify relevant research, the *Database of Abstracts of Reviews of Effectiveness (DARE)*, and *The Cochrane Database of Systematic Reviews*. Many databases can now also be accessed via the Internet.

Initiatives aimed at improving the readability of research reports

This issue was acknowledged as a problem by the Taskforce on the Strategy for Research in Nursing, Midwifery and Health Visiting, which suggested that 'researchers might be given a financial incentive for producing readable material, possibly equivalent to the costs of hiring someone else to do it' (DoH 1993d).

Initiatives to overcome individual barriers

Educational opportunities

A variety of educational opportunities exist both nationally and locally which not only address the conduct of research, but also consider the complex and messy business of interpreting research findings and putting them into practice. Research appreciation and awareness courses, conferences, study days and seminars are a valuable way of developing research-mindedness with the added bonus of peer support and opportunities for networking.

Community nurses interviewed by Luker and Kenrick (1992) listed study days as their main way of keeping up to date. Possible links between attendance on research-based courses and positive attitudes towards research or involvement in research activities have also been suggested in studies by Champion and Leach (1989), Coyle and Sokop (1990), Rizutto *et al* (1994), Pearcey (1995) and McDonnell *et al* (1997).

Whilst funding to attend courses and conferences remains a perennial problem for many nurses and midwives and the implications of Post Registration Education and Practice Project, UKCC 1994 (PREPP) are still to be fully realized, the need for research awareness and application modules at a range of academic levels is now recognized by many departments and schools of nursing.

Collaboration between practitioners and researchers to put research into practice

The need for researchers to play an active role in the implementation of research findings is often advocated. Alexander and Orton (1988) describe **action learning** as a way of bringing together researchers and clinicians to implement the findings of research on the role of the ward sister. Triads of nurses, consisting of the ward sister, his/her manager and a nurse teacher with links to the clinical area, were invited to a King's Fund conference where the research was presented. These nurses were subsequently supported to innovate and implement changes based on the research through a series of workshops with positive benefits, including putting research into practice, reported for all participants. Clearly, this kind of approach to dissemination and implementation of research findings produces active interest and involvement in research. However, there are resource implications.

Luker and Kenrick (1995) describe an alternative method of disseminating research-based information to nurses. They outline the development and evaluation of a clinical information pack on leg ulcers for community nurses. Having previously explored how the nurses preferred to receive information, efforts were made to present the pack in a jargon-free format which was appealing to practitioners. Given the response of some nurses to material produced by pharmaceutical companies, a grant was obtained from a commercial company who oversaw production of the packs. The impact of the pack on reported practice was assessed through an experimental study design. The information pack produced a significant increase in the knowledge scores of the experimental group.

An alternative approach to researcher–clinician collaboration is called for by Wilson-Barnett *et al* (1990). They advocate the introduction of **researcher teachers** in practice areas as a way of identifying relevant topics and providing education and support to change practice, followed by an evaluation of the effects. They report on two studies where previous research had revealed nurses' knowledge base and confidence to be low; in caring for patients with tracheal stomas (De Carle 1985) and in dealing with cancer patients (Corner 1988). In both studies the researchers were actively involved in producing and implementing teaching packages for clinical staff and evaluating their success.

Collaboration between clinicians and researchers to carry out research

Collaborative research of this nature is seen by many as a surefire way to ensure that subsequent research findings are seen as relevant by practitioners and therefore applied in practice. Many successful attempts at collaborative research are reported in the literature. For example, Tierney and Taylor (1991) describe the collaboration between researcher and ward sister on a specialist breast care unit, to devise and conduct a research study on the effects of scalp cooling on patients undergoing chemotherapy. In contrast to the much reported research–practice divide discussed earlier, the authors report that their respective contributions to the research process were naturally complementary rather than in conflict.

Much of the documented collaboration between clinicians and

researchers involves innovations in clinical practice and the evaluation of change and is described under the heading of *action research*. Although one of the principal features of action research is collaboration, the term also has other implications. Action research implies a different philosophical approach to research, where research questions are generated by practitioners in response to problems 'on the ground' and local solutions are sought through the collaboration and participation of clinicians and researchers. Participation in the research process is thus seen as empowering for clinicians.

Action research is seen by many as a particularly appropriate approach to nursing research not least because research results are immediately available and relevant to practitioners. Its advocates include Greenwood (1984) and Webb (1989). Nursing studies using action research methods are reported by Hunt (1987) (changing mouth care and preoperative fasting) and Webb (1990) who used action research methods to evaluate the introduction of team nursing in an elderly care ward.

Action research as a method has its critics, largely on the basis that research findings may not be generalizable across a wider population, the findings only being useful locally. Nonetheless, this approach represents a powerful way of ensuring that research is not only useful to clinicians in terms of the results produced but also in terms of the questions it seeks to answer. Action research is also discussed in Chapters 5 and 6.

Secondment of clinicians to research teams to acquire skills

Given the need for more nurses to undertake research training highlighted in the Taskforce report (DoH 1993c), secondments for practitioners to academic departments to participate in funded research projects may provide valuable learning opportunities. Not only is it likely that these nurses will become more active in using research themselves, it is possible that they will become advocates for research in their own practice area, thus providing a further impetus for research-based practice. Two nationally funded research projects recently completed within my own school – an evaluation of the effects of educational programmes in nursing on promoting autonomy and independence in older people and an investigation of the role of the practice nurse in the prevention of cardiovascular disease and stroke – have involved the secondment of a staff nurse from a local NHS trust as a research assistant in order to provide a research training opportunity.

Initiatives to overcome barriers related to the setting

Policy initiatives

The policy context of health care research has changed markedly over recent years and is fully discussed by Sue Read in Chapter 2 of this book. The greater emphasis on the implementation as well as on the conduct of research is reflected not only in research strategy documents such as *Research for Health* (DoH 1993a) but explicitly in a wider policy context in the form of Targets 8 and 9 of *A Vision for the Future* (DoH 1993e).

Appointment of facilitators to promote research-based practice

The need for clinical leadership in the form of a named facilitator to promote and support research based practice is often cited. Hunt (1987) and Armitage (1990) provide two examples of this kind of approach. Many NHS Trusts employ practice development nurses with the promotion of research-based practice forming part of their remit. Some see the clinical nurse specialist (CNS) as ideally suited to implementing research findings within his or her sphere of expertise. However, as Waterworth (1990) points out, there is evidence (Markham 1980) to suggest that CNSs have experienced difficulties with the research component of their role, possibly due to lack of research experience. The lecturer–practitioner may also have the potential to facilitate research-based practice, given the nature of their remit to narrow the theory–practice gap. A detailed examination of all these roles is beyond the scope of this text. However, it is important to highlight the value of positive role models and practical support for all clinicians wishing to make their practice as research-based as possible.

Establishment of research interest groups

In attempts to tackle research implementation 'on the ground', some practitioners are involved in journal clubs or research interest groups. McCloughlin *et al* (1993) describe how hospital and community nurses in County Antrim, Northern Ireland set up a research interest group to overcome barriers such as lack of research knowledge and inaccessibility of research. A key step was to negotiate with managers to provide time off for nurses to attend workshops and seminars and administrative and secretarial support for the group. Lack of knowledge about the research process was addressed through a series of workshops organised in conjunction with outside bodies such as the local college of nursing.

Journal clubs, where clinicians meet on a regular basis and take turns in presenting either a paper from a journal or an overview of a particular edition of a journal, represent a simple yet effective way of keeping up to date. Journal clubs can provide peer support and provide a means of accessing literature and expertise within the group. When facilitated by members with the skills to critically evaluate research findings, they can provide a powerful springboard for ideas and increase the drive towards research-based care.

There are many other simple steps which can improve accessibility to research findings such as providing journals in clinical areas, keeping a file of relevant research reports, and presentation of research at staff meetings or as part of a ward-based teaching programme. All of these can contribute to a more positive climate for evidence-based health care.

Local development and implementation

In the USA, the government have funded a number of nursing research utilization programmes – notably the Western Interstate Commission for Higher Education (the WICHE programme) and the Conduct and Utilization of Research in Nursing project (the CURN project).

The WICHE programme carried out in the 1970s and reported by Loomis (1985) and Closs and Cheater (1994) involved collaborative workshops between researchers and clinicians at a number of sites. The intention was to identify patient care problems and work towards research-based solutions through planned change. Interestingly, the WICHE researchers note that the major barrier was lack of access to good nursing research and concluded that no further large scale research utilization projects should be attempted until current research was made more accessible.

The CURN project viewed research utilization as an organizational rather than an individual process (Horsley *et al* 1983). Project staff developed ten research-based protocols for use in general hospital settings. Innovation teams from seventeen hospitals then participated in a series of collaborative workshops including researchers and clinicians, to implement the protocols in practice with some success. Goode *et al* (1987) and Titler *et al* (1994) document similar organizational approaches to research utilization in the USA.

There are few published examples of organizational approaches to research implementation in the UK, although one example is provided by Hunt (1987). Hunt's attempts to change mouth care and preoperative fasting procedures and the organizational difficulties she faced serve as a salutary reminder of the bureaucratic obstacles that may stand in the way of planned organizational change.

Chapter conclusion

Whose responsibility is it?

This chapter has concentrated on presenting information which practising nurses might find helpful in their quest to make research-based care a reality and to enhance their understanding of the issues involved. Related issues such as the nature of change and ways of managing change will be considered in Chapter 12.

Nurses in particular often castigate themselves for their failure to implement research findings. The onus on individual health care practitioners to base their practice on scientific knowledge rather than on outdated rituals is enormous. However, having examined the evidence, it becomes apparent that criticizing individual practitioners for their lack of research awareness or clinical managers for the low level of research utilization in their area belies a simplistic approach to the problem. Overcoming the barriers to research utilization is neither simple nor straightforward but is rather complex and messy. Furthermore, research utilization should be viewed not merely as an individual responsibility but an organizational responsibility in the widest sense of the word. There is a responsibility on the NHS, clearly recognized in the current Research and Development strategy (DoH 1993a), to embrace not only an evidence-based culture, but to create effective strategies to enable meaningful knowledge to be generated. We also need to probe much further into the complex issues surrounding research utilization to find out which implementation strategies are most effective and why.

Within *individual* institutions, we overlook organizational and cultural barriers to change at our peril! Without managerial support, both personal and structural, individual enthusiasm for innovation is squandered.

Finally, clinicians have a right to look to researchers to disseminate the results of their work effectively. If the message is so deeply encoded that it is incomprehensible or so zealously guarded that it is only revealed in élite forums, one can hardly blame clinicians for not receiving it. New guidelines for dissemination to be issued by the NHS Centre for Reviews and Dissemination may prove a positive step in this direction.

The responsibility for research-based practice is one that is shared by all health professionals whatever their sphere of responsibility, from policy makers to those at the clinical workface. Given the nature of the barriers that need to be overcome, many might wonder why we are still struggling on and chasing the holy grail of research-based care. The answer must lie in the fact that in spite of the difficulties, as health professionals we share a common conviction that the ultimate goal of best practice is worth the struggle.

Exercise 11.4
- What do you think you as an individual can do to become more 'research-minded'?
- What can your organization do?
- What educational opportunities exist in your area for research appreciation/application?
- How could you access these?

Further reading   Bulechek GM and McCloskey JC (1992) *Interventions* (2nd edn). Philadelphia: WB Saunders.

This book covers a wide range of nursing interventions and the research base for these.

Pritchard AP and David JA (1992) (eds) *The Royal Marsden Hospital Manual of Clinical Nursing Procedures*, 3rd edn. Oxford: Blackwell.

This manual, whilst describing clinical nursing procedures, provides a rationale for each step and includes relevant research findings which support or inform the process.

Vaughan B and Edwards M (1995) *Interface Between Research and Practice: Some Working Models*. London: King's Fund Centre.

This book arose through the practical experience of promoting evidence-based practice in a number of Nursing Development Units. The strengths and difficulties of six models of research utilization are discussed.

Wilson-Barnett J and Batehup L (1988) *Patient Problems: A Research Base for Nursing Care*. London: Scutari Press.

This book covers a variety of patient problems, e.g. pain, sleep disturbance, and describes the research which assists in the assessment, intervention and evaluation of interventions for these problems.

References

Alexander MF and Orton HD (1988) Research in action. *Nursing Times* **84**: 8, 38–41.

Anglia and Oxford RHA Cholesterol Screening. *Bandolier* 1994; **5**: 1–6.

Antman EM, Lau J, Kopelnik B, Nosteller F and Chalmers TC (1992) Comparison of results of meta-analyses of randomized controlled trials and recommendations of clinical experts. *Journal of the American Medical Association* **268**: 240–248.

Armitage S (1990) Research utilization in practice. *Nurse Education Today* **10**(1): 10–15.

Baier M (1988) Why research doesn't yield treatment. *Journal of Psychosocial Nursing* **26**(5): 29–33.

Luckenbill-Brett J (1987) Use of nursing practice research findings. *Nursing Research* **36**(6): 344–349.

Bostrom AC, Malnight M, MacDougall J and Hargis D (1989) Staff nurses' attitudes towards nursing research: a descriptive survey. *Journal of Advanced Nursing* **14**: 915–922.

Bostrum J and Suter WN (1993) Research utilisation. Making the link to practice. *Journal of Nursing Staff Development* **9**: 28–34.

Carper BA (1978) Fundamental patterns of knowing in nursing. *Advances in Nursing Science* **1**(1): 13–23.

Champion VL and Leach A (1989) Variables related to research utilization in nursing. *Journal of Advanced Nursing* **14**: 705–710.

Closs SJ and Cheater FM (1994) Utilization of nursing research. Culture, interest and support. *Journal of Advanced Nursing* **19**: 762–773.

Corner J (1988) Assessment of nurses' attitudes towards cancer: a critical view of research methods. *Journal of Advanced Nursing* **13**: 640–648.

Coyle LA and Sokop AG (1990) Innovation behaviour among nurses. Nursing Research **39**(3): 176–180.

De Carle B (1985) Tracheostomy care. *Nursing Times* **81**: Occasional Paper 6, 50–54.

DoH (1992) *Assessing the Effects of Health*

Technologies. Principles, Practice, Proposals. London: HMSO.

DoH (1993a) *Research for Health.* London: HMSO.

DoH (1993b) *Key Area Handbook: Coronary Heart Disease and Stroke.* London: HMSO.

DoH (1993c) *Report of the Taskforce on the Strategy for Research in Nursing, Midwifery and Health Visiting.* London: HMSO.

DoH (1993d). *Strategy for Research in Nursing, Midwifery and Health Visiting.* Annexes 1–4. London: RCN & RCM.

DoH (1993e) *A Vision for the Future: the Nursing, Midwifery and Health Visiting Contribution to Health and Health Care.* London: HMSO.

DoH (1994) *Research and Development in Occupational Therapy, Physiotherapy and Speech and Language Therapy: A Position Statement.* London: HMSO.

Dukes J (1993) *Patient Protocols – A Review for Those Who Commission, Design and Use Them.* Oxford: Templeton College.

Funk SG, Champagne MT, Weise RA and Tornquist EM (1991) Barriers: barriers to using research findings in practice: the clinicians' perspective. *Applied Nursing Research* 4(2): 90–95.

Goode CJ, Lovett MK, Hayes JE and Butcher LA (1987) Use of research based knowledge in clinical practice. *Journal of Nursing Administration* 17(12): 11–18.

Gould (1986) Pressure sore prevention and treatment: an example of nurses' failure to implement research findings. *Journal of Advanced Nursing* 11: 389–394.

Greenwood J (1984) Nursing research: a position paper. *Journal of Advanced Nursing* 9: 77–82.

Grimshaw JE and Russell IT (1993) Effect of clinical guidelines on medical practice: a systematic review of rigorous evaluations. *The Lancet* 342: 1317–1321.

Hicks C (1995) The shortfall in published research: a study of nurses' research and publication activities. *Journal of Advanced Nursing* 21: 594–604.

Hinshaw AS and Heinrich J (1990) New initiatives in nursing: a national perspective. In Bergman R (ed) *Nursing Research for Nursing Practice. An International Perspective.* London: Chapman & Hall.

Horsley JA, Crane J, Crabtree MK and Wood DJ (1983) *Using Research to Improve Nursing Practice: A Guide.* New York: Grune and Stratton.

Hull J (1995) Do nurses get involved in research? *Nursing Times* 91(4): 11–12.

Hunt J (1981) Indicators for nursing practice: the use of research findings. *Journal of Advanced Nursing* 6(3): 189–194.

Hunt M (1987) The process of translating research findings into nursing practice. *Journal of Advanced Nursing* 12: 101–110.

Ketefian S (1975) Application of selected nursing research findings into nursing practice: a pilot study. *Nursing Research* 24: 89–92.

Kimberly JR and Evanisko MJ (1981) Organizational innovation. The influence of individual, organizational and contextual factors on hospital adoption of technological and administrative innovations. *Academy of Management Journal* 24: 689–713.

Kirchoff KT (1982) A diffusion survey of coronary precautions. *Nursing Research* 31: 196–201.

Kreuger JC (1982) Using research in practice. A survey of research utilization in Community Health Nursing. *Western Journal of Nursing Research* 4(2): 244–248.

Lacey AE (1994) Research utilization in nursing practice – a pilot study. *Journal of Advanced Nursing* 19: 987–995.

Loomis ME (1985) Knowledge utilisation and research utilisation in nursing. *Image – the Journal of Nursing Scholarship* 17(2): 35–39.

Luker KA and Kenrick M (1992) An exploratory study of the sources of influence on the clinical decisions of community nurses. *Journal of Advanced Nursing* 17: 457–466.

Luker KA and Kenrick M (1995) Towards knowledge-based practice; an evaluation of a method of dissemination. *International Journal of Nursing Studies* 32(1): 59–67.

Mander R (1988) Encouraging students to be research minded. *Nurse Education Today* 8: 30–35.

Markham G (1988) Special cases. *Nursing Times* 84(26): 29–30.

Murray Y (1988) Tradition rather than cure? *Nursing Times* 84(38): 75–80.

McCloughlin NA, Aitcheson S and Irvine H (1993)

The appliance of science. *Nursing Times* **89**(39): 52–53.

McDonnell A, Davies S, Brown J, Shewan J and Crookes P (1997) A detailed investigation of factors associated with the implementation of research-based knowledge by practice nurses in the prevention of cardiovascular disease and stroke. Final report to the NHS Development Executive (Cardiovascular Disease and Stroke). Sheffield: University of Sheffield.

McIntosh J (1995) Barriers to research implementation. *Nurse Researcher* **2**(4): 83–91.

Myco F (1980) Nursing research information; are nurse educators and practitioners seeking it out? *Journal of Advanced Nursing* **6**: 51–58.

Pearcey P (1995) Achieving research-based practice. *Journal of Advanced Nursing* **22**: 33–39.

Peters DA (1992) Implementation of research findings. *Health Bulletin* **50**(1): 68–77.

Rizzuto C, Bostrom J, Suter WN and Chenitz WC (1994) Predictors of nurses' involvement in research activities. *Western Journal of Nursing Research* **16**(2): 193–204.

Rodgers S (1994) An exploratory study of research utilization by nurses in general medical and surgical wards. *Journal of Advanced Nursing* **20**: 904–911.

Sheldon T, Freemantle N, Grimshaw J and Russell I (1994) The good guide to guides. *Health Services Journal* **8**: 34–35.

Sleep J (1992) Research and the practice of midwifery. *Journal of Advanced Nursing* **17**: 1465–1471.

Stetler CB and DiMaggio G (1991) Research utilization among clinical nurse specialists. *Clinical Nurse Specialist* **5**(3): 151–155.

Tierney AJ and Taylor J (1991) Research in practice; 'an experiment' in researcher-practitioner collaboration. *Journal of Advanced Nursing* **16**: 506–510.

Titler MG, Kleiber C, Steelman V, Goode C, Rakel B, Barry-Walker J, Small S and Buckwalter K (1994) Infusing research into practice to promote quality care. *Nursing Research* **43**(5): 307–313.

Trent RHA. (1993) *The Health Gain Investment Programme: Coronary Heart Disease and Stroke*. Sheffield: Trent RHA.

Tunstall-Pedoe H (1991) The Dundee coronary risk disk for management of change in risk factors. *British Medical Journal* **303**: 744–747.

United Kingdom Central Council for Nursing, Midwifery and Health Visiting (1994). The Future of Professional Practice: the Council's Standards for Education and Practice. London: UKCC.

Walsh M and Ford P (1989) *Nursing rituals: Research and Rational Actions*. Oxford: Heinemann.

Waterworth S (1990) Basing practice on research. *Nursing Standard* **5**(11): 30–33.

Webb C (1989) Action research: philosophy, methods and personal experience. *Journal of Advanced Nursing* **14**: 403–410.

Webb C (1990) Partners in research. *Nursing Times* **86**(32): 40–44.

Webb C and Mackenzie J (1993) Where are we now? Research-mindedness in the 1990s. *Journal of Clinical Nursing* **2**(3): 129–133.

Williamson P (1992) From dissemination to use: management and organizational barriers to the application of health services research findings. *Health Bulletin* **50**(1): 78–86.

Wilson-Barnett J, Corner J and De-Carle B (1990) Integrating nursing research and practice – the role of the researcher as teacher. *Journal of Advanced Nursing* **15**(5): 621–625.

12 Techniques and strategies for translating research findings into health care practice

Patrick Crookes

Once the decision has been made about whether a body of research is rigorous and worthy of application to practice, plans need to be made regarding how best to go about introducing, managing and evaluating its implementation – even the best ideas are not self-executing. In Chapter 11, Ann McDonnell discussed barriers to research utilization, along with some solutions. In this chapter, I argue the need for a planned approach when implementing change of any kind. This is a view I hold from personal experience and the reviews of innovation research undertaken by authors such as Rogers (1962), Rogers and Shoemaker (1971) and Havelock (1972).

From my reading, it would appear that in health care, systematic planning based on a clear theoretical framework is rather rare. The nursing journals are full of examples of keen and committed nurses attempting to change and improve systems for patients and professionals alike, yet rarely do they overtly utilize any particular model of change to inform and structure their efforts. One of the principles of this chapter, therefore, is that much of the theory of 'managing change' *can* and *should be* applied to the implementation of research findings within health care settings.

The five essential factors for change, identified within the document *Managing Change in Nursing Education* (ENB 1987) will be used as the framework for much of the rest of the chapter. Content will be categorized under the headings of:

- The attributes of the environment where change is to take place
- The users of proposed innovation
- The attributes of the innovation itself
- Change agents
- Change strategies (including models of change).

The justification for this approach is twofold. The first is that this model provides a clear structure for the presentation of the material.

The second is that it is work which itself has an empirical basis, which is important in a text which advocates the use of research-based knowledge wherever possible.

The overall intention for the chapter, is to inform the reader about the variety of issues necessary for the change agent to consider, when devising a strategy for change in their *own* practice environment. It should be acknowledged, however, that this is not a book about management and so further useful reading will be recommended where relevant.

Key issues

- The role of change agents in introducing and managing change
- The importance of a systematic approach to successful innovation
- The use of models of change

Background

I became particularly interested in the management of change when working as a tutor on English National Board (ENB) clinical courses for registered nurses. It became apparent to me that the courses were having the desired *educational* impact, in that participants were invariably more questioning of practice (theirs and that of others) and wished to 'make a difference' when they went back to the institutions which seconded them. However, within months or even weeks, having had little success in engendering any degree of support amongst peers and supervisors for their 'new' ideas, they would invariably have regressed to a point where they saw no point in trying to change the status quo. They had developed, or perhaps returned to, a state of 'learned helplessness' (Seligman 1975, Larson 1987) which has been defined as 'a behavioural state and personality of a person who believes he or she is ineffectual, responses are futile, and control over the environment has been lost' (*Mosby's Medical Dictionary* 1990).

In talking to these nurses it quickly became apparent to me that this should perhaps come as no surprise, since invariably they had not sought to use any well thought-through strategy to initiate change. Instead they had rather naively presumed that because *they* were enthusiastic about the need for change in a given area of care, then *ipso facto* everyone else would be. Rarely had any more planning taken place than the decision to leave copies of relevant literature in staff common rooms, in the rather forlorn hope that this would engender support. I determined at that point that I would try to do something about this apparent gap in research skills, i.e. *research application*, in my future work as a nurse educator and researcher.

I can make a difference

In the above introduction, I pointed out that *much of* the chapter would be based on five essential factors said to be crucial to the accomplishment of change (ENB 1987). I emphasised the *much of* because for me they do not tell the whole story. The 'five factors' model works well when considering an intended innovation that has been clearly thought out to start with, usually by someone who – by virtue of their job description – has a responsibility to initiate change. However, the model inherently ignores the importance of the mental set of the innovator(s), as well as the need for a clear picture of what they want to achieve. I believe these are fundamental issues which need to be discussed in a textbook which seeks to inform readers who may be new to managing change. Hence my decision to cover them separately and in some detail.

In order to successfully occupy the role of change agent, an individual needs both to perceive the need for change, and to possess the belief that they can effect it – that they can make a difference. Harvey (1990: 19) offers the adage 'if you say you can, or if you say you cannot, you are right'. This perception of self-efficacy is perhaps the key step in becoming an innovator. Mabbett (1987) suggests a number of reasons why some people become, and remain, focused and motivated professionals, who are open and supportive of positive change to improve patient care, whilst others do not. She refers to such individuals as 'positive energy people' and suggests that what Maslow (1971) refers to as 'transcendent values' – the possession of a sense of purpose which is greater than merely self-interest – is a major factor in their continued positive outlook. Wortman and Brehm's theory of 'reactance' (1975) also has relevance here – reactance being the antithesis of 'learned helplessness'. You are advised to access this material for further detail, not least because it identifies why some people retain a sense of self-efficacy even in the face of great opposition, while others readily adopt a position of 'there's no point in trying'.

For many of the clinical course participants referred to earlier, the impetus to change things seemed to be the enhancement of their skills of reflection on practice (Schon 1987) using critical incident analysis as an educational tool, along with 'time-out' of their clinical area to engage in reflection. This typically led them to identify a 'problem with care' which they sought to 'solve' or change.

Invariably this was the point of failure. Often what they sought to change was not 'a problem' *per se* but rather a situation made up of a myriad of interconnecting issues, personalities and vested interests, all of which needed to be considered and resolved if change was to be successful. They were attempting to 'problem solve' when often what they should have been following was the process of 'problem resolution'. The story in Box 12.1 seeks to explicate this concept more fully.

Box 12.1
Oliver's Wall

Oliver is marooned on a beach. Behind him is an uncrossable ocean, in front a wall. This wall is very well built, stretches as far as the eye can see and is very high. Oliver knows that to survive he needs to get to the other side of the wall. So what does he do? Well, after panicking for a while he starts to review the situation. There is no escape and he needs to get through the wall. On closer inspection he sees that the wall is not as well built as first appeared and that some of the mortar is a little loose. He sets to work on them and over time manages to put several small holes in the structure – enough to destabilize it and send the wall crashing down.

Oliver's wall therefore encompasses several important issues related to the processes of change. First, the benefit of analyzing what 'the problem' actually is, perhaps followed by breaking it into manageable parts. Second, the need to feel that you *can* do something no matter how small, even if it only adds to a personal sense of achievement and well-being. Finally that whilst planned innovation is perceived to be the ideal, for many 'chipping away' is the most realistic way that they will make a difference.

Unfortunately, it appears to be much more common for people to try to problem solve rather than resolve. I previously ran a course called 'innovation in clinical practice'. Part of the programme required students to reflect on the relevance of the concept of problem resolution to innovation attempts they had been involved with in the past. Almost without fail they came to the conclusion that those involved (often themselves) had not clearly 'diagnozed' exactly what the 'problem' was, and as a result had put a lot of time and effort into solving the wrong problem. For example, a sister from a casualty department was concerned about the level of recording of wound assessment and dressings used in the minor injuries clinic of her unit. Her answer was to introduce a wound assessment card to be used on an ongoing basis for all patients attending this clinic for follow-up dressings. The tool was not completed adequately and the innovation was deemed a failure. However, on reflection, she came to realize that this was because the majority of staff had little or no idea about objective wound assessment. What was really needed was a period of staff updating in this area, followed by a re-launch of the wound assessment system. This was subsequently done – successfully.

As well as aiding diagnosis of the true nature of 'the problem' by providing a cognitive mechanism for clarifying its various components, problem resolution also offers the would-be innovator an insight into those aspects which are potentially solvable within their sphere of influence and those which aren't. In doing so, such thought processes not only maximize the chances of success of any proposed innovation, but also allow even the most junior of personnel to perceive *realistically* that they can make a difference – even if the impact is relatively small in the greater scheme of things. As Harvey (1990: 25) points out 'you only learn to walk by taking baby steps'.

In practice, the clarification of what 'the problem' actually is can only take place if a thorough analysis of the *need* for a change has also been carried out. That is, not merely an examination of the attributes of the innovation (Rogers and Shoemaker 1971) to be discussed later, but rather a clear understanding of the problem that requires the change to be made and a consideration of *why* it needs to take place. If this diagnostic work has been done then the innovator should be in possession of a clearly defined and focused statement of what they wish to change and why, which can then be shared coherently with others. Havelock and Zlotolow (1995) provide a useful model of such activity, as does Lewin's Force Field Analysis, discussed later. This preparatory work should also ensure that the change(s) they make addresses the true problem. Finally it means that they will find themselves at a point where the 'five essential factors' of change (ENB 1987) are of real relevance and use to them.

Summary

In order to occupy the role of change agent successfully, an individual needs both to perceive the need for change, and to possess the belief that they can effect it – that they can make a difference.

One-dimensional 'problems' rarely exist. Instead we are usually confronted by amalgamations of inter-related issues. As a result, problem resolution should be seen as an alternative to problem solving as a basis for identifying the true nature of problems – including what should be the focus of innovation.

Exercise 12.1

Think about the following questions in relation to your own practice:

- Do you perceive the need for change within your area of work?
- Do you perceive that it is possible for you to effect any of these changes?
- Think about the concept of 'problem resolution' and apply it to an issue that you view as 'a problem'. Try to identify the component parts of 'the problem' and some possible solutions to them.

Five factors crucial to the success of change management

If you take the time to read the ENB *Managing Change* document, you will see that its authors discuss the five factors in a different order to the one I am using. Most notable is that they cover the attributes of the innovation first. I have chosen to discuss the situation where it is intended that change will take place (the change environment), and the people within it (the users) first. This is because it seems more logical to me to consider the importance of diagnozing a situation (e.g. a workplace) and the people within it (perhaps to the point of involving them in the processes of problem resolution and identification), before discussing the attributes of any solutions put forward (the innovation). In writing this it occurs to me that perhaps a consideration of the environment and those who will be affected by change, is perhaps where the innovator should start. Otherwise there will always be a tendency to try to start the process at the point of implementation, rather than at the point of assessment and diagnosis. Models of change typically attempt to steer innovators away from this trap – a major indication for their use.

Attributes of the environment

No-one has yet come up with the definitive work on 'innovative environments' or what essentially characterizes a workplace where a 'research culture' can be said to exist. The team who developed the ENB document *Managing Change in Nursing Education* (1987) suggest that an environment is ripe for change when five conditions co-exist:

- Openness
- Interpersonal and information linkages
- Freedom from organizational constraints
- Supportive leadership
- Trust.

Openness

This relates to the need for people within an organization to be willing to question the status quo and be prepared to accept that there is benefit in recognizing and constantly exploring the idea that there is always scope for improvement. Furthermore, they need to recognize that there is rarely only one answer to any particular question – what Pirsig (1974) refers to as 'value rigidity'. It is crucial that these 'truths' are recognized by staff at all levels of the hierarchy. Those at the top have a responsibility to encourage reflection, personal initiative and innovation, not least by avoiding the tendency to dismiss ideas and suggestions put forward by more junior colleagues. Meanwhile, those in subordinate positions need to accept that they have a responsibility to do more than 'just the job'. Such an ethos could be engendered in a number of ways, including the formation of quality circles to review and develop policies and procedures (Crocker *et al* 1984, Hatfield *et al* 1987, King's Fund 1992) and the development of participatory action research groups (Street 1995).

Interpersonal and information linkages

Effective channels of communication (both formal – meetings, team briefings, memos – and informal) need to exist. If they don't, then openness in the form of sharing of ideas and information, along with the opportunity to give and receive support and discuss issues openly, is lost. Numerous health authorities and trusts have formal mechanisms for cascading information throughout the organization. Perhaps more effort needs to be put into facilitating upward motion of feedback and ideas – again through quality circles and research groups, for example.

Freedom from organizational constraints

This again is a two-edged sword, in that organizations (in the form of managers) need to function in such ways that individuals and groups are encouraged *and rewarded* for initiative, self-directedness and innovation. At the same time 'subordinates' must acknowledge the imperative that they accept the burdens of increased autonomy, responsibility and accountability.

Supportive leadership

The leadership within an organization must support innovation and be *seen* to be doing so by those in subordinate positions. Indeed, as stated above, they need to encourage and reward innovative thought and action. Fullan (1986: 77) sees leaders as being central to successful change, either in the role of supporter or as a director of the change effort. For individual innovation attempts, leaders can also help by exerting their influence and authority to sustain motivation and impetus, until such a time as the change has become 'custom and practice'. Argyris (1983) offers other interesting suggestions for managers on ways in which they can be more supportive of change. What appears to be fundamental from his point of view is the need for managers to acknowledge that they can and should learn from those around them, that they neither have, nor do they need to have, the answer to every problem.

It is perhaps useful to point out here that leadership and authority may not always be a function of seniority. Rogers and Shoemaker (1971) and Havelock and Zlotolow (1995) identify that opinion leaders can be from any echelon of an organization. They also make the point that any would-be innovator should attempt to ensure that such people are 'on board' early on in their planning, so as to benefit from their input and influence as well as avoiding the potential risk of being covertly undermined by them.

Trust

Change leads to an uncertain and unsettling time for most people, even those leading the way. If an air of trust and collegiality exists, then staff involved will be more likely to collaborate constructively and effectively towards achieving common goals. If it doesn't, then vested interests, rivalries and 'office politics' will conspire to ensure failure.

Summary

A supportive environment is crucial to the nurture of a climate of innovation. Such an environment needs leaders who can facilitate and sustain a sense of personal and professional responsibility among subordinates. They must encourage and invite staff to put forward innovative ideas. Perhaps above all they need to trust and respect their staff. Meanwhile, subordinates need to be ready, willing and able to take up the challenge to be more autonomous and accountable – to be expert and advanced practitioners (Benner 1984), as well as having a positive 'I can make a difference' attitude.

Health care culture – a possible obstruction to innovative environments

Unfortunately, as Ann McDonnell outlined in Chapter 11, in many health care environments (particularly those where nursing care is delivered) both staff and managers can erect barriers to innovation and change. This can be explained in terms of culture. A culture has been defined as:

> '... a complex of more or less shared ideas about what is known, how things ought to be, and how things ought to be done which can be transmitted from one generation to the next'
>
> (Waters and Crook 1990: 29)

A perusal of almost any text or article which considers aspects of the sociology of nursing will invariably lead the reader to conclude that nursing and health care 'culture' tends to minimize the chances of nurses working in an environment which supports innovation. Examples include:

- The assimilation of initiates into nursing (Green 1988, Salvage 1985)
- Managerialism in nursing (Coxon 1990, Farmer 1993)
- The concept of 'horizontal violence' between nurses as a manifestation of oppressed group behaviour (Freire 1971, Roberts 1983, Speedy 1987 (see Box 12.2)).

Neither does the literature on nurse–physician relationships suggest that doctors are likely to support innovation on the part of their nurse colleagues.

Box 12.2
Oppressed group behaviour

Horizontal violence is said to be an example of oppressed group behaviour – a concept first expounded by Freire (1971) in his text *The Pedagogy of the Oppressed*. Freire points out that the major characteristics of oppressed behaviour stem from the ability of dominant groups (D) to impress and enforce their norms and values, their world view, onto others – the oppressed (O). Examples commonly cited include: white people (D) and non-white people (O) in predominantly white societies; men (D) and women (O); and doctors (D) and nurses (O). Horizontal violence occurs because the oppressed feel powerless to criticize or question those in power, or they fear change (even though the status quo is so oppressive) and so they vent their aggression on those within their own group. In nursing this leads to lack of perceived support from peers and supervisors.

A second issue is that to progress personally, a member of an oppressed group is typically required to adopt the demeanour and outlook of a member of the dominant group. In nursing this leads to the development of 'queen bees' (Grissum and Spengler, 1976) who because of the rewards they receive, do not feel any animosity towards the system. They blame nurses for the relatively powerless position they are in, rather than history and gender politics. Finally they do not value, and indeed may actively denigrate, nurses and nursing values and skills.

Based on Roberts (1983)

A perusal of the material referenced above suggests that the nursing profession has a tendency to 'browbeat' those new to the job, to inculcate 'desirable' attributes such as obedience and deference to more senior peers (Coxon 1990, Farmer 1993). The literature presents the view that in many cases, progression through clinical ranks and into management posts, may lead to the development of nurse managers who do not value the views and ideas of their junior colleagues (Roberts 1983, Speedy 1987). It would also suggest that the ethic of nurses caring for others does not necessarily extend to supporting and caring for other nurses (Crookes 1996, Whitehouse 1991, Skevington 1984).

Meanwhile, the literature on nurse–physician relationships would seem to suggest that at best doctors would have little interest in nurse-led innovation, and at worst would seek to ridicule and/or block it. Which of these scenarios would apply in a given set of circumstances is presumably a function of whether or not the innovation encroaches upon the domain of the medical profession (Richman 1987).

As a result one could venture to say that many nurses may find themselves in an environment that is lacking with regards to the attributes identified by Rogers and Shoemaker (1971). It is against this fairly negative backdrop of nursing and health care culture that the would-be innovator has to work. Box 12.3 quotes from a 16th century work by Machiavelli which encapsulates much of what I have said about possible forces of opposition to innovation. It is also sobering to recognize that the human response to change does not appear to have altered since the 16th century.

Box 12.3
Machiavelli on change

> Machiavelli was a courtier to the Doges of Venice in the 16th century. It was his job to educate the princes of good families in the ways of getting and maintaining power for the benefit of themselves and their families. He said:
>
> 'There is nothing more difficult to carry out, nor more doubtful of success, nor more dangerous to handle, than to initiate a new order of things. For the reformer has enemies from all who profit by the old order, and only lukewarm defenders in all those who will profit from the new order. This lukewarmness arises partly from fear of their adversaries, who have law in their favour, and partly from the incredulity of mankind who do not truly believe in anything new until they have had actual experience of it'
>
> Machiavelli (1513)

It is because the health care environment has been so unsupportive of innovation led by anyone other than physicians and managers, that I believe that change agents within health care need to consider their environment perhaps even before they decide on any particular change they would like to make. It is important that they become attuned to the internal and external political climate, so that they can react quickly and positively to opportunities (Milio 1988). In doing so they may find themselves in a position where they can inform and lead policy rather than merely react to changes in it. These issues are covered in greater detail elsewhere within a discussion of 'the politics of health care' (Crookes 1992).

In closing this section on nursing and health care culture, which to this point has been fairly negative, I feel that it is important to indicate that there are positive signs of change with regard to innovation, particularly within the British National Health Service. A number of the policy documents which Sue Read discussed in Chapter 2 contain recommendations aimed at generating innovative cultures and the application of research findings within clinical practice. In Chapter

11 Ann McDonnell discusses a whole array of solutions to blocks to research utilization. In his text *Changing Nursing Practice* (1989) Steve Wright presents similar material to the present chapter in a very optimistic though realistic manner. Politically it is a fairly good time to be an innovator: what nurses and other health professionals need is a positive attitude based on the theory of reactance and a deeper understanding of the processes of planned change.

Summary

The nature of health care culture is such that innovators cannot always rely on the support of peers, managers and colleagues. However, the chances of success are increased if the innovator is aware of the physical and human environment of their area.

Exercise 12.2

- Consider the environment in which you work. Does it have the 'attributes of an environment' conducive to innovation and change identified above?
- What could/should be done to make it an environment more conducive to change?
- Consider ways in which you might be able to become more involved in the development of policy and practice relating to your clinical area, rather than merely reacting to changes in policy.

The users of the innovation

From the above discussion of the 'innovative environment', it almost seems redundant to consider the 'users' of an innovation, given that the concept refers in the main to the social, as opposed to the physical, environment. However, I believe the difference between the two is that the former reflects a somewhat proactive and institutional view of things – characteristics that need to be right to facilitate the generation and sharing of good ideas. On the other hand, consideration of the 'users' is more concerned with a recognition and a consideration of how people involved in, and affected by the innovation, will *react*.

Based on the evaluation of numerous studies of innovative behaviour in health, education and the social sciences over a number of years, Rogers and Shoemaker (1971) suggest that in any group or organization where change is being considered, the people affected will tend to react in fairly predictable ways. Their reaction also allows them to be categorized under a number of headings, seen as points along a continuum, as shown in Figure 12.1.

The work of Havelock and Huberman (1978) allows expansion of this perspective on how and why people respond to change in the way(s) that they do, including the imperative to provide 'users' with information and support during the change process. This is supplemented by an excellent discussion of the same issue by Havelock

Figure 12.1 *Adopter categorization on the basis of innovativeness*

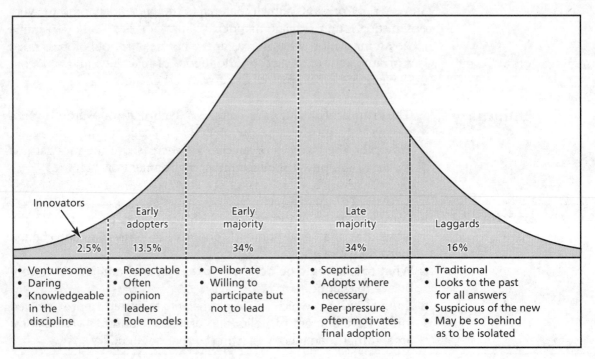

Innovators	Early adopters	Early majority	Late majority	Laggards
2.5%	13.5%	34%	34%	16%
• Venturesome • Daring • Knowledgeable in the discipline	• Respectable • Often opinion leaders • Role models	• Deliberate • Willing to participate but not to lead	• Sceptical • Adopts where necessary • Peer pressure often motivates final adoption	• Traditional • Looks to the past for all answers • Suspicious of the new • May be so behind as to be isolated

(Developed from Rogers and Shoemaker 1971)

and Zlotolow in their text *The Change Agents Guide* (1995). The benefits of enlisting the support of 'opinion leaders' were alluded to earlier. However, all these authors also highlight the imperative of generating and maintaining a sense of ownership of any change if it is to be adopted and if slipping back to old ways is to be resisted. In the main they suggest that this can be achieved by involving 'the users' of any innovation in the processes of diagnosis in both formal and informal settings as suggested within point 3 (interpersonal and information linkages) of Rogers and Shoemaker's requirements for an innovative environment (1971).

An interesting article by Cornwell (1996) demonstrates this inter-relationship between an environment supportive of innovation, the people who work within it and a lasting change. In this paper he discusses the processes which staff in a psychogeriatric hospital went through to review and subsequently modify practices for lifting and moving patients, including those with challenging behaviours. An example of a positive outcome was a reduction in the incidence of back injuries – not surprising since the new protocols which were developed led to the total weight being moved manually each morning *on one ward alone* to be reduced from over three tonnes to less than one tonne. Riding on the wave of enthusiasm from this success, the staff then turned their energies to reviewing and improving their practices of restraint – an issue which took on importance from observations made during the review of lifting and handling practices. Nothing breeds success like success! Other important issues related to 'users' are discussed by Ann McDonnell in Chapter 11.

Summary

People tend to react in fairly predictable ways when confronted by change. The change agent needs to be aware of this and be proactive in enlisting the help of opinion leaders as well as minimizing the negative effects of laggards and rejecters. Participation in the processes of planning and implementation of change is seen as a major factor in the success of any innovation.

Exercise 12.3

Take some time to think about an innovation you have been involved with, either as a change agent or a 'user'. Consider the following questions:

■ What was the range of reactions elicited by the change and who experienced them?
■ What was their impact on the innovation?
■ Where would you consider yourself to be along Rogers and Shoemaker's scale of innovativeness (Figure 12.1)?
■ Was a sense of ownership developed within the users of the change?
■ If so, how?
■ To what degree were opinion leaders involved in the processes of change?
■ What information and support was available to the 'users' of the innovation during the time of this change?
■ In considering these questions, what insights, if any, have you gained into why the particular innovation succeeded or failed?

Attributes of the innovation

Having considered the environment in which innovation is intended, as well as issues related to the potential 'users' of innovation, the ENB model leads me to discuss the attributes of an innovation which will tend to mitigate against failure. Rogers and Shoemaker (1971), having considered research on the diffusion of innovations in a number of settings and disciplines including health (page 3); marketing and mass media (page 118); agriculture (page 117); and education (page 157), identified five key attributes which tend to be found in successful attempts at innovation. These are:

- Relative advantage
- Compatibility
- Complexity
- Trialability
- Observability.

The ENB team added communicability and relevance to the list. You will note in the discussion below that I do not differentiate between communicability and complexity. I do however add another attribute to the list – credibility.

The first 10 chapters of this textbook are aimed at informing you the reader, so that you can become more discerning of research reports and research-based literature and are able to evaluate its credibility. Perhaps we should *hope* for the failure of any intended innovation which is not grounded on sound empirical evidence or a credible theoretical basis, not least because we cannot be sure that it will be beneficial.

Relative advantage

Relative advantage is the need for any change to be demonstrably better than the *status quo*. Perhaps even more crucial is that the important perception of relative advantage is *not* that of the person(s) seeking to initiate the change, but those most affected by it. In some ways this can be seen to relate to the clinical course graduates I referred to earlier, in that they typically perceived clear 'relative advantage' in the changes they sought to make. Unfortunately it was also often the case that, for a variety of reasons, their colleagues (the 'users') did not. Being able to 'sell' an idea (Wright 1989) is therefore an important attribute for anyone wishing to innovate (there is further discussion of this under the heading 'change agents' on page 296).

Compatibility

Compatibility refers to the degree of congruence between a proposed change and existing custom and practice. The ENB working party (1987) make the valuable point that this compatibility must prevail at both the philosophical and pragmatic levels. A practical example of this would be a situation where a nurse or group of nurses, decided that patient care would improve if 'moist wound' dressings and techniques formed the basis of practice. At a philosophical or theoretical level, they might convince colleagues and managers of the desirability or benefits of such a move. However, if funding for staff training and – perhaps more importantly – the relevant products are not available, then for purely pragmatic reasons the innovation will be unsuccessful.

If the proposed change appears congruent on these two levels, then it would seem obvious that it has a greater chance of adoption. Furthermore, the nearer the elements of the change are to existing values and practices, the easier the change will be to implement. In some ways this can be seen to relate to the issues of problem resolution and diagnosis discussed earlier. Therefore, a sensible and strategic way forward is for an innovator to proceed with small but definite steps, whilst never losing sight of the 'bigger picture' – what they wish to achieve in time.

Complexity and communicability

These relate to the ease with which the idea of an innovation can be shared with others. From their evaluation of numerous innovation attempts, Rogers and Shoemaker (1971: 154) identify that rate of adoption of an innovation is negatively related to its complexity. Communicability is therefore affected by the content of the innovation as well as the abilities of the change agent(s) in terms of clarity of thought and exposition. No matter what the relative advantage of a proposed change may be, if the change agent cannot convey its benefit to the 'users', then it is doomed to failure. The imperative to move slowly but surely, using small steps, is again demonstrated here as the ideas behind small, relatively simple incremental changes will inevitably be easier to communicate to the users than larger more complex ones.

Trialability

Triability is the degree to which an innovation may be experimented with on a limited basis. Rogers and Shoemaker (1971) are of the view that innovations that can be tried on an instalment plan will generally be adopted more rapidly than innovations which are not divisible (page 155). In practical terms this could be in the form of trialling an innovation in one clinical area, before expanding to others. Alternatively it could be that a set period of time is put forward, during which the proposed innovation will be piloted. Both offer benefits, such as allowing opportunities to deal with any teething troubles which arise in practice (no plan will ever be perfect). They also mean that should a change be found to have had unforeseen negative consequences, then a return to the status quo is not precluded.

Having a trial period can also present a less threatening face to a proposed change. If 'users' (particularly laggards and rejecters – see Figure 12.1) can be assured that the changes are not 'set in stone' and that if unsuccessful, things will revert back to 'normal', then at least overt rejection can be minimized. If the change proves successful, however, then the innovators and the 'early and later adopters' (Rogers and Shoemaker 1971) (Figure 12.1) who could be said to equate to the 'luke-warm supporters' referred to by Machiavelli (Box 12.3, page 290) will have had their chance to see and experience the change in reality and so become protagonists.

Observability

The observability of a proposed change refers to how visible its results – and perhaps more importantly its benefits and drawbacks – are to both participants and observers. It goes without saying that the more obvious benefits (relative advantage) that can be observed, the greater the chance of success. Rogers and Shoemaker (1971) take the issue of observability to the point of suggesting that physical observation of the change in action or its effects, in itself aids adoption by other people. In other words, 'seeing is believing'.

Relevance

The relevance of an innovation also improves the chances of its acceptance by 'users'. The relevance may be serendipitous, i.e. the change just happens to appear relevant to them. Or it may be as a result of political astuteness on the part of the innovator, in that they may have had ideas and plans 'on hold' until such times as they took on relevance in the light of policy changes. It may even be that they have been so politically effective that they have been able to engender and inform such policy changes.

Summary

Any innovation should be credible in that it should be a change based upon rigorous research or theory. Other key 'attributes' of an innovation which will affect its success revolve around the benefits to be accrued by those who will be most affected by it – the 'users'. Being able to 'sell' an innovation is therefore an important facet of the change agent's role.

Exercise 12.4

Identify an innovation you have seen or been involved with and rate it against each of the criteria discussed above:
  – Relative advantage
  – Compatibility
  – Complexity
  – Trialability
  – Observability.
Come to some conclusion as to why it succeeded or failed based on its attributes as an innovation.

Change agents

Vaughan and Pillmoor (1992) characterize change agents as people (or groups of people) who can take an idea for change from the drawing board, carry it through all the stages of its implementation and finally evaluate its success (or failure). Given this view, without a change agent innovation will not take place. This can even be seen to be the case in action research (see Chapter 4) where the team can be considered change agents.

  In organizations such as the modern National Health Service, the responsibility for the role of change agent is typically invested with clinical and general managers. This is not accidental. Change agents do not necessarily need to be senior but this can certainly help, not least because the ability to initiate and implement change is often a function of power. This is not to say that power is merely linked to position or rank and the ability to control resources. Charisma (personal power) and expertise (power of authority) also confer power to those who possess these traits or attributes (Handy 1986). Whatever the source, it seems reasonable to suggest that a change agent needs power to implement change (Allen 1993), even if it is conferred vicariously through the support of someone with power.

However, it should be recognized that power is not the be all and end all to leading successful innovation, not least because of the need for collaboration and ownership of the change by its 'users'. I have already discussed, for example, the importance of the innovator's 'mental set' (I can make a difference, page 283) along with the imperative to have a clear vision of the problem and what they want to achieve. Again, having reviewed a range of studies, Rogers and Shoemaker (1971: 183–191) identify other attributes of effective change agents related to the success or otherwise of innovation. Interestingly, these relate less to the need for power (though credibility or 'authority' in the eyes of users is seen as crucial), and more to their willingness to value and include input from prospective users of the innovation.

Specific attributes demonstrated by successful innovators include their empathy with users, along with the points encompassed within earlier discussions of the first three 'essentials for change' (ENB 1987). Another interesting point raised by Rogers and Shoemaker (1971: 183) is the issue of venturesomeness – the eagerness to take risks and try new ideas, while at the same time being willing to accept the occasional setback when one of the new ideas proves unsuccessful. This relates to the issue of 'reactance' discussed earlier in the chapter.

Lancaster and Lancaster (1982) take a slightly different tack. In addition to the above, they highlight the need for a sound knowledge of human behaviour and group processes (pages 2 and 20), along with good interpersonal skills (both verbal expression and listening, page 3). They reiterate the need for the change agent to possess an awareness of the general feel of the change environment and the users within it (as in preceding discussions). In particular, they emphasize the need to be able to engender an atmosphere of trust and a willingness to work through the processes of change systematically and with clarity of mind – preferably with clear objectives and a strategic plan. Finally they and others (e.g. The Open University 1991) make the crucial point that change agents must recognize that there are any number of factors outside their control which can influence the success or failure of any innovation. They therefore need to be politically astute, resilient, flexible and perhaps most important of all, lucky.

See *Change strategies and models of change*, page 299

Lancaster and Lancaster (1982: 20–23 and Chapter 6 on Leadership), Hunt (1986) and Havelock and Zlotolow (1995) all present excellent further reading, in the form of research-based discussions of the attributes of leaders and change agents.

The merits of being a change agent

Earlier in this chapter in discussing health care culture and its possible ramifications for innovation, a fairly negative picture was painted of the change agent's lot. This was followed by a suggestion of indicators that this may slowly be changing in the light of policy shifts at the highest levels, for example the increasing emphasis on innovation and evidence-based practice within purchasing agreements between health authorities and health providers.

It should also be acknowledged that being successful as an agent of change – being vindicated in the belief that you can indeed make a difference – is a heady potion. It does wonders for self-esteem and may even enhance the level of regard you are held in by others – peers, managers and even prospective employers. It also makes any job more interesting and fulfilling, leading to a sense of self-efficacy and worth. This brings us back to the issue of oppressed group behaviour (Freire 1971) which I discussed earlier in relation to 'culture'. It is interesting that those who offer solutions to the vicious cycle of horizontal violence and marginalization in nursing (Roberts 1983), rather than merely exposing and bemoaning it (Speedy 1987, Farmer 1993), suggest that such behaviours will disappear only when a critical mass of nurses possess such self-esteem and pride in their work and their profession.

See Box 12.2, page 289

Summary

Power to initiate and/or enforce change is a useful tool for any change agent. If this is combined with a clear sense of purpose, along with a willingness to invite and value input from the potential 'users' of the innovation, then the chances of success are increased.

Being a successful change agent can lead to a sense of personal well-being and self-efficacy. However, it should also be recognized that seeking to change the established order of things can lead to conflict, and the change agent may become the focus of antagonism. Prospective innovators should be prepared for both eventualities.

Exercise 12.5

■ Familiarize yourself with the managerial and/or committee structure of the organization in which you work, then try to identify ways in which you could have more of an input into these levels of activity (**hint:** what about putting yourself forward for election onto a committee?)

■ In light of the discussion in this chapter, think about whether you feel prepared to take on the role of change agent. If not, what needs to happen before you will feel prepared for the role? (**hint:** reading the texts referred to might be a good start).

Change strategies and models of change

The ENB text (ENB 1987), along with Wright (1989) discuss the strategies for change first put forward by Bennis *et al* in 1976. These are:

- Getting people to change by *telling* them that they must (the power-coercive approach, P-C)
- *Selling* them the idea so that they come to perceive the need for change (the rational-empirical approach, R-E)
- *Delegating* responsibility for the change to users (the normative re-educative approach, N-R) with the belief that such *participation* (a combination of R-E and N-R) will lead to ownership and so more lasting change.

More detailed description of these strategies along with exemplar case studies in both clinical and educational settings are presented by Wright (1989). I will therefore not present them here but I do encourage you to read this item, because these strategies play a part in the management of any change. The readings regarding action research in chapter 4 can also be usefully accessed to identify how this approach could be used to initiate and plan change.

Here I will present a short discussion of the perceived benefits of using a model of change to structure and inform planning for innovation, along with a brief overview and comparison of two different models of change – Lewin (1951) and Lippitt (1973).

Benefits of using a model of change

Several times in this chapter, I have re-visited the imperative for change agents to be systematic and to follow some sort of plan if they wish to maximize their chances of success. This has ranged from a discussion of the need for diagnosis of environments and 'the problem' at the outset (what you want to change), through to the processes of innovation (how you intend to change it), and finally evaluation (how successful have you been?). I decided to expand the coverage of 'change strategies' as cited by the ENB (1987) to incorporate models of change because change agents, particularly those new to the role, need more structure to their thoughts and actions than Bennis *et al* provide. To a degree, these models can be seen as recipes to follow, when trying to manage change, and as such offer far more detail than the indication that 'telling', 'selling' and 'participating' are all important facets of change management.

There are a number of benefits associated with following a model of change. One is that these frameworks invariably encourage some degree of formal diagnostic work, both of the environment and the users. Some even extend to the provision of criteria or check points for such work, e.g. Lewin's Force Field Analysis technique (see Figure 12.2). Another is that they provide structure (to varying degrees) for the action aspects of the innovation.

Figure 12.2
*Lewin Force Field
Analysis*

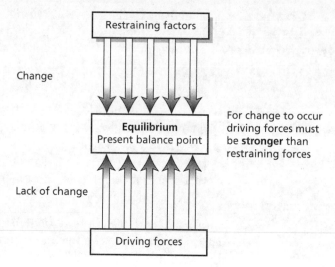

(Adapted from Lewin 1951)

Finally, they highlight the importance, indeed necessity, of re-stabilizing the change environment and evaluating the success of the innovation attempt, preferably against some objective criteria, once the process has ended. The fact that a time-frame needs to be identified and agreed is in itself beneficial to the neophyte change agent.

Overview and comparison of models of change

A perusal of the literature on models of change identifies a marked degree of agreement amongst theorists about key aspects of the change process. Kurt Lewin is seen as the father of change theory. Miles (1995) is of the view that it was Lewin's work in the 1940s which led to the development of a systematic, scientific study of planned change. Lewin (1951) suggests that the first step in any proposed innovation is to carry out a detailed analysis of the situation, to allow the identification of forces considered supportive (driving) and obstructive (restraining) to the proposed innovation (Figure 12.2). This can be seen as the diagnostic phase of this model. The result of this exercise can be to indicate to the innovator that restraining forces outweigh driving forces, so their chances of success are slim and they may be better served using their energies in some other ways.

However, if driving forces outweigh restraining forces the change agent may reasonably embark upon the first phase of the action plan – **unfreezing**. Allen (1993) describes this as a period where the users of the innovation come to recognize the need for change, diagnoze the problem and select a solution. Once this has been achieved the **moving** phase begins. Essentially this involves enacting the solution, a movement from 'old' practice to 'new'. Having done that, all that is left to do is to **re-freeze** the change environment, to allow a period of consolidation and evaluation.

You may note a sense of irony in what I have just written. This was intended. The beauty of Lewin's model is its apparent simplicity, but just how would you go about unfreezing a situation? Just what would you do to get things moving? How do you re-freeze the situation and the people within it? Ollikainen (1987) presents a case study of her use of this model to introduce the nursing process into a hospital setting. She indicates that she had a fair degree of success. However, it is also apparent that she had to expend an immense amount of creative energy translating the words into meaningful actions. Laight (1995) and Wilkinson (1994) used Lewin's model to help introduce change into separate intensive care units (ICUs). Laight was concerned with standardizing eye care and Wilkinson with changing the nursing model used in her unit. Both provide excellent examples of the benefits of diagnozing the situation with a force field analysis exercise. Wilkinson's is shown in Table 12.1 as an example. Unfortunately from there on, as with Ollikainen, they were both left with little else to base their future plans upon and so held meetings, tried to canvass support by being as communicative as possible and encouraged participation in the process. This should not be seen as a criticism of these nurses. Though neither author was able to indicate how successful they had been with their innovation, they gave the impression that they had been as systematic as possible. Watkins (1997) also used Lewin's model to introduce bedside handover reports. What is interesting about her account is that she also reflects on other possible theories she could have used – essentially Rogers and Lippitt (see below). She concludes that she used Lewin's model because she was most familiar with it, however, she could see that on reflection she also followed steps to be found in the other models – albeit 'accidentally'. This reinforces the point that a more structured model of change can make things far simpler for the change agent.

In 1962, Everett Rogers (of Rogers and Shoemaker) expanded on Lewin's three phase theory by emphasizing that the backgrounds of the potential users and the environment in which change is proposed are other issues to be considered in planning change. This is the basis of Rogers' five phase theory of 'change diffusion'. Figure 12.3 shows these phases and their relationship to Lewin's work. I will not be discussing this theory in any detail here, as not only has Rogers written a text (1962) which does this in great detail, but also it does not offer a great deal more structure to follow than Lewin's model. This is a view shared by Hagerman and Tiffany (1994) who, after using a tool developed by Lutjens and Tiffany (1994) to evaluate change theories, concluded that Rogers' diffusion model is not really a planned change theory and is only really of use in tracking the adoption of previous innovations rather than informing the process of new ones, not least because it 'pays scant attention to the processes of change' (Hagerman and Tiffany 1994).

A useful alternative to both Lewin and Rogers is the change model identified by Lippitt (1973). In comparison, Lippitt's model provides far greater structure to the processes of change. It does this by identifying key aspects of the change cycle, which is very useful to anyone new to the role of change agent. Figure 12.3 indicates the relationships between Lewin's, Rogers' and Lippitt's theories (developed from Lancaster and Lancaster 1982).

The strong parallels between Lippitt and the work of Lewin and Rogers and Shoemaker affords further credibility to Lippitt's model. This relationship should perhaps not be surprising given the fact that Lippit worked with Lewin at the National Training Laboratories in the USA in the 1940s. These laboratories were designed to develop researchers to work in the area of interpersonal and group behaviour (Hagerman and Tiffany 1994), focusing particularly on change and changing behaviour. A brief description of the stages of the theory explicates this relationship further. Reading this will also reveal the parallels between Lippitt's model and the content of this chapter. The author acknowledges the work of Gordon Lippitt (1973) and Lancaster and Lancaster (1982: 10–12) as the basis of this discussion.

Table 12.1
An example of force field analysis of factors affecting the introduction of change into an ICU

Driving forces	Restraining forces
Minimal finance required	Financial cost of printing documents
Partial knowledge base of the new model already established	Deficiency of knowledge for some staff
Inherent motivation – change not imposed 'from above'	Lack of time available to prepare and educate staff
Staff dissatisfied with existing model of care	Scepticism about nursing models in general
Less paperwork and so more time available for patient and family	Perception of increase in work load
Desire to change from staff	Emotional cost of change on nursing staff
Successful pilot and evaluation	

Wilkinson (1994)

Figure 12.3 *A comparison between Rogers', Lewin's and Lippitt's phases of the change process*

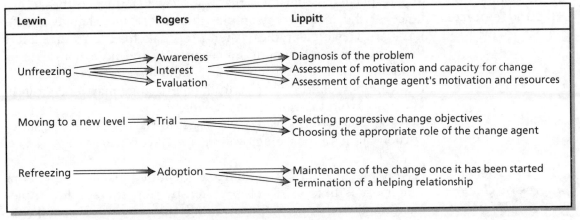

Lewin	Rogers	Lippitt
Unfreezing	Awareness Interest Evaluation	Diagnosis of the problem Assessment of motivation and capacity for change Assessment of change agent's motivation and resources
Moving to a new level	Trial	Selecting progressive change objectives Choosing the appropriate role of the change agent
Refreezing	Adoption	Maintenance of the change once it has been started Termination of a helping relationship

(Adapted from Lancaster and Lancaster 1982, with kind permission of Mosby)

The stages of change, based on Lippitt's model

Stage 1: Diagnosing the problem

This requires that participants keep an open mind and avoid jumping to conclusions before all possible causes have been considered. The first step of data collection and problem identification is critical. Ideally, all who will be involved in the change process or affected by the change should be included in this phase. They also need to be kept informed and should feel free to raise questions and make suggestions. The more information the change agent has, the more likely an accurate assessment and problem identification will be made. Key people, especially those with considerable power and authority in the organization, need to be involved in the change process as much and as early as possible. This stage needs to include a clear statement of 'the problem(s)', perhaps after a process of problem resolution (discussed earlier). An evaluation of the current situation is also necessary. This can be seen as collecting base-line data, against which the effects of the change can be measured.

Stage 2: Assessment of the motivation and capacity for change

Successful planned change generally involves considerable hard work and commitment to the project. During this stage it is necessary to assess both the people involved and the environment in which the proposed change is to take place – the equivalent of Lewin's Force Field Analysis. Factors such as resources, constraints and helpers must be identified. Since the majority of nursing practice takes place within agencies or institutions, the organizational structure must be examined to determine whether the rules, policies, norms, and people involved will either help or hinder the change process. It is also necessary to think about the availability or limitations of financial resources and the views of those who control them.

Stage 3: Assessment of the change agent's motivation and resources

This requires honest and critical self-assessment on the part of the change agent. The degree to which the change agent is trusted and respected within the organization will influence the acceptance of the idea. For example, if many of the change agent's ideas are viewed as radical, then proposals for change are likely to be viewed with scepticism, especially by more conservative members of the establishment. It should also be recognized that knowing how hard it may be to initiate change may lead an individual to avoid the role of change agent.

To reiterate, using this model we get to stage 3 before the introduction of the proposed innovation is even considered.

Stage 4: Selecting progressive change objectives

Having diagnosed the problem and identified resources and constraints, it is time to develop a step-by-step strategy for implementing the change. This planning stage must be specific in terms of the steps to be taken, by whom, and when. Deadlines are especially helpful and a trial period could be instituted at this time. Goals can be re-evaluated based on the trial experience, and alterations made to the plan as necessary. It is important that clear indications of what will constitute success are included as steps in this plan, so as to help you to keep on track.

Stage 5: Choosing the appropriate change agent role

The change agent may choose to be an expert role model, catalyst, teacher or group leader. The change agent may actively gather information and demonstrate new procedures or may serve more as a motivator for others who will actually implement the project. It helps the change process if both the participants and the change agent have similar conceptions of the change agent's role.

Stage 6: Maintenance of the change

Once a change has been instituted, the interest and enthusiasm seen during the developmental phase may wane, and old methods may re-emerge. Once the change has been implemented it is necessary to keep the lines of communication open so that questions, concerns, and ideas can receive attention. It is also helpful to provide frequent reports about the change to supervisory personnel as well as to participants. When the change has been successfully instituted, plans must be made for the diffusion of information, since other people in the organization may wish to become involved in a similar initiative. Members of the original change group may serve as resource people to other units, keeping in mind that the actual design of a change project may require modification to meet the unique needs of a different setting. Also, each setting has unique personality and structural qualities that may necessitate modification of the original plan. A clear statement of 'the problem(s)' and a clear evaluation of the 'state of affairs' at the outset (as outlined earlier in this chapter) help greatly in the maintenance of the change. If it can be clearly demonstrated that positive outcomes have been achieved by the change, then positive attributes of the change can be reinforced. It is also the case that such information can be used to indicate that a return to the status quo is advisable. Such information can therefore be seen to relate closely with Rogers and Shoemaker's (1971) attributes of an innovation. In essence, meaningful audit pre and post change is of the utmost importance.

Stage 7: Termination of the helping relationship

During this stage the change agent, following a prescribed plan, withdraws from the situation. This should be accomplished gradually so that participants can increasingly take more responsibility for the maintenance functions. The change agent may continue to serve as a consultant or resource person but should actively encourage autonomy on the part of the change implementers.

Lippitt's model therefore provides far more detailed information about *how* a change agent might go about initiating and enacting change than does Lewin or Rogers. However, it can be seen that in many ways Lippitt's work reflects and builds upon their work and that of others. The choice is yours . . .

Summary

A number of models of change exist, though the literature would suggest that few are regularly used in practice. They all present some degree of structure for planning, implementing and evaluating change, though some provide more than others. Perhaps *the* most important thing they offer is the advice that detailed assessments of the prospective users of the innovation and the environment in which they work, using a tool such as the Force Field Analysis, is a vital first step in the process of managing planned change.

Exercise 12.6

■ What change strategies and/or models of change have you used or seen in use in your work environment?

■ Identify a change you would like to see introduced into your workplace and use Lewin's or Lippitt's model to structure an action plan.

Chapter summary

I stated at the beginning of this chapter that it is vital for any would-be innovator to feel that they can make a difference. With such a mind-set, the change agent then needs to be cognisant of change theory so as to benefit from the experiences of those who have gone before and so maximize their chances of success. I have used the ENB document *Managing Change in Nursing Education* (1987) as the basis for presenting this material, but incorporated other points – most importantly the importance of pre-innovation assessment and the benefits of problem resolution. Models of change were presented as a formal framework for organizing such activities, particularly for the person new to innovation.

I hope that I have helped you, the reader, in terms of both motivation and knowledge base. Happy Innovating!

Exercise 12.7   A checklist for change

This exercise is intended to link together the various parts of the 'five essential factors for change' (ENB 1987) model used in this chapter. Think of an innovation you have been involved with either as a change agent or an innovation 'user'. Compare it against the following checklist and identify where you think the planning was sound and where it was found wanting.

1. Assess the 'ripeness for change' of the environment into which the attempted change was introduced. Was there evidence of:

- Openness?
- Interpersonal and informational linkages?
- Freedom from organizational constraints?
- Supportive leadership?
- Trust?

If the innovation failed on one or more of these counts, there may be problems in the environment that will hinder any future attempts at innovation. Make a note of any personal or organizational barriers to change which you identify from this exercise.

2. Assess the 'users' of the innovation in terms of their readiness to change. What proportion, and who, were:

- Innovators?
- Early adopters?
- Early majority?
- Later majority?
- Laggards?
- Rejecters?

3. To what extent do you think users' readiness to adopt the innovation was affected by:

- Their sense of ownership (or lack of it) of the change?
- Their informal personal contacts (or lack of them) over the change?
- The involvement (or lack of it) of opinion leaders?
- The information and support (or lack of it) that they received in connection with the change?

Based on this, do you perceive that on balance you work with an innovative group of people or not?

4. Assess the attributes of the innovation you are recalling, in terms of its:

- Credibility
- Relative advantage
- Compatibility
- Complexity and communicability
- Trialability
- Observability
- Relevance.

Did the innovation fail on one, or several, of these counts? Looking back, could the innovation have been better conceived?

5. Assess the success of the change agent(s) involved in the innovation. How well did they perform in terms of:

- Diagnozing the problem and situation?
- Identifying and clarifying goals?
- Developing appropriate strategies and tactics?
- Developing good working relationships with users?
- Their use of any source of power open to them?

What personal characteristics did they possess which appeared to help or hinder the change process? For example, were they:

- Credible?
- Resilient?
- Empathic?
- Approachable?
- Supportive?
- Charismatic?

What effects (if any) did these characteristics have on the success of the innovation?

6. Was a recognized model of change utilized?

- Which?
- Was it used effectively in your opinion?

Having considered the intended change using this checklist, you should be in a position to identify the impact of the five essential factors for change on the overall success or failure of the innovation attempt.

- Do you feel that the innovation could have been better planned?
- What would you have done differently in the light of the theory presented in this chapter, and the benefit of hindsight?

Adapted from Wright (1989) *Changing Nursing Practice* Edward Arnold, with kind permission

References

Allen A (1993) Changing theory in nursing practice. *Senior Nurse* **13**(1): 43–45.

Argyris C (1983) In Pugh DS, Hickson J, Hinings CR (eds) *Writers on Organisations,* 3rd edn. Harmondsworth: Penguin Business Books, pp 167–170.

Benner P (1984) *From Novice to Expert: Excellence and Power in Clinical Nursing Practice.* Menlo Park, CA: Addison Wesley.

Bennis WG, Benne KD, Chin R and Corey KE (1976) *The Planning of Change.* London: Holt Rinehart and Winston.

Cornwell T (1996) Manual handling and the elderly. *The Lamp* **53**(2): 40–41, 44–45.

Coxon T (1990) Ritualised repression. *Nursing Times* **86**(31): 35–36.

Crocker OL, Chiu JSK and Charney C (1984) *Quality Circles: a Guide to Participation and Productivity.* New York: Methuen Publications.

Crookes PA (1992) The Politics of Health Care. In Boddy J and Rice V (eds) *Health: Perspectives and Practices.* The Dunmore Press.

Crookes PA (1996) *Personal Bereavement in Registered General Nurses* (Unpublished PhD Thesis). Hull: University of Hull.

English National Board for Nursing, Midwifery and Health Visiting Working Group (1987) *Managing Change in Nursing Education.* London: ENB.

Farmer B (1993) The use and abuse of power in nursing. *Nursing Standard* **7**(23): 33–36.

Freire P (1971) *Pedagogy of the Oppressed.* New York: Continuum.

Fullan MG (1986) The management of change. In Hoyle E and McMahon A (eds) *The World Yearbook of Education.* Kogan Page, 73–86.

Green GJ (1988) Relationships between role models and role perceptions of new graduate nurses. *Nursing Research* **37**(4): 245–248.

Grissum M and Spengler C (1976) *Women, Power and Health Care.* Boston: Little, Brown and Company.

Hagerman ZT and Tiffany CR (1994) Evaluation of two planned change theories. *Nursing Management* **25**(4): 57–62.

Handy J (1986) Considering organisations in organisational stress research: a rejoinder to Glowinkowski and Cooper to Duckworth. *Bulletin of the British Psychological Society* **39**: 205–210.

Harvey TR (1990) *Checklist For Change: a Pragmatic Approach to Creating and Controlling Change.* Boston, MA: Allyn and Bacon.

Hatfield B and Campbell D (1987) Quality circles: tapping people power. *Nursing Management* **18**: 94.

Havelock R (1972) *Bibliography on Knowledge Utilisation and Dissemination.* Ann Arbor, MI: Institute for Social Research.

Havelock RG and Huberman M (1978) *Solving Educational Problems*: the theory and reality of innovation in developing countries: a study prepared for the International Bureau of Education. Paris and Toronto: UNESCO.

Havelock RG and Zlotolow S (1995) *The Change Agent's Guide to Innovation in Education,* 2nd edn. Eaglewood Cliffs, NJ: Educational Technology Publications.

Hunt JW (1986) Changing organisations. In *Managing People At Work,* 2nd edn. London: The Institute of Personnel Management.

King's Fund Centre (1992) *Nursing Developments Network.* Guidance notes. London: King's Fund.

Laight SE (1995) A vision for eye care: a brief study of the change process. *Intensive and Critical Care Nursing* **11**: 217–222.

Lancaster J and Lancaster L (1982) *Concepts for Advanced Nursing Practice: the Nurse as a Change Agent.* St Louis, MO: Mosby.

Larson DG (1987) Internal stressors in nursing: helper secrets. *Journal of Psychosocial Nursing* **25**(4): 20–27.

Lewin K (1951) cited in Lancaster J and Lancaster L (eds) (1982) *Concepts for Advanced Nursing Practice: the Nurse as a Change Agent.* St Louis, MO: Mosby.

Lippitt GL (1973) *Visualizing Change: Model Building and the Change Process.* Fairfax VA: NTL – Learning Resources Corporation.

Lutjens LRJ and Tiffany CR (1994) Evaluating planned change theories. *Nursing Management* **25**(3): 54–57.

Mabbett P (1987) From burned out to turned on: skills of personal energy management and 'caring'. *Canadian. Nurse* **83**(3): 15–19.

Machiavelli N (1513) *The Prince.* Translated by Bull G (1961). Harmondsworth: Penguin.

Maslow AH (1971) *Attaining the Farther Reaches of Human Nature*. New York: Penguin.

Miles MB (1995) Foreword to Havelock RG and Zlotolow S (1995) *The Change Agent's Guide to Innovation in Education,* 2nd edn. New Jersey: Educational Technology Publications.

Milio N (1998) Strategic lessons for health-promoting policy. A meta-study of national case studies. A paper prepared for presentation at the 2nd international conference on health promotion. WHO and Commonwealth of Australia, 3–10 April 1988, Adelaide.

Mosby's Medical, Nursing and Allied Health Dictionary (1990), Glauze WD (ed), 3rd edn. St Louis, MO: Mosby.

Ollikainen L (1986) Towards a change in nursing practice. *International Nursing Review* **33**(2): 40–43.

Pirsig RM (1974) *Zen and the Art of Motorcycle Maintenance*. London: Vintage.

Richman J (1987) *Medicine and Health*. London: Longman.

Roberts SJ (1983) Oppressed group behaviour: implications for nursing. *Advances in Nursing Science* **5**(4): 21–30.

Rogers EM (1962) *Diffusion of Innovations*. New York: The Free Press.

Rogers EM and Shoemaker FF (1971) *Communication of Innovations: a Cross-cultural Approach*. New York: The Free Press.

Salvage J (1985) *The Politics of Nursing*. London: Heinemann.

Seligman MEP (1975) *Helplessness: on Depression, Development and Death*. New York: WH Freeman.

Schon D (1987) *Educating the Reflective Practitioner*. San Francisco, CA: Jossey-Bass.

Skevington S (1984) *Understanding Nurses*. Chichester: John Wiley.

Speedy S (1987) Feminism and the Profession of Nursing. *Australian Journal of Nursing* **4**(2): 20–28.

Street A (1995) *Nursing Replay: Researching Nursing Culture Together*. Melbourne: Churchill Livingstone.

Taylor SE (1979) Hospital patient behaviour: reactance, helplessness or control? *Journal of Social Issues* **35**: 156–184.

The Open University (1991) Managing Health Services, Book 9 *Managing Change*. MK: The Open University Press.

Vaughan B and Pillmoor M (1992) *Managing Nursing Work*. London: Scutari Press.

Waters M and Crook R (1990) *Sociology One: Principles of Sociological Analysis for Australians*, 2nd edn. Melbourne: Longman Cheshire.

Watkins S (1997) Introducing bedside handover reports. *Professional Nurse* **12**(4): 270–273.

Whitehouse DM (1991) Games of one-upmanship and sabotage. *Nursing Management* **2**(6): 46–50.

Wilkinson P (1994) Introducing a change of nursing model in a general intensive therapy unit. *Intensive and Critical Care Nursing* **10**: 267–231.

Wortman CB and Brehm JW (1975) Responses to uncontrollable outcomes: an integration of reactance theory and the learned helplessness model. In Berkowitz L (ed) *Advances in Experimental Social Psychology,* Vol 8. New York: Academic Press.

Wright SG (1989) *Changing Nursing Practice*. London: Edward Arnold.

Glossary

With grateful thanks to W.B. Saunders Company for permission to reproduce adapted extracts from the glossary in Burns N., Grove S.K. (1997) *The Practice of Nursing Research: Conduct, Critique and Utilization, 3rd edn.*

A

abstract. Clear, concise summary of a study, usually limited to 100–250 words.

abstract thinking. Oriented towards the development of an idea without application to, or association with, a particular instance and is independent of time and space. Abstract thinkers tend to look for meaning, patterns, relationships, and philosophical implications.

accessible population. Portion of the target population to which the researcher has reasonable access.

accidental or convenience sampling. Subjects are included in the study because they happened to be in the right place at the right time; available subjects are simply entered into the study until the desired sample size is reached.

across-method triangulation. Combining research methods or strategies from two or more research traditions in the same study.

alpha (α). Level of significance or cut-off point used to determine whether the samples being tested are members of the same population or of different populations; alpha is commonly set at .05, .01, or .001.

alternate form reliability. Comparing the equivalence of two versions of the same instrument.

analysis of covariance (ANCOVA). Statistical procedure designed to reduce the error term (or variance within groups) by partialing out the variance due to a confounding variable by performing regression analysis before performing ANOVA.

analysis of variance (ANOVA). Statistical technique used to examine differences among two or more groups by comparing the variability between the groups with the variability within the groups.

analytic induction. Qualitative research technique that includes enumerative induction, in which a number and variety of instances are collected that verify the model, and eliminative induction, which requires that the hypothesis be tested against alternatives.

anonymity. Subject's identity cannot be linked, even by the researcher, with his or her individual responses.

applied research. Scientific investigations conducted to generate knowledge that will directly influence or improve practice.

associated key words. A set of words that could be allied with the topic area concerned.

associative relationship. Identifies variables or concepts that occur or exist together in the real world; thus, when one variable changes, the other variable changes.

assumptions. Statements taken for granted or considered true, even though they have not been scientifically tested.

attrition. The loss of participants during the course of a study: can introduce an unknown amount of bias by changing the composition of the sample initially drawn – particularly if more subjects are lost from one group than another; can thereby be a threat to the internal validity of a study.

auditability. Rigorous development of a decision trail that is reported in sufficient detail to allow a second researcher, using the original data and the decision trail, to arrive at conclusions similar to those of the original researcher.

B

backward stepwise regression analysis. Type of stepwise regression analysis where all the independent variables are initially included in the analysis. Then, one variable at a time is removed from the equation and the effect of that removal on variance is evaluated.

baseline measure. The measurement of the dependent variable before the introduction of an experimental intervention.

beneficence, principle of. Encourages the researcher to do good and above all, do no harm.

benefit–risk ratio. Researchers and reviewers of research weigh potential benefits and risks in a study to promote the conduct of ethical research.

bias. Any influence or action in a study that distorts the findings or slants them away from the true or expected.

bibliography. A list of references, either computer- or text-based.

bivariate analysis. Statistical procedures that involve the comparison of summary values from two groups of the same variable or of two variables within a group.

bivariate correlation. Analysis techniques that measure the extent of the linear relationship between two variables.

body of knowledge. Information, principles and theories that are organized by the beliefs accepted in a discipline at a given time.

borrowing. Appropriation and use of knowledge from other disciplines to guide nursing practice.

box-and-whisker plots. Exploratory data analysis technique to provide visualization of some of the major characteristics of the data, such as the spread, symmetry, and outliers.

bracketing. Qualitative research technique of suspending or laying aside what is known about an experience being studied.

breach of confidentiality. Accidental or direct action that allows an unauthorized person to have access to raw study data.

broad brush approach. An approach to searching the literature identified by Burnard (1995) and meaning searching the library indexes for any information that could be related to the topic area.

C

canonical correlation. Extension of multiple regression with more than one dependent variable.

case study design. Intensive exploration of a single unit of study, such as a person, family, group, community, or institution.

catalogue. Identifies what is available in the library.

causal hypothesis or relationship. Identifies a cause-and-effect interaction between two or more variables, which are referred to as independent and dependent variables.

causal relationship. Relationship between two variables where one variable (independent variable) is thought to cause or determine the presence of the other variable (dependent variable).

causality. Includes three conditions: (1) must be a strong correlation between the proposed cause and effect, (2) proposed cause must precede the effect in time, and (3) cause has to be present whenever the effect occurs.

cell. Intersection between the row and column in a table where a specific numerical value is inserted.

census. A survey covering an entire population.

central limit theorem. States that even when statistics, such as means, come from a population with a skewed (asymmetrical) distribution, the sampling distribution developed from multiple means obtained from that skewed population will tend to fit the pattern of the normal curve.

central tendency. A statistical index of the 'typicalness' of a set of scores that come from the centre of the distribution of scores. The three most common indices of central tendency are the mode, the median, and the mean.

change agent. Professional outside a system who enters the system to promote adoption of an innovation.

chi-square (χ^2) test. Used to analyze nominal data to determine significance of differences between observed frequencies within the data and frequencies that were expected.

citation. A word that means that an author is being used to support the statement as in the sentence above. Burnard (1995) is being cited.

citation indexes. Written and computer indexes that cross reference the authors that writers are citing.

chronology. A type of unstructured observation that provides a detailed description of an individual's behaviour in a natural environment.

cleaning data. Checking raw data to determine errors in data recording, coding, or entry.

cluster sampling. A form of multistage sampling in which large groupings ('clusters') are selected first (e.g. nursing schools), with successive subsampling of smaller units (e.g. nursing students).

Cochran Q test. Nonparametric test that is an extension of the McNemar test for two related samples.

codebook. Identifies and defines each variable in a study and includes an abbreviated variable name (limited to 6–8 characters), a descriptive variable label, and the range of possible numerical values of every variable entered into a computer file.

coding. Process of transforming qualitative data into numerical symbols that can be computerized.

coercion. An overt threat of harm or excessive reward intentionally presented by one person to another in order to obtain compliance, such as offering subjects a large sum of money to participate in a dangerous research project.

coefficient of determination (R^2). Computed from a matrix of correlation coefficients and provides important information on multicollinearity. This value indicates the degree of linear dependencies among the variables.

cohorts. Samples in time-dimensional studies within the field of epidemiology.

comparative descriptive design. Used to describe differences in variables in two or more groups in a natural setting.

comparison group. The group not receiving a treatment or receiving the usual treatment (standard care) when non-random sampling methods are used.

complete observer. The researcher is passive and has no direct social interaction in the setting.

compatibility. The degree to which the innovation is perceived to be consistent with current values, past experience, and priority of needs.

complete participation. The researcher becomes a member of the group and conceals the researcher role.

complex hypothesis. Predicts the relationship (associative or causal) among three or more variables; thus, the hypothesis could include two (or more) independent and/or two (or more) dependent variables.

computerized database. A structured compilation of information that can be scanned, retrieved and analyzed by computer and can be used for decisions, reports, and research.

computer searches. Conducted to scan the citations in different databases and identify sources relevant to a research problem.

concept. A term that abstractly describes and names an object or phenomenon, thus providing it with a separate identity or meaning.

conceptual definition. Provides a variable or concept with connotative (abstract, comprehensive, theoretical) meaning and is established through concept analysis, concept derivation, or concept synthesis.

conceptual framework. A set of highly abstract, related constructs that broadly explains phenomena of interest, expresses assumptions, and reflects a philosophical stance.

conclusions. Synthesis and clarification of the meaning of study findings.

concurrent validity. The degree to which scores on an instrument are correlated with some external criterion, measured at the same time.

confidence interval. A range where the value of the parameter is estimated to be.

confidentiality. Management of data in research so subjects' identities are not linked with their responses.

confounding variables. Variables recognized before the study is initiated but cannot be controlled, or variables not recognized until the study is in process, which may have an effect on the dependent variable.

consent form. A written form, tape-record-ing, or videotape used to document a subject's agreement to participate in a study.

consent rate. The percentage of people that indicate a willingness to participate in a study based on the total number of people approached.

constructs. Concepts at very high levels of abstraction that have general meanings.

construct validity. Examines the fit between conceptual and operational definitions of variables and determines if the instrument actually measures the theoretical construct it purports to measure.

content analysis. Qualitative analysis technique to classify words in a text into a few categories chosen because of their theoretical importance.

content validity. Examines the extent to which the method of measurement includes all the major elements relevant to the construct being measured.

context. The body, the world and the concerns unique to each person within which that person can be understood.

contingency tables. Cross-tabulation tables that allow visual comparison of summary data output related to two variables within a sample.

control. Imposing of rules by the researcher to decrease the possibility of error and increase the probability that the study's findings are an accurate reflection of reality.

control group. The group of elements or subjects not exposed to the experimental treatment.

convenience or accidental sampling. Subjects are included in the study because they happen to be in the right place at the right time; available subjects are simply entered into the study until the desired sample size is reached.

correlation. A tendency for variation in one variable to be related to variation in another variable.

correlation coefficient. Indicates the degree of relationship between two variables; the coefficients range in value from +1.00 (perfect positive relationship) to 0.00 (no relationship) to −1.00 (perfect negative or inverse relationship).

correlational analysis. Statistical procedure conducted to determine the direction (positive or negative) and magnitude (or strength) of the relationship between two variables.

correlational research. Systematic investigation of relationships between two or more variables to explain the nature of relationships in the world and not to examine cause and effect.

cost–benefit analysis. Analysis technique used in outcomes research that examines costs and benefits of alternative ways of using resources as assessed in monetary terms and the use that produces the greatest net benefit.

cost-effectiveness analyses. Type of outcomes research where the costs and benefits are compared for different ways of accomplishing a clinical goal, such as diagnosing a condition, treating an illness, or providing a service. Goal of cost-effectiveness analyses is to identify the strategy that provides the most value for the money.

covert data collection. Occurs when subjects are unaware that research data are being collected.

Cramer's V. Analysis technique for nominal data that is a modification of phi for contingency tables larger than 2×2.

criterion-referenced testing. Comparison of a subject's score with a criterion of achievement that includes the definition of target behaviours. When the behaviours are mastered, the subject is considered proficient in these behaviours.

critical analysis of studies. Minute examination of the merits, faults, meaning, and significance of studies.

critical incident technique. A method of obtaining data from study participants by in-depth exploration of specific incidents and behaviours related to the matter under investigation.

critical social theory. Qualitative research methodology guided by critical social theory; the researcher seeks to understand how people communicate and develop symbolic meanings in a society.

critique. An objective, critical and balanced appraisal of a research report's various dimensions (e.g. conceptual, methodological and ethical). It requires detailed critical analysis based on a fairly sophisticated level of knowledge about research.

crossover design. Includes the administration of more than one treatment to each subject and the treatments are provided sequentially, rather than concurrently, and comparisons are then made of the effects of the different treatments on the same subjects.

cross-sectional designs. Used to examine groups of subjects in various stages of development simultaneously with the intent of inferring trends over time.

cross-tabulation. A determination of the number of cases occurring when simultaneous consideration is given to the values of two or more variables (e.g., sex – male/female – cross-tabulated with smoking status – smoker/non-smoker). The results are typically presented in a table with rows and columns divided according to the values of the variables.

cultural immersion. Used in ethnographic research for gaining increased familiarity with such things as language, sociocultural norms, and traditions in a culture.

curvilinear relationship. The relationship between two variables varies depending on the relative values of the variables. The graph of the relationship is a curved line rather than a straight one.

D

data. Pieces of information that are collected during a study.

database. *See* computerized databases.

data analysis. Conducted to reduce, organize, and give meaning to data.

data coding sheet. A sheet for organizing and recording data for rapid entry into a computer.

data collection. Precise, systematic gathering of information relevant to the research purpose or the specific objectives, questions, or hypotheses of a study.

data entry. The process of entering data (usually in coded form) onto an input medium for computer analysis.

data reduction. Technique for analyzing qualitative data that focuses on decreasing the volume of data to facilitate examination.

data transformation. A step often undertaken prior to the analysis of research data, to put the data in a form that can be meaningfully analyzed (e.g., recoding of values).

data triangulation. Collection of data from multiple sources in the same study.

debriefing. Complete disclosure of the study purpose and results at the end of a study.

deception. Misinforming subjects for research purposes.

decision theory. Theory that is inductive in nature and is based on assumptions associated with the theoretical normal curve. The theory is applied when testing for differences between groups with the expectation that all of the groups are members of the same population.

decision trail. *See* auditability.

Declaration of Helsinki. Ethical code based on the Nuremberg code that differentiated therapeutic from non-therapeutic research.

deductive reasoning. Reasoning from the general to the specific or from a general premise to a particular situation.

degrees of freedom (df). The freedom of a score's value to vary given the other existing scores' values and the established sum of these scores ($df = N - 1$).

Delphi technique. A method of measuring the judgments of a group of experts for assessing priorities or making forecasts.

demographic variables. Characteristics or attributes of the subjects that are collected to describe the sample.

dependent variable. The response, behaviour, or outcome that is predicted or explained in research; changes in the dependent variable are presumed to be caused by the independent variable.

description. Involves identifying the nature and attributes of nursing phenomena and sometimes the relationships among these phenomena.

descriptive codes. Terms used to organize and classify qualitative data.

descriptive correlational design. Used to describe variables and examine relationships that exist in a situation.

descriptive design. Used to identify a phenomenon of interest, identify variables within the phenomenon, develop conceptual and operational definitions of variables, and describe variables.

descriptive research. Provides an accurate portrayal or account of characteristics of a particular individual, event, or group in real-life situations for the purpose of discovering new meaning, describing what exists, determining the frequency with which something occurs, and categorizing information.

descriptive statistics. Statistics that allow the researcher to organize the data in ways that give meaning and facilitate insight, such as frequency distributions and measures of central tendency and dispersion.

design. Blueprint for conducting a study that maximizes control over factors that could interfere with the validity of the findings.

dialectic reasoning. Involves the holistic perspective, where the whole is greater than the sum of the parts, and examining factors that are opposites and making sense of them by merging them into a single unit or idea, greater than either alone.

diary. Record of events kept by a subject over time that is collected and analyzed by a researcher.

diffusion. Process of communicating research findings (innovations) through certain channels over time among the members of a discipline.

directional hypothesis. States the specific nature of the interaction or relationship between two or more variables.

discriminant analysis. Designed to allow the researcher to identify characteristics associated with group membership and to predict group membership.

disproportionate stratified sampling. A sampling strategy wherein the researcher samples differing proportions of subjects from different strata in the population to ensure adequate representation of subjects from strata that are comparatively smaller.

dissemination of research findings. The diffusion or communication of research findings.

double-blind experiment. An experiment in which neither the subjects nor those who administer the treatment know who is in the experimental or control group.

dummy variables. Categorical or dichotomous variables used in regression analysis.

E

early adopters of innovations. Opinion leaders in a social system who learn about new ideas rapidly, utilize them, and serve as role models for their use in nursing practice.

effect size. A statistical expression of the magnitude between two variables, or the magnitude of the difference between two groups, with regard to some attribute of interest.

eigen values. Numerical values generated with factor analysis that are the sum of the squared weights for each factor.

element of a study. A person (subject), event, behaviour, or any other single unit of a study.

emic approach. Anthropological research approach of studying behaviours from within the culture.

empirical generalization. Statements that have been repeatedly tested through research and have not been disproved. Scientific theories have empirical generalizations.

empirical literature. Includes relevant studies published in journals and books as well as unpublished studies, such as master's theses and doctoral dissertations.

empirical world. Experienced through our senses and is the concrete portion of our existence.

epistemology. The philosophical theory of knowledge. Epistemology seeks to define the nature, derivation, scope and reliability of the claims of knowledge.

equivalence. Type of reliability testing that involves comparing two versions of the same instrument or two observers measuring the same event.

error score. Amount of random error in the measurement process.

ethical inquiry. Intellectual analysis of ethical problems related to obligation, rights, duty, right and wrong, conscience, choice, intention, and responsibility to obtain desirable, rational ends.

ethical principles. Principles of respect for persons, beneficence, and justice relevant to the conduct of research.

ethical rigour. Requires recognition and discussion by the researcher of the ethical implications related to the conduct of the study.

ethics. The quality of research procedures with respect to their adherence to professional, legal, and social obligations to the research subjects.

ethnographic research. A qualitative research methodology for investigating cultures that involves collection, description, and analysis of data to develop a theory of cultural behaviour.

ethnomethodology. A research approach which aims to increase the understanding of taken-for-granted or implicit practices in a society, particularly in relation to social interaction. An ethnomethodological study usually uses documents and audio-visual taped materials that focus on everyday events as the source of the data.

etic approach. Anthropological research approach of studying behaviour from outside the culture and examining similarities and differences across cultures.

event sampling. In observational studies a sampling plan that involves the selection of integral behaviours or events.

exclusion criteria. Sampling requirements identified by the researcher that eliminate or exclude an element or subject from being in a sample. Exclusion criteria are exceptions to the inclusion sampling criteria.

execution errors. Errors that occur because of a defect in the data collection procedure.

experimental designs. Designs that provide the greatest amount of control possible in order to more closely examine causality.

experimental group. The subjects who are exposed to the experimental treatment.

experimental research. Objective, systematic, controlled investigation to examine probability and causality among selected variables for the purpose of predicting and controlling phenomena.

explanation. Achieved when research clarifies the relationships among phenomena and identifies why certain events occur.

explanatory codes. Developed late in the data collection process after theoretical ideas from the qualitative study have begun to emerge.

exploratory data analysis. Examining the data descriptively, to become as familiar as possible with the nature of the data.

exploratory factor analysis. Similar to stepwise regression in which the variance of the first factor is partialed out before analysis is begun on the second factor. It is performed when the researcher has few prior expectations about the factor structure.

exploratory regression analysis. Used when the researcher may not have sufficient information to determine which independent variables are effective predictors of the dependent variable; thus, many variables may be entered into the analysis simultaneously. This is the most commonly used regression analysis strategy in nursing studies.

external validity. The extent to which study findings can be generalized beyond the sample used in the study.

extraneous variables. Exist in all studies and can affect the measurement of study variables and the relationships among these variables.

F

face validity. Verifies that the instrument looked like or gave the appearance of measuring the content.

factor analysis. Analysis that examines inter-relationships among large numbers of variables and disentangles those relationships to identify clusters of variables that are most closely linked together. Two types of factor analysis are exploratory and confirmatory factor analysis.

factor rotation. An aspect of factor analysis where the factors are mathematically adjusted or rotated to reduce the factor structure and clarify the meaning.

factorial analysis of variance. Mathematically the analysis technique is simply a specialized version of multiple regression; a number of types of factorial ANOVAs have been developed to analyze data from specific experimental designs.

factorial design. Study design that includes two or more different characteristics, treatments, or events that are independently varied within a study.

fatigue effect. When a subject becomes tired or bored with a study.

feasibility of a study. Determined by examining the time and money commitment; the researcher's expertise; availability of subjects, facility, and equipment; cooperation of others; and the study's ethical considerations.

field research. The activity of collecting the data that requires taking extensive notes in ethnographic research.

findings. The translated and interpreted results from a study.

focus group interview. An interview in which the respondents are a group of individuals assembled to answer questions on a given topic.

forced choice. Response set for items in a scale that have an even number of choices, such as four or six, where the respondents cannot choose an uncertain or neutral response and must indicate support for or against the topic measured.

forward stepwise regression analysis. Type of stepwise regression analysis where the independent variables are entered into the analysis one at a time and an analysis is made of the effect of including that variable on R^2.

framework. The abstract, logical structure of meaning that guides the development of the study and enables the researcher to link the findings to a body of knowledge.

fraudulent publications. There is documentation or testimony from co-authors that the publication did not reflect what had actually been done.

frequency distribution. A statistical procedure that involves listing all possible measures of a variable and tallying each datum on the listing. There are two types of frequency distributions, ungrouped and grouped.

frequency polygon. Graphic display of a frequency distribution, in which dots connected by a straight line indicate the number of times a score value occurs in a set of data.

Friedman two-way analysis of variance by ranks. Non-parametric test used with matched samples or in repeated measures.

G

generalization. Extends the implications of the findings from the sample that was studied to the larger population or from the situation studied to a larger situation.

gestalt. Organization of knowledge about a particular phenomenon into a cluster of linked ideas. The clustering and interrelatedness enhances the meaning of the ideas.

going native. In ethnographic research, when the researcher becomes a part of the culture and loses all objectivity, and, with it, the ability to observe clearly.

grounded theory research. An inductive research technique based on symbolic interaction theory, which is conducted to discover what problems exist in a social scene and the process persons use to handle them. The research process involves formulation, testing and redevelopment of propositions until a theory is developed.

Guttman scale. A method of measuring attitudes that makes use of a set of cumulative (monotone) items with which respondents are asked to agree or disagree.

H

hard copy. A written or typed paper copy of what is listed or written in a computer.

Hawthorne effect. A psychological response in which subjects change their behaviour simply because they are subjects in a study, not because of the research treatment.

heterogeneity. The researcher's attempt to obtain subjects with a wide variety of characteristics to reduce the risk of bias in studies not using random sampling.

historical research. A narrative description or analysis of events that occurred in the remote or recent past.

history effect. An event that is not related to the planned study but occurs during the time of the study and could influence the responses of subjects to the treatment.

homogeneity. The degree to which objects are similar or a form of equivalence, such as limiting subjects to only one level of an extraneous variable to reduce its impact on the study findings.

human rights. Claims and demands that have been justified in the eyes of an individual or by the consensus of a group of individuals and are protected in research.

hypothesis. Formal statement of the expected relationship between two or more variables in a specified population.

I

immersed in the culture. Involves gaining increasing familiarity with such things as language, sociocultural norms, traditions, communication patterns, religion, work patterns, and expression of emotion in a selected culture.

implications. The meaning of research conclusions for the body of knowledge, theory and practice.

inclusion criteria. Sampling requirements identified by the researcher that must be present for the element or subject to be included in the sample.

incomplete disclosure. Subjects are not completely informed about the purpose of a study because that knowledge might alter the subjects' actions. Following the study, the subjects must be debriefed.

incremental searching. A searching strat-

egy identified by Burnard (1995) which suggests that a single piece of literature should be examined for its references. These references should then be found and examined for relevance and their references examined. This should occur until the searcher is satisfied that all the relevant pieces have been found.

independent groups. Groups where the selection of one subject is totally unrelated to the selection of other subjects. An example is when subjects are randomly assigned to the treatment and control groups.

independent variable. The treatment or experimental activity that is manipulated or varied by the researcher to create an effect on the dependent variable.

index. A list of references often to be found in a library. It can either be written or computer-based. Provides assistance in identifying journal articles and other publications relevant to a topic of interest.

indirect measurement. Used with abstract concepts, when the concepts are not measured directly but, rather, indicators or attributes of the concepts are used to represent the abstraction.

inductive reasoning. Reasoning from the specific to the general where particular instances are observed and then combined into a larger whole or general statement.

inferential statistics. Statistics designed to allow inference from a sample statistic to a population parameter; commonly used to test hypotheses of similarities and differences in subsets of the sample under study.

inferred causality. A cause-and-effect relationship is identified from numerous studies conducted over time to determine risk factors or causal factors in selected situations.

informed consent. The prospective subject's agreement to voluntarily participate in a study, which is reached after assimilation of essential information about the study.

innovation. An idea, practice, or object that is perceived as new by an individual or other unit of adoption.

innovators. Individuals who actively seek out new ideas.

institutional review. A process of examining studies for ethical concerns by a committee of peers.

instrumentation. A component of measurement that involves the application of specific rules to develop a measurement device or instrument.

interlibrary loan department. Department that locates books and articles in other libraries and provides the sources within a designated time.

internal validity. The extent to which the effects detected in the study are a true reflection on reality, rather than being the result of the effects of extraneous variables.

interpretative codes. Organizational system developed late in the qualitative data collection and analysis process as the researcher gains some insight into the processes occurring.

inter-rater reliability. The degree of consistency between two raters who are independently assigning ratings to a variable or attribute being investigated.

interrupted time-series designs. These designs are similar to descriptive time designs except that a treatment is applied at some point in the observations.

interval-scale measurement. Interval scales have equal numerical distances between intervals of the scale in addition to following rules of mutual exclusive categories, exhaustive categories, and rank ordering, such as temperature.

interviews. Structured or unstructured verbal communication between the researcher and subject, during which information is obtained for a study.

inverse linear relationship. Indicates that as one variable or concept changes, the other variable or concept changes in the opposite direction. Also referred to as a negative linear relationship.

investigator triangulation. Exists when two or more research-trained investigators with divergent backgrounds explore the same phenomenon.

J

justice, principle of. States that human subjects should be treated fairly.

K

Kendall's tau. Non-parametric test to determine correlation used when both variables have been measured at the ordinal level.

Kolmogorov–Smirnov two-sample test. Non-parametric test used to determine whether two independent samples have been drawn from the same population.

Kruskal–Wallis test. Most powerful non-parametric analysis technique for examining three independent groups for differences.

kurtosis. The degree of peakedness of the curve shape that is related to the spread or variance of scores.

L

laggards. Individuals who are security-oriented, tend to cling to the past, and are often isolated without a strong support system. Term used to describe persons who are reluctant or refuse to adopt innovations.

lambda. Analysis technique that measures the degree of association (or relationship) between two nominal level variables.

Likert scale. An instrument designed to determine the opinion or attitude of a subject; it contains a number of declarative statements with a scale after each statement.

limitations. Theoretical and methodological restrictions in a study that may decrease the generalizability of the findings.

linear relationship. The relationship between two variables or concepts will remain consistent regardless of the values of each of the variables or concepts.

logical positivism. The philosophy underlying the traditional scientific approach. The meaning of a proposition is in the method of its verification and any proposition which is not verified by observation is meaningless.

longitudinal study. A study designed to collect data at more than one point in time, in contrast to a cross-sectional study.

M

manipulation. To move around or to control the movement of a variable or treatment.

Mann–Whitney _U_ test. Used to analyze ordinal data with 95% of the power of the t-test to detect differences between groups of normally distributed populations.

matching. This technique is used when an experimental subject is randomly selected and a subject similar in relation to important extraneous variables is randomly selected for inclusion in the control group.

maturation effect. Unplanned and unrecognized changes experienced during a study, such as growing older, wiser, stronger, hungrier, or more tired, that can influence the findings of a study.

McNemar test. Non-parametric test to analyze the changes that occur in dichotomous variables using a 2×2 table.

mean. The value obtained by summing all the scores and dividing that total by the number of scores being summed.

measurement. The process of assigning numbers to objects, events, or situations in accord with some rule.

measurement error. The difference between what exists in reality and what is measured by a research instrument.

measures of central tendency. Statistical procedures (mode, median and mean) for determining the centre of a distribution of scores or a typical value.

measures of dispersion. Statistical procedures (range, difference scores, sum of squares, variance and standard deviation) for examining how scores vary or are dispersed around the mean.

median. The score at the exact centre of the ungrouped frequency distribution.

memo. Developed by the researcher to record insights or ideas related to notes, transcripts, or codes during qualitative data analysis.

meta-analysis design. Merging of findings from several completed studies to determine what is known about a particular phenomenon.

method of least squares. Procedure in regression analysis for developing the line of best fit.

methodological limitations. Restrictions in the study design that limit the credibility of the findings and the population to which the findings can be generalized.

methodological triangulation. The use of two or more research methods or procedures, such as different designs, instruments and data collection procedures, in a study.

modal percentage. Appropriate for nominal data and indicates the relationship of a number of data scores represented by the mode to the total number of data scores.

mode. The numerical value or score that occurs with the greatest frequency in a distribution; but it does not necessarily indicate the centre of the data set.

mortality. Subjects drop out of a study before completion, which creates a threat to the internal validity.

multicausality. The recognition that a number of inter-relating variables can be involved in causing a particular effect.

multilevel analysis. Used in epidemiology to study how environmental factors and individual attributes and behaviours interact to influence individual-level health behaviours and disease risks.

multiple regression analysis. Extension of simple linear regression with more than one independent variable entered into the analysis.

multivariate analysis techniques. Used to analyze data from complex research projects. *See also* multiple regression, factorial analysis of variance, analysis of covariance, factor analysis, discriminant analysis, canonical correlation, structural equation modelling, and time-series analysis.

N

natural settings. Field settings or uncontrolled, real-life situations examined in research.

negative linear relationship. *See* inverse linear relationship.

networking. A process of developing channels of communication between people with common interests throughout the country.

network sampling. Snowballing technique that takes advantage of social networks and the fact that friends tend to hold characteristics in common. Subjects meeting the sample criteria are asked to assist in locating others with similar characteristics.

nominal-scale measurement. Lowest level of measurement that is used when data can be organized into categories that are exclusive and exhaustive, but the categories cannot be compared, such as gender, race, marital status, and nursing diagnoses.

non-directional hypothesis. States that a relationship exists but does not predict the exact nature of the relationship.

non-equivalent control group designs. Designs in which the control group is not selected by random means, such as the one-group post-test-only design, post-test-only design with non-equivalent groups, and one-group pretest–post-test design.

non-parametric statistics. Statistical techniques used when the assumptions of parametric statistics are not met and most commonly used to analyze nominal- and ordinal-level data.

non-probability sampling. Not every element of the population has an opportunity for selection in the sample, such as convenience (accidental) sampling, quota sampling, purposive sampling, and network sampling.

non-therapeutic research. Research conducted to generate knowledge for a discipline, and the results from the study might benefit future patients but will probably not benefit those acting as research subjects.

normal curve. A symmetrical, unimodal bell-shaped curve that is a theoretical distribution of all possible scores, but no real distribution exactly fits the normal curve.

null hypothesis. States that there is no relationship between the variables being studied; a statistical hypothesis used for statistical testing and interpreting statistical outcomes.

Nuremberg Code. Ethical code of conduct to guide investigators in conducting research.

O

oblique rotation. A type of rotation in factor analysis used to accomplish the best fit (best factor solution) and the factors are allowed to be correlated.

observed score. The actual score or value obtained for a subject on a measurement tool.

observer-as-participant. The researcher's time is spent observing and interviewing subjects and less in the participation role.

one-tailed test of significance. An analysis used with directional hypotheses where extreme statistical values of interest are thought to occur in a single tail of the curve.

ontology. The theory of what really exists as opposed to what appears to exist. It is the primary element in metaphysics. It is contrasted with epistemology, the study of knowing, rather than being.

operational definition. Description of how variables or concepts will be measured or manipulated in a study.

operationalization. The process of translating research concepts into observable and/or measurable phenomena.

ordinal-scale measurement. Yields data that can be ranked but the intervals between the ranked data are not necessarily equal, such as levels of coping.

outcomes research. Important scientific methodology that was developed to examine the end results of patient care. The strategies used in outcomes research are a departure from the traditional scientific endeavours and incorporate evaluation research, epidemiology, and economic theory perspectives.

outliers. The extreme scores or values in a set of data.

P

***p* value.** In statistical testing, the probability that the obtained results result from chance alone.

paradigm. A way of looking at natural phenomena that encompasses a set of philosophical assumptions and that guides one's approach to inquiry.

parallel-forms reliability. *See* alternate forms reliability.

parameter. A measure or numerical value of a population.

parametric statistical analyses. Statistical techniques used when three assumptions are met: (1) the sample was drawn from a population for which the variance can be calculated, the distribution is expected to be normal or approximately normal; (2) the level of measurement should be interval or ratio with an approximately normal distribution; and (3) the data can be treated as random samples.

participant-as-observer. A special form of observation where researchers immerse themselves in the setting so they can hear, see, and experience the reality as the participants do. But the participants are aware of the dual roles of the researcher (participant and observer).

path coefficient. The effect of the independent variable on the dependent variable that is determined through path analysis.

Pearson's product-moment correlation coefficient. Parametric test used to determine the relationship between variables.

percent of variance. The value obtained by squaring the Pearson's correlation coefficient (r) and that is the amount of variability explained by the linear relationship.

phenomenology. An approach to human inquiry that emphasizes the complexity of human experience and the need to study that experience holistically as it is actually lived. In sociology, phenomenology is used to investigate people's assumptions involved in everyday social life.

phenomenological research. Inductive, descriptive qualitative methodology developed from phenomenological philosophy for the purpose of describing experiences as they are lived by the study participants.

phi coefficient. Analysis technique to determine relationships in dichotomous, nominal data.

philosophical inquiry. Research using intellectual analyses to clarify meanings, make values manifest, identify ethics, and study the nature of knowledge.

philosophy. A broad, global explanation of the world.

pilot study. A smaller version of a proposed study conducted to develop and/or refine the methodology, such as the treatment, instrument, or data collection process.

population. All elements (individuals, objects, or events) that meet sample criteria for inclusion in a study. Sometimes referred to as a target population.

positive linear relationship. Indicates that as one variable changes (value of the variable increases or decreases), the second variable will also change in the same direction.

poster session. Visual presentation of a study, using pictures, tables, and illustrations on a display board.

power. The probability that a statistical test will detect a significant difference that exists; power analysis is used to determine the power of a study.

power analysis. Used to determine the risk of a Type II error, so the study can be modified to decrease the risk if necessary.

practice effect. Occurs when subjects improve as they become more familiar with the experimental protocol.

precision. The accuracy with which the population parameters have been estimated within a study. Also used to describe the degree of consistency or reproducibility of measurements.

prediction. The ability to estimate the probability of a specific outcome in a given situation that can be achieved through research.

predictive validity. The degree to which an instrument can predict some criterion observed at a future time.

primary source. A source that is written by the person who originated or is responsible for generating the ideas published.

principal component analysis. The second step in exploratory factor analysis that provides preliminary information needed by the researcher in order for decisions to be made prior to the final factoring.

principal investigator (PI). In a research grant, the individual who will have primary responsibility for administering the grant and interacting with the funding agency.

probability sampling. Random sampling techniques in which each member (element) in the population should have a greater than zero opportunity to be selected for the sample; examples include simple random sampling, stratified random sampling, cluster sampling, and systematic sampling.

probability theory. Addresses statistical analysis from the perspective of the extent of a relationship or the probability of accurately predicting an event.

probing. Technique used by the interviewer to obtain more information in a specific area of the interview.

process-outcome matrix. Qualitative analysis technique that allows the researcher to trace the processes that led to differing outcomes.

proposal, research. Written plan identifying the major elements of a study, such as the problem, purpose, and framework, and outlining the methods to conduct the study. A formal way to communicate ideas about a proposed study to receive approval to conduct the study and to seek funding.

proposition. An abstract statement that further clarifies the relationship between two concepts.

prospective cohort study. An epidemiologic study in which a group of people are identified who are at risk for experiencing a particular event.

purposive sampling. Judgmental sampling that involves the conscious selection by the researcher of certain subjects or elements to include in a study.

Q

Q-sort methodology. A technique of comparative rating where a subject sorts cards with statements on them into designated piles (usually 7 to 10 piles in the distribution of a normal curve) that might range from best to worst.

qualitative research. A systematic, interactive, subjective approach used to describe life experiences and give them meaning.

quantitative research. A formal, objective, systematic process to describe, test relationships, and examine cause and effect interactions among variables.

quasi-experimental designs. Designs with limited control that were developed to provide alternate means for examining causality in situations not conducive to experimental controls.

quasi-experimental research. A type of quantitative research conducted to explain relationships, clarify why certain events happen, and examine causality between selected independent and dependent variables.

questionnaire. A printed self-report form designed to elicit information that can be obtained through written responses of the subject.

quota sampling. A convenience sampling technique with an added strategy to ensure the inclusion of subject types that are likely to be under-represented in the convenience sample, such as women, minority groups, and the under-educated.

R

R^2 (coefficient of determination). Computed from a matrix of correlation coefficients and provides important information on multicollinearity. This value indicates the degree of linear dependencies among the variables.

random assignment to groups. (Also known as random allocation or randomization.) A procedure used to assign subjects to the treatment or control groups, where the subjects have an equal opportunity to be assigned to either group.

random error. An error that causes individuals' observed scores to vary haphazardly around their true score.

randomized controlled trials. Classic means of examining the effects of various treatments where the effects of a treatment are examined by comparing the treatment group with the no-treatment group.

random number table. A table of digits from 0 to 9 set up in such a way that each number is equally likely to follow any other. Used in randomization or random sampling.

random sampling. *See* probability sampling.

random variation. The expected difference in values that occurs when one examines different subjects from the same sample.

range. The simplest measure of dispersion obtained by subtracting the lowest score from the highest score.

rating scales. Crudest form of measure using scaling techniques that include a list of an ordered series of categories of a variable, assumed to be based on an underlying continuum.

ratio-level measurement. Highest measurement form that meets all the rules of other forms of measure: mutually exclusive categories, exhaustive categories, rank ordering, equal spacing between intervals, and a continuum of values and also has an absolute zero, such as weight.

refereed journal. Uses referees or expert reviewers to determine whether a manuscript will be accepted for publication.

references. This word has two meanings. (1) A list of the books and articles that have been referred to in the main body of writing. (2) A list of books and journals available in a library.

reflexive thought. Critically thinking through the dynamic interaction between the self and the data occurring during analysis of qualitative data. During this process, the researcher explores personal feelings and experiences that may influence the study and integrates this understanding into the study.

regression line. The line that best represents the values of the raw scores plotted on a scatter diagram and the procedure for developing the line of best fit is the method of least squares.

relational statement. Declares that a relationship of some kind exists between two or more concepts.

reliability. Represents the consistency of the measure obtained.

reliability testing. A measure of the amount of random error in the measurement technique.

replication. Reproducing or repeating a study to determine whether similar findings will be obtained.

representativeness of sample. A sample must be like the population in as many ways as possible.

research. Diligent, systematic inquiry or investigation to validate and refine existing knowledge and generate new knowledge.

research hypothesis. The alternative hypothesis to the null hypothesis that states there is a relationship between two or more variables.

research objectives. Clear, concise, declarative statements that are expressed to direct a study and are focused on identification and description of variables and/or determination of the relationships amongst variables.

research problem. A situation in need of a solution, improvement, or alteration, or a discrepancy between the way things are and the way they ought to be.

research proposal. *See* proposal, research.

research purpose. A concise, clear statement of the specific goal or aim of the study that is generated from the problem.

research questions. Concise, interrogative statements developed to direct studies that are focused on description of variables, examination of relationships among variables, and determination of differences between two or more groups.

research topics. Concepts or broad problem areas that provide the basis for generating numerous questions and research problems.

research tradition. A programme of research that is important for building a body of knowledge related to the phenomena explained by a particular conceptual model.

respect for persons, principle of. Indicates that persons have the right to self-determination and the freedom to participate or not participate in research.

response set. The parameters within which the question or item is to be answered in a questionnaire.

results. The outcomes from data analysis that are generated for each research objective, question, or hypothesis.

retrospective cohort study. An epidemiologic study in which a group of people are identified who have experienced a particular event; for example, studying occupational exposure to chemicals.

review of relevant literature. An analysis and synthesis of research sources to generate a picture of what is known about a particular situation and the knowledge gaps that exist in the situation.

rigour. The striving for excellence in research through the use of discipline, scrupulous adherence to detail, and strict accuracy.

risk–benefit ratio. Researchers and reviewers of research weigh potential benefits and risks in a study to promote the conduct of ethical research.

S

sample. A subset of the population that is selected for a study.

sampling. Includes selecting groups of people, events, behaviours, or other elements with which to conduct a study.

sampling criteria. A list of the characteristics essential for membership in the target population.

sampling distribution. Developed using

statistical values (such as means) of many samples obtained from the same population.

sampling error. The difference between a sample statistic used to estimate a parameter and the actual but unknown value of the parameter.

sampling frame. Listing of every member of the population using the sampling criteria to define membership.

sampling method. The process of selecting a group of people, events, behaviours, or other elements that are representative of the population being studied.

sampling plan. Describes the strategies that will be used to obtain a sample for a study and may include either probability or non-probability sampling methods.

scale. A self-report form of measurement that is composed of several items that are thought to measure the construct being studied and the subject responds to each item on the continuum or scale provided.

scatter plot. A graphic representation of the relationship between two variables.

science. A coherent body of knowledge composed of research findings, tested theories, scientific principles, and laws for a discipline.

scientific method. Incorporates all procedures that scientists have used, currently use, or may use in the future to pursue knowledge, such as quantitative research, qualitative research, and outcomes research.

secondary analysis design. Involves studying data previously collected in another study; data are re-examined using different organizations of the data and different statistical analyses.

secondary source. A source that summarizes or quotes content from primary sources.

selection bias (self-selection). A threat to the internal validity of the study resulting from pre-existing differences between the groups under study. The differences affect the dependent variable in ways extraneous to the effect of the independent variable.

self-determination. Based on the ethical principle of respect for persons, which states that humans are capable of controlling their own destiny. Right to self-determination is violated through the use of coercion, covert data collection, and deception.

semantic differential scale. An instrument that consists of two opposite adjectives with a seven-point scale between them. The subject selects one point on the scale that best describes his or her view of the concept being examined.

sensitivity. In measurement, the ability of the measuring tool to make fine discriminations between objects with differing amounts of the attribute being measured.

serendipity. The accidental discovery of something valuable or useful during the conduct of a study.

sets. A set of key words or words that can be associated with one topic area. This word is often used when searching for information on a computer.

setting. Location for conducting research, such as a natural, partially controlled, or highly controlled setting.

sign test. A non-parametric analysis technique developed for data that it is difficult to assign numerical values to, but the data can be ranked on some dimension.

simple hypothesis. States the relationship (associative or causal) between two variables.

simple linear regression. Parametric analysis technique that provides a means to estimate the value of a dependent variable based on the value of an independent variable.

simple random sampling. Elements are selected at random from the sampling frame for inclusion in a study. Each study element has a probability greater than zero of being selected for inclusion in the study.

skewness. A curve that is asymmetrical (positively or negatively skewed) that is developed from an asymmetrical distribution of scores.

skim reading. A way of rapidly reading a piece of literature or a book to see if it is relevant to the topic area.

slope. Determines the direction and angle of the regression line within the graph. The value is represented by the letter *b*.

snowball sampling. The selection of subjects by means of nominations or referrals from earlier subjects.

Solomon four-group design. An experimental design that uses a before–after design for one pair of experimental/control groups, and an after–only design for a second pair.

Spearman rank-order correlation coefficient. A non-parametric analysis technique for ordinal data that is an adaptation of the Pearson's product-moment correlation used to examine relationships amongst variables in a study.

split-half reliability. Used to determine the homogeneity of an instrument's items, where the items are split in half, and a correlational procedure is performed between the two halves.

stability. Aspect of reliability testing that is concerned with the consistency of repeated measures.

standard deviation. A measure of dispersion that is calculated by taking the square root of the variance.

standard scores. Used to express deviations from the mean (difference scores) in terms of standard deviation units, such as *Z* scores where the mean is zero and the standard deviation is 1.

statistic. A numerical value obtained from a sample used to estimate the parameters of a population.

statistical regression. The movement or regression of extreme scores toward the mean in studies using a pretest–post-test design.

statistical significance. A term indicating that the results obtained in an analysis of sample data are unlikely to have been caused by chance, at some specified level of probability.

stem-and-leaf displays. Type of exploratory data analysis where the scores are visually presented to obtain insights.

stepwise regression analysis. Type of exploratory regression analysis where the independent variables are entered into or removed from the analysis one at a time.

stratified random sampling. Used when the researcher knows some of the variables in the population that are critical to achieving representativeness. The sample is divided into strata or groups using these identified variables.

strength of relationship. The amount of variation that is explained by the relationship.

structural equation modelling. Analysis technique designed to test theories.

structured interviews. Use of strategies that provide increasing amount of control by the researcher over the content of the interview.

structured observation. Clearly identifying what is to be observed and precisely defining how the observations are to be made, recorded, and coded.

subjects. Individuals participating in a study.

subject terms. A list of key words associated with a specific subject area. These words are often used when searching using a computer index.

substantive theory. A theory recognized within the discipline as useful for explaining important phenomena.

sum of squares. Mathematical manipulation that involves summing the squares of the difference scores and part of the analysis process for calculating the standard deviation.

survey. Technique of data collection using questionnaires or personal interviews to gather data about an identified population.

survey design. A design to describe a phenomenon by collecting data from a large sample using questionnaires or personal interviews.

symmetrical relationship. Complex relationship that consists of two statements: If A occurs (or changes), B will occur (or change); if B occurs (or changes), A will occur (or change); A ↔ B.

systematic bias or variation. A consequence of selecting subjects whose measurement values are different or vary in some way from the population.

systematic error. Measurement error that is not random but occurs consistently, such as a scale that inaccurately weighs subjects three pounds heavy.

systematic sampling. Conducted when an ordered list of all members of the population is available and involves selecting every *n*th individual on the list, using a starting point that is selected randomly.

T

tails. Extremes of the normal curve where the significant statistical values exist.

target population. A group of individuals who meet the sampling criteria.

test–retest reliability. Determination of the stability or consistency of a measurement technique by correlating the scores obtained from repeated measures.

theoretical limitations. Weaknesses in the study framework and conceptual and operational definitions that restrict the abstract generalization of the findings.

theoretical literature. Includes concept analyses, maps, theories and conceptual frameworks that support a selected research problem and purpose.

theoretical triangulation. The use of two or more frameworks or theoretical perspectives in the same study, and the hypotheses are developed based on the different theoretical perspectives and tested using the same data set.

theory. Consists of an integrated set of defined concepts and relational statements that present a view of a phenomenon and can be used to describe, explain, predict and/or control that phenomenon.

theoretical notes. In field studies, notes about the observer's interpretations of observed activities.

therapeutic research. Research that provides the patient an opportunity to receive an experimental treatment that might have beneficial results.

thesaurus. A book or computer programme which groups together words that have similar meanings.

Thurstone scale. A type of attitude scale in which a panel of judges first rates the degree of favourability of a set of statements about some attitudinal object (e.g., abortion), and then subjects identify with the statements with which they agree.

time sampling. In observational research, the selection of time periods during which observations will take place.

time-series analysis. A technique designed to analyze changes in a variable across time and thus to uncover patterns in the data.

traditions. Truths or beliefs that are based on customs and past trends and provide a way of acquiring knowledge.

transformation of ideas. Movement of ideas across levels of abstraction to determine the existing knowledge base in an area of study.

translation. Involves transforming from one language to another to facilitate understanding and is part of the process of interpreting research outcomes where results are translated and interpreted into findings.

treatment. The independent variable that is manipulated in a study to produce an effect on the dependent variable. The treatment or independent variable is usually detailed in a protocol to ensure consistent implementation in the study.

trialability. The extent to which an individual or agency can try out the idea on a limited basis with the option of returning to previous practices.

trial and error. An approach with unknown outcomes used in a situation of uncertainty, where other sources of knowledge are unavailable.

triangulation. The use of two or more theories, methods, data sources, investigators, or analysis methods in a study.

true score. Score that would be obtained if there were no error in measurement but there is always some measurement error.

t-test. A parametric analysis technique used to determine significant differences between measures of two samples; t-test analysis techniques exist for dependent and independent groups.

two-tailed test of significance. The analysis used for a non-directional hypothesis where the researcher assumes that an extreme score can occur in either tail.

Type I error. Occurs when the researcher concludes that the samples tested are from different populations (there is a significant difference between groups) when, in fact, the samples are from the same population (there is no significant difference between groups). The null hypothesis is rejected when it is true.

Type II error. Occurs when the researcher concludes that there is no significant difference between the samples examined when, in fact, a difference exists. The null hypothesis is regarded as true when it is false.

U

unstructured interviews. Initiated with a broad question and subjects are usually encouraged to further elaborate on particular dimensions of a topic.

unstructured observations. Involve spontaneously observing and recording what is seen with a minimum of prior planning.

unsubstantiated statements. Statements that are argumentative and unsupported by the literature.

utilization of research findings. The use of knowledge generated through research to guide practice.

V

validity, design. The strength of a design to produce accurate results or findings may be determined by examining statistical conclusion validity, internal validity, construct validity, and external validity.

validity, instrument. Determining the extent to which the instrument actually reflects the abstract construct being examined.

variables. Qualities, properties, or characteristics of persons, things, or situations that change or vary and are manipulated or measured in research.

varimax rotation. A type of rotation in factor analysis used to accomplish the best fit (best factor solution) and the factors are uncorrelated.

vignette. A brief description of an event, person, or situation to which respondents are asked to react.

visual analogue scale. A line of 100 mm in length with right angle stops at each end, where subjects are asked to record their response to a study variable.

voluntary consent. The prospective subject has decided to take part in a study of his or her own volition without coercion or any undue influence.

W

weighting. A correction procedure used to arrive at population values when a disproportional sampling design has been used.

Wilcoxon matched-pairs signed-ranks test. Non-parametric analysis technique used to examine changes that occur in pretest/post-test measures or matched-pairs measures.

Z

z-scores. The standardized scores developed based on the normal curve.

Index

Numbers in bold refer to tables or illustrations; numbers in italics refer to glossary entries.

A

Abstracts 67, *311*
Abuse of research participants 204
Accessibility of research
 improving 270–2
 lack of 265–7
Accessible population 183
Accidental sampling *see*
 Convenience sampling
Action
 learning 272–3
 research 5, **90**, 93–4, 131–2,
  154, 274
Aesthetics 8–9
Alpha coefficients 145, *311*
American Journal of Nursing,
 International Nursing Index 64,
 78
Analytic induction 175–6, *311*
ANOVA (analysis of variance) test
 163, 164, 165, *311*
Artistry, professional 14, 15
*Assessing the Effects of Health
 Technologies*, DoH 33
ASSIA database **78**
Attitudes to research 267–8
Attrition 200, *312*
Audiotaping 155
Authority to change procedures 269
Autonomy 207–14
 consent 207–8
  'broad consent' 209, 212, 213
  to treatment/to participate in
   research 208–9

exercise and discussion 222–5,
  226, 228
 voluntariness 213–14
 see also English National Board
  (ENB): older people,
  autonomy and
  independence research
  project

B

Bandolier 271
Barriers to ultilization, research
 findings 264–70
Becker's health belief model 112
'Before-and-after' studies 124, 128
Beneficence and non-maleficence
 214–18, *312*
 exercises and discussion 222–5,
  226–7, 228
Benner's model 2, 11–13, 15
Between method triangulation 153
Bias 201, 210, *312*
 attrition rate 200
 cultural 63
 publication 221
 social response 211
 sources of sampling 198–9
Bibiographic software packages
 71–2, 239
Bradshaw's taxonomy of social
 need 103
Breast Cancer Screening
 Questionnaire (BCSQ) 145
British Paediatric Association,
 consent guidelines 213
British Reference Library 66
'Broad consent' 209, 212, 213

C

Card indexes 70–1
Career opportunities, therapy
 professionals 39
Carper, types of knowledge 7, 8–9,
 11
Case studies 132–3, *312*
 data analysis 176
 data collection 156–7
Censuses 127
Central R&D committee (CRDC) 30
 Standing Group on HTA 31
Centre for Policy in Nursing
 Research 46
Centre for Practice Research 48
Centre for Reviews and
 Dissemination (CRD) 30, 37,
 234, 269, 275
 CRD databases **78**
*The Challenges for Nursing and
 Midwifery in the 21st Century*,
 DoH 44, 49
Champion's Health Belief Model
 Scale 145
Change management xvii, 281, 282
 attributes of innovation 293–6
 change agents 294–6, *313*
 merits 298
 checklist for change 306–7
 essential factors for 281, 286–8
 health culture as obstruction to
  innovative environment
  288–91
 making a difference 283–5
 models of change 299–305
  benefits of 299–300
  overview and comparison
   300–**303**

Change management – *contd*
  users of innovation 291–93
  see also Critical theory
Chi-square (χ^2) test 165, *313*
Children
  informed consent 213
  vulnerability 220
CINAHL database 59, 60, 61, **79**
  search strategy record **63**
Citation indexes 64, **83**, *313*
Clinical
  expertise, Benner's model 2,
    11–13, 15
  guidelines initiative, RCN 271
  information packs 273
  nurse specialists 275
Cluster sampling **184**, 187–8, *313*
Cochrane Collaboration 30, 48, 234,
    270–1
  Cochrane Database of
    Systematic Reviews **79**, 271,
    272
  Cochrane Pregnancy &
    Childbirth Database **79**, 271
Code of Professional Conduct,
  UKCC 42, 43, 49, 116
Coercion 213, *313*
Cognitive competence, informed
  consent 212
Cohens's Kappa (K coefficient)
  144
Collaboration, interdisciplinary
  28
  between clinicians and
    researchers 273–4
  between practitioners and
    researchers 272–3
Communication, effective channels
  of 287
Comparative need 103
Computers
  computer card file index 70–1,
    72
  recording information, literature
    review 239–40
Concepts *314*
  identifying in literature review
    237
Conceptual
  frameworks **102**, 103, 106, 110,
    314
    exercises 112–13
    identifying in literature
      review 237

*Potential causal routes of
  complicated grief
  reactions in nurses and
  midwives* 103-**4**
  relationship between
    theoretical and 108
  maps 57
Conduct and Utilization of Research
  in Nursing (CURN project)
  274
Confidence intervals 167, *312*
Confidentiality 216
Confirmability, qualitative data
  collection 152–3
Confounding variables 148, 149,
  168, 169–70, *313*
Consensus methods 156
Consent 207–8
  broad consent 209, 212, 213
  client's understanding 212–13
    making randomization easier
      to explain **217**
  form 209, *314*
  independent observer 210
  randomized controlled trials
    (RCTs) 126, 211, 218
  to treatment/to participate in
    research 208–9
Consistency of findings 201
Constant comparative methods
  174–6
Construct validity 147, *314*
Content validity 145, *314*
Context, health care research xiv,
  23–51
  international 49
  NHS research and development
    (R&D) 29–33
    from 1994: 39–42
    strategy for research 34–9
    recent developments 42–9
    UK variations 47–9
  reflective exercises 33, 50–1
  research in nursing before 1980:
    24–9
  strategy for research 34–9
Convenience sampling 142, 148,
  189–90, *311, 314*
Convergent validity 146, 147
Correlation coefficients 144, *314-15*
Council of Europe 49
Credibility, qualitative data
  collection 152
CRIB database **79**

Crisis theory, framework exercise
  112
Criterion validity 146
Critical
  analysis 55, 73–6, 77, 241, *315*
    definition 73–4
    reading 55
    theory paradigm 6, 88, **90**, 92–4
Criticism, historical research 131
Critiquing research 74, 76, *315*
  ethical issues 204–29
  methodological critique 244–7
  samples 199–201
  theoretical critique 241, 243–4
Cronbach's alpha 145
Cross case analysis 133
Cross-over studies 125, *315*
Cross-sectional design 128, *315*
Cultural bias 63
Culture
  definition 288
  health care 288–90
Culyer Report 41–2
Cumulative Index of Nursing and
  Allied Health Literature *see*
  CINAHL
Current Research in Britain *see*
  CRIB database
Customer/contractor relationship 29

D
Data analysis xvi, 162–78, *316*
  independent and dependent
    variables 148, 168–70, *316*
  qualitative 173–7
  quantitative 162–7
  sample size 197
  statistical flow chart **166**
Data collection xv-xvi, 139–58, *316*
  approach to measurement 140
  degree of structure 139
  historical research 131
  objectivity 140
  observation, effects of 140
  qualitative methods 139, 153–7,
    158
    sampling issues 150–1, 189–93
    validity and reliability 151–3
  quantitative methods 139,
    141–3, 157–8
    reliability 144–5
    sampling issues 147–50, 158,
      182–9
    validity 145–7

Deception in research *316*
    acceptability 211
    scientific fraud 220–1
Deductive
    boundary setting 182
    reasoning 95, 96, 97, 176–7, *316*
        and theory testing 98
Delphi technique 156, *316*
Dependability, qualitative data
        collection 152
Dependent variables 148, 168–70,
    316
Description 73, *316*
    critical analysis 75
    research design 117, *316*
Descriptive surveys 127
Design of research xv, 116, 139,
    316
    bridging the gap 129–33
    factors influencing choice
        116–19
    qualitative approaches 119–23
    quantitative approaches 123–9
DHSS-DATA **80**
Director of R&D, NHS 32, 33
Disclosure/non-disclosure of
        information 208, 209–10
Discriminant validity 147
Dissemination of research 37, 39,
    44, *315*
    conferences or workshops 266,
        273
Distributive justice 218–19
Doctors, barrier to research
        utilization by nurses 269
Dreyfus model 11, 13
Drug studies, volunteer participants
    214

E
Education and training 46, 272
    early degree courses 25
    Strategy for Research
        recommendations 36
    therapy professionals 39
Educational research 213–14
Effect size 171–2, *317*
Effective Health Care Bulletin 271
Elaboration, confounding variables
    168
Electronic databases 58, 59, 60, 61,
    62, **78-83**
EMBASE **80**

Empirical knowledge 8
    see also Scientific knowledge
English National Board (ENB) 46
    Health Care Database 66, **80**
    *Managing Change in Nursing
        Education* 281, 286, 299
    older people, autonomy and
        independence research
        project 233, 243–4
        key concepts 248
        methodological matrix 245,
            246, 247
        summary of literature review
            250–2
        theme matrix **242**
Environment, innovative 286–8, 292
    health care culture as
        obstruction 288–91
Epidemiological research 210, 216
Epistemology *317*
    epistemological questions 4
    extended 16
ERIC database **80**
Ethical issues xvi, 204–29
    autonomy 207–14
    beneficence and non-
        maleficence 214–18
    the challenge for health workers
        205–6
    exercises 222–4
        discussion of 224–9
    Four Principles plus Scope of
        Application approach 205,
        206–7
    guidelines
        British 229–30
        international 230–1
    justice 218–22
    unethical studies, using findings
        204–5
Ethics 9
Ethnography 120–1, 195, *317–18*
Ethnomethodology 121, *318*
Ethology 121
Event sampling 193–4, *318*
Evidence-based practice (EBP) 44–5
Experiential knowledge 6, 10, 11,
    19
Experimental research 88, 124–6,
    210, *318*
Explanatory surveys 127–8
Exploration, research design 117,
    118
Expressed need 103

External validity 124

F
Face validity 145, 146, *318*
Factorial design *319*
    randomized control trials (RCTs)
        126
    surveys 128
Felt need 103
Feminist research 5
Field notes, qualitative research
    154, 155
First principles 4
Focus groups 155–6
Force field analysis **302**, 305
    Lewin 299, **300**, 301
    Wilkinson 301, **312**
Four Principles plus Scope of
    Application approach 205,
    206–7, 222–3
Frames of reference 86, 101–13,
    113–14
    definition 101, 102
    frameworks exercise 112–13
    origin of 103–5
    presentation 105
    relationship between levels of
        research and 105–8
    what to look for in framework
        section of study 110
    where to find 109
*A Framework for R&D for Nursing
    for Wales*, Welsh Office 48
Fraud, scientific 220–1
'Free text' search 58
Funding
    NHS R&D, criteria for assessing
        32
    sources of 28
    Strategy for Research
        recommendations 36

G
General Health Questionnaire
    (GHQ) 141, 146
Generation of theory 97, 98, 119
'Gestalt' perspective 91, *319*
Glossary *311–32*
'Grey literature' 265–6
Griffiths inquiry 28
Grounded theory 122–3, 196–7,
    319
    case studies 156–7
    data analysis 173–4

Guidelines
clinical guidelines initiative 271
critiquing samples 199–200
ethical issues 229–31

H
'Hawthorne effect' 125, 152, *319–20*
Heading levels, literature review 247–8
Health belief model
Becker, framework exercise 112
Champion's scale 145
Health care culture 288–91
Health Education Authority database **81**
The Health of the Nation 30
Health technology assessment (HTA) 31
advisory group, research utilization 264
HEALTHPLAN database **81**
Heathrow debate 44, 49
HELMIS database **81**
Historical research 129–31, *320*
Homogeneity of population 196, *320*
'Horizontal violence' 288, 289, 298
House of Lords Select Committee on Science and Technology 29
Hypotheses
hypothesis validity 147
null hypothesis 164, 170, 171, 172, *323*
one and two tailed 164–5

I
Inclusion and exclusion criteria 217–18, *320*
Incremental literature searching 62–4, *320*
Independent variables 148, 168–70, *320*
Index of Nursing Research 26
Indexes *320*
card index recording system 70–1, 72
literature searching 58, 59–60, 61
citation indexes 64
Indicators for practice, identifying in literature review 237
Inductive reasoning 95, 96, 97, 176–7, *320*
and theory generation 98

Information
disclosure/non-disclosure 208, 209–10
local sources 65
national sources 65–6
selective non-disclosure 210–11
Informed consent *320–21*
see also Consent
Innovation
attributes 293–6
compatibility 294–5
complexity and communicability 295
observability 295–6
relative advantage 294
relevance 296
trialability 295
environment for 288–91, 292
users of 291–93
Innovativeness, adopter categorization 291, **292**
Internal
reliability 144–5
validity 124, *321*
International Council of Nurses (ICN) 49
International Nursing Index, AJN 64, **78**
Internet 66
Interobserver reliability 144
Interval data 163
non-parametric tests 165, 167
Interviews 154–5, *321*
Introduction
books and journals 67, 69
literature review 249
Intuition 17, 19

J
Journal
clubs 275–6
publications 266
'skimming' 67–8
Judgemental sampling 191–2
Justice 218–22, *321*
discussions of exercise 225, 227, 228–9

K
K coefficient 144
Key words 57, 58, 60, 72
keeping records 62, **63**
linear presentation **59**

King's Fund 66
database **81**
'Knower', types of 7, 8
Knowledge 1–2, 17
accessing 55–83
critical analysis 73–6
see also Critical analysis; Critiquing research
literature searching 55, 56–67
reading literature 67–72
changing 2–4
concept of knowing xiv
ways of knowing 19
achieving a balance 16–19
major contributors 11–16
overview 7–11
reality, knowing and method 4–7
Knowledge Scales of Dickson's Breast Cancer Screening Inventory 145
Kogan Old People Scale 243

L
Language, research reports 266, 272
Leadership, supportive 287
Learned helplessness 282
theory, framework exercise 112
Lewin's
Force Field Analysis 299, **300**, 301
phases of change **303**
Library facilities
British Reference Library 66
lack of access to 266
Lippitt's model of change 302, **303**
stages of change 303–5
Literature review, definition 235
see also Reviewing research
Literature searching 55, 56–67
choosing an index 61
defining and refining the topic 57–8, 60–1
further refining, search terms 58, 59–60
incremental searching 62–4
integrated approach 65
local and national sources of information 65–6
systematic searching 57
time involved 62
where to start 56–7
Local research ethics committees (LRECs) 205, 209, 210, 215, 222

Longitudinal studies 128, *322*
Lord Rothschild's review 28–9

M
Machiavelli, veiws on change 290
Management change, effect of
    implementation 28
Managers, lack of cooperation from
    269
*Managing the New NHS: Functions
    and Responsibilities*, DOH
    39–40
Mann-Whitney test 165, *322*
Maslow's theory of motivation,
    framework exercise 113
Master of Stress Instrument 142
Matched pair design 128
Medical model of care 87
Medical Research Council (MRC),
    health services research 27
MEDLINE database 60, 61, **82**
Mental illness, informed consent
    212–13
Meta-analysis 221, 235–6, *322*
Methodological
    critique 244–7
        guiding questions, evaluating
            non-research sources 247
        methodological matrix 245,
            246, 247
    questions 4
    triangulation *see* Triangulation
MIDIRS (Midwives Information and
    Resource Service) database **82**
MIRIAD database 272
Models 11, 26–7
    Becker 112
    Benner 2, 11–13, 15
    Carper 7, 8–9, 11
    of change xvii, 299–305
        benefits 299–301
        overview and comparison
            300–**303**
        stages of change, Lippett
            303–5
    Dreyfus 11, 13
    Prochaska and Diclemente 112
    Schön 2, 13–15, 17–18
Module, Research Appreciation and
    Application xi–xiii
Monetary gain 213
Moral knowledge 9
Multidimensional Health Locus of
    Control Scale 142–3

Multidisciplinary research units
    37–8

N
National
    forum, NHS R&D 41
    project register 30
National Board for Northern Ireland
    (NBNI) 48–9
'The naturalistic paradigm' 6, 87,
    89, **90**, 91–2
Need for change 281–3
Network sampling 192, *323*
Neutrality of researcher 91
Newsheets, research-based 271–72
NHS Centre for Reviews and
    Dissemination (CRD) 30, 37,
    234, 271, 277
    CRD databases **78**
NHS Research and Development
    (R&D) strategy 3, 29–33, 260,
    272, 277
    from 1994: 39–42
    for Scotland 47–8
    see also Strategy for Research in
        Nursing Midwifery and
        Health Visiting
Nightingale, Florence 24, 34
Nominal data 163, 165
Non-maleficence and beneficence
    214–18
Non-numerical Unstructured Data
    Indexing, Searching and
    Theorising computer
    programme *see* NUDIST
    computer programme
Non-parametric
    statistics 163, *323*
    tests 163, 164, 165
        interval data 165, 167
Non-probability (non random)
    sampling 182, *323*
Non-response 200
    bias on studies 198–9
Non-verbal behaviour, description
    of *see* Ethology
Normative need 103
Northern Ireland, health care
    research 48–9
Notes
    field 154, 155
    keeping 70–2
Notes on Hospitals, Nightingale 24
NUDIST computer programme 174

Null hypothesis (H0) 164, 170, 171,
    172, *323*
Nurse-physician relationship 288,
    289
Nursing
    models *see* Models
    practice, nature of 261
    research officer, Ministry of
        Health 25
    systems 26
Nursing Research Abstracts, (DHSS)
    25, 26
Nursing Research Initiative for
    Scotland (NRIS) 47

O
Observational methods, data
    collection 153–4
    risk-benefit ratio 216
Oliver's Wall 282
One shot surveys 128
Ontological questions 4
Openness, change management
    286–7
Opportunistic sampling 142, 148,
    189–90, *311*
Oppressed group behaviour 288,
    289, 298
Oral history 131
Ordinal data 163, 165
Orem, theory of self-care 103, 104
    framework exercise 112–13
Organizational
    barriers to change 268–9, 277
    constraints, freedom from 287
Orientation of study 196–7
Original hypothesis (H1) 164
OSH-ROM database **82**
Outcome measurement 31
Ownership
    of change 292, 297
    of research 93

P
P-value 165, 167
Palmore's Facts on Ageing Scale
    243
Panel studies 128
Paradigms 4–5, 85, 87, *324*
    comparison of **90**
    critical theory paradigm 6, 88,
        90, 92–4
    'the naturalistic paradigm' 6, 87,
        89, **90**, 91–2

Paradigms – *contd*
'the positivist paradigm' 5, 87,
88–9, **90**
Parametric statistics 163, *324*
Participant observation 153, 154,
324
Pearson correlation coefficient 144
Personal
knowledge 6, 9, 10
reactivity 198
Phenomenology 119–20, 122, *324*
Philosophical underpinnings of
research xv, 85, 86–94, 113
paradigms in research 5, 6, 85,
87, 88–94
implications for reader 94
philosophy and research 86–8
Photocopier, use of 62
Pilot studies 143, *324*
Placebo controlled trials 211
double-blind 124–5
Policy initiatives 23–4, 274–5
see also NHS Research and
Development (R&D) strategy
Populations 182–3, *325*
characteristics, bias 199
homogeneity 196
measuring whole **182**
vulnerable
informed consent 212
justice 219–20
'Positive energy people' 283
'The positivist paradigm' 5, 87,
88–9, **90**
Postregistration
courses, recognition of research
26, 27
Post Registration Education and
Practice (PREPP) 272
Power *325*
of change agent 296–7
of profession 9
of researcher 6
statistical 149, 150, 170, 171, 172
power analysis 197, *325*
Practical knowledge 10, 11, 17, 18
see also Experiential knowledge
Practice development nurses 275
Predicitve convergent validity 146,
325
Prediction, research design 117
Preregistration courses, recognition
of research 26, 27, 43
Prima facie moral principles 206–7

Primary sources *325*
historical research 130
Privacy, upholding 216
Probability (random) sampling 182,
183–8, 201, *325*
description, advantages and
disadvantages **184**
Problem resolution, process of
283–5
Procedural bias 198
Prochaska and Diclemente,
readiness to change model 112
Psychometric testing of
questionnaire 141–2
Psycinfo/Psyclit database **82**
Publication bias 221
Publications, research-based 271–72
journals 266
journal clubs 275–6
Purposive sampling 191, 192, *325*

Q
Qualitative research xvi, 5, 6, 118,
326
critiquing samples 200, 201
data analysis 173–7
data collection
methods 139, 153–7, 158
sampling 150–1, 189–93
validity and reliability 151–3
designs 119–23
the qualitative paradigm 4–5, 6,
89, **90**, 91–2
risk-benefit ratio 215–16
using existing data 123
'Qualitative versus quantitative
debate' 87–8, 94
Quantitative research xvi, 5, 6, 118,
326
critiquing samples 200, 201
data analysis 162–7, 176
data collection
methods 139, 141–3, 157
sampling 147–50, 158, 182–9
validity and reliability 144–7
designs 123–9
see also The positivist paradigm
'Queen bees' 289
Queen's Institute of District Nursing
(QIDN) 25
Questionnaires 141–3, *326*
development of 142
reliability

internal/split-half 144–5
interobserver 144
test/retest 144
validity
construct (hypothesis) 147
content 145, 146
convergent 146
Questions, nature of research 117,
118
Quota sampling 188, *326*

R
Random sampling 148–9, 219
cluster **184**, 187–8
simple **184**, 185–6
stratified **184**, 186–7
systematic **184**, 186
Randomized controlled trials (RCTs)
124–6
flow chart **126**
informed consent 126, 211, 218
patient's understanding of
randomization **217**
RAPID database **83**
Ratio data 163
Reactance, theory of 283, 297
Readiness to change model,
framework exercise 112
Reading the literature 67–72
Reality, nature of 4
Reasoning skills 17
Records 70–2
References 72, *324*
examining 68, 69
Harvard system 70, 72
in literature review 253, 254
'Reflection-in-action' 15, 17–18
Reforms in NHS 43
Regional Office R&D Directorates
30, 40, 42
Regression line 144, *327*
Reliability *325*
qualitative data collection 151–3
quantitative data collection
144–5
relationship with validity **146**
Reorganizations in NHS 28
Repeated contact design 128
Representative sampling 149
Research
findings, translating into
practice *see* Change
management
interest groups 275–6

Research – *contd*
  liaison groups, DHSS 29
  processes *see* Design of
    research
Research Appreciation and
  Application module xi–xiii
*Research and Development:
  Towards an Evidence-based
  health Service*, DOH 40
*Research and Development in the
  New NHS: Functions and
  Responsibilities*, DOH 40
Research and Development (R&D)
  Information Systems Strategy,
  DOH 30, 33, 37
Research for Health, DOH 32, 33,
  39, 42
Research Highlights, ENB 46
Researcher teachers 271
Reviewing research xvii, 233–55
  common pitfalls, literature
    reviews 234
  criteria for evaluation 253
  examples, literature reviews 255
  methodology 238–47
    classifying material 240
    methodological critique
      244–7
    recording information
      239–40
    stages in process 238–9
    systematic approach,
      importance 238
    theme matrix, developing
      241, **242**
    theoretical critique 241,
      243–4
  purposes of literature review
    236–8
  putting it all together 247–54
    aims and objectives 247
    points about style 252–4
    putting reviews into practice
      254
    structure 247–52
  types of review 234–6
Rigour *327*
  comparison, quantitative and
    qualitative research 152–3
Risks
  indentifying unknown 210
  minimal and substantial 215
  risk-benefit ratio 215–16, *327*
Roger's five phase theory of

'change diffusion' 301, **303**
Roper, conceptual frameworks for
  nursing 103, 104
Royal College of Nursing (RCN)
  45–6, 66
  clinical guidelines initiative
    271
  early research publications 24–5
  NURSE ROM database **83**
  The Study of Nursing Care
    project 25, 45

S
Samples *325*
  critique 199–201
  distributive justice 218–19
  inclusion and exclusion criteria
    217–18
  reasons for taking 181–2
  size 195–8
    confidence intervals 167
    and effect size 171–2
    practical considerations 198
    quantitative research 147–50
  types of 182
Sampling *327*
  bias, sources of 198–9
  by setting 195
  error 183, 196, 198, *328*
  event 193–4
  interval 186
  qualitative research 189–93
    convenience 189–90
    purposive 191–2
    snowball 192
    theoretical in data analysis
      150, 174–5, 191
  quantitative research 182–9
    cluster **184**, 187–8
    quota 188
    simple random **184**, 185–6
    stratified 149, **184**, 186–7
    systematic **184**, 186
    time 193, 194
Schön's model 2, 13–15, 17–18
Science Citation Index **83**
Scientific
  fraud 220–1
  knowledge 3, 6, 8, 9–10
Scotland, health care research 47–8
Scottish National Board (SNB) 47–8
Secondary sources *328*
  historical research 130

Secondment to research teams 274
Self-care, Orem's theory of 112–13
Self-confidence, research utilization
  268
Self-efficacy, perception of 283
'Sense of belonging' (SOBI)
  questionnaire 142
Sentence construction, critical
  analysis 74–6
Setting, sampling by 195
Sheffield Centre for Health and
  Related Research (SCHARR)
  27
Shotgun research 261
Simple random sampling **184**,
  185–6
'Simpson's paradox' 168
Skim reading 67, *329*
  books 68–9
  journals 67–8
Snowball sampling 192, *329*
Social
  and behavioural research 211
  need, Bradshaw's taxonomy,
    103
  world 5–6
Social Science Citation Index *83*
Socially desirable response 211
Specification, confounding
  variables 168
Speed reading 55, 67–70
Spelling 59
Spider diagrams 57, *58*
Split-half reliability 144–5, *329*
Statistical
  power 149, 150, 170, 171, 172
  records 130–1
  significance **170**, 171, **173**,
    329
Statutory professional bodies, role
  of 45–9
*Strategy for the Development of
  Research in Nursing in Wales*,
  Welsh Office 48
Strategy for Nursing, DOH 43
Strategy for Nursing Research,
  Scottish Office 47
Strategy for Research in Nursing
  Midwifery and Health Visiting
  Taskforce Report xi, xii, 3, 34–8,
  270
    key recommendations 36–7
Stratified random sampling 148,
  184, 186–7, *329*

Structure
    literature review 247–52
        introduction 249
        critical review, themes and
            concepts 249
        summary 250–2
    and organization, Strategy for
        Research recommendations
        36
The Study of Nursing Care project,
    RCN 25, 45
Subject terms see Key words
Summary, literature review 250
    example 250–2
Supporting Research and
    Development in the NHS 41–2
Surveys 117, 127–8, 330
Systematic
    non-probability samples 150
    reviews 235
    sampling **184**, 186, 330

T
T-tests 147, 163, 165, 331
Target population 183, 330
Test/retest reliability 144–5
Theme matrix, development 241,
    242
Theoretical
    critique 241, 243–4
    frameworks 106, **107**, 108, 111
        exercises 112–13
        identifying in literature
            review 237
        relationship between
            conceptual and 108
    knowledge 3, 10, 16–17, 18
        see also Scientific knowledge
    sampling 150, 174–5, 191
Theory xv, 85, 86, 95–101, 113, 330
    development, contribution of
        research processes 96–8
    generation 97, 98, 119
    inductive reasoning 98
    implications for reader of
        research 100–1
    meaning and characteristics 95
    purpose of 95–6
    relationship with research
        99–101
    testing, deductive reasoning 97,
        98
    see also Grounded theory

Therapeutic privilege, doctrine of
    210
Therapy professions 45
    Therapy Professions Research
        Group 38, 39, 45
Thesaurus facility, online indexes
    59
Time
    sampling 193, 194, 330
    series (trend design) 128, 330
Transferability, qualitative data
    collection 152
Trialability 293, 331
Triangulation 133, 151, 153, 157,
    176, 331
    between method 153
    within method 153
Trust, change management 287–8
Tuskagee Study 210, 220
Type I error 171, 331
Type II error 170, 171, 172, 331

U
UK Clearing House on Health
    Outcomes Literature Database
    83
Unethical studies, using findings
    204–5
United Kingdom Central Council
    (UKCC) 46, 47
    Code of Professional Conduct
        42, 43, 49
User friendliness, research reports
    266–7
Utilization, research findings xvii,
    37, 257–76, 331
    American studies 263
    barriers to 264–70
        accessibility of research
            265–7
        related to individual 267–8
        related to setting 268–9
        why nurses don't use
            research findings 264–5
    current state of knowledge,
        nursing practice 260–1
    inappropriate use 262
    levels of utilization 261–2
    possible solutions 270–6
        improving accessibility
            270–2
        overcoming barriers related
            to setting 274–6

        overcoming individual
            barriers 272–4
    responsibility for
        implementation 276–7
    UK studies 264

V
Validity 331
    establishing in action research
        94
    external and internal 124
    qualitative data collection 151,
        152–3
    quantitative data collection
        145–7
'Value rigidity' 286
Variables 331
    confounding 148, 149, 168,
        169–70, 314
    controlling for 124
    dependent and independent
        148, 168–70
Video recordings 121
A Vision for the Future, DOH 43–4,
    49
Voluntariness 213–214
Volunteer sampling see
    Convenience sampling
Vulnerability of subjects
    informed consent 212
    justice, 219–20

W
Wales, health care research **48**
Welsh National Board (WNB) 48
Western Interstate Commission for
    Higher Education (WICHE
    programme) 276
Wilcoxon test 165, 332
Wilkinson's force field analysis 301,
    302
Within case analysis 133
Within method triangulation 153
Women, vulnerability 219–20
Workgroup of European Nurse
    Researchers (WENR) 49
World Wide Web 66
Writing style
    literature review 252–4
    sentence construction, critical
        analysis 74–6

X
χ^2 (chi-square) test 165, 313